10 Minute ENT Consult

10 Minute ENT Consult

Hamid R. Djalilian, MD

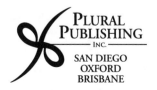

PLURAL
PUBLISHING
INC.

SAN DIEGO
OXFORD
BRISBANE

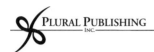

PLURAL PUBLISHING
INC.

5521 Ruffin Road
San Diego, CA 92123

e-mail: info@pluralpublishing.com
Web site: http://www.pluralpublishing.com

49 Bath Street
Abingdon, Oxfordshire OX14 1EA
United Kingdom

FSC
Mixed Sources
Product group from well-managed
forests and other controlled sources

Cert no. SW-COC-002283
www.fsc.org
© 1996 Forest Stewardship Council

Library of Congress Cataloging-in-Publication Data

10 minute ENT consult / [edited by] Hamid Djalilian.
       p. ; cm.
  Includes bibliographical references and index.
  ISBN-13: 978-1-59756-255-3 (alk. paper)
  ISBN-10: 1-59756-255-6 (alk. paper)
  1.   Otolaryngology—Handbooks, manuals, etc. 2.   Medical history taking—
Handbooks, manuals, etc.   I. Djalilian, Hamid. II. Title: Ten minute ENT con-
sult.
  [DNLM: 1.   Otorhinolaryngologic Diseases—diagnosis—Handbooks. 2.
Medical History Taking—methods—Handbooks. 3.   Physical Examination—
methods—Handbooks.   WV 39 Z99 2009]
  RF56.T46 2009
  617.5'1075—dc22

                                                            2008039881

Contents

Foreword

The practice of medicine for the family physician has always required well-crafted and updated written resource material. Amidst a landscape of burgeoning knowledge and unwavering complexities of a health care structure, this need is certainly critical for the physician who embraces the newer concept of the medical home. This philosophical approach to care espouses efficient primary care for common problems and expertise at coordinated referral for specialty care. It is refreshing that this book is designed to offer an expedited guide to diagnosis and treatment of many of the common otolaryngologic problems seen by the primary care physician. Top 20 lists of common problems seen by the family physician typically include four to five presenting symptoms related to head and neck pathology or disease.

The organization of this text by symptom, rather than by disease, is definitely the main strength of this text. The broader organizational categories of disease of the ear, dizziness, and facial paralysis; diseases of the nose and sinuses; and diseases of the mouth, throat, and neck offer ease in referencing for the busy physician. The discussion of each symptom, including background information, description of common disorders, and recommendations regarding appropriate tests, treatment, and need for specialty referral, allow for a focus on common problems, which is often more challenging in books with listings of diseases where there is not an emphasis on the commonness of a particular entity. The reader is also visually guided in these reviews by clinical algorithms.

There are several welcomed features of this book that merit particular emphasis. The constellation of the clinically focused symptom discussion, diagnostic flow diagrams, and recommendations for test ordering and treatment do indeed provide for a rapid (10-minute) evaluation, but without compromise of the quality of the process. The author appropriately provides backup references for each symptom and associated diseases. Two other features of note are the symptom-based indications for specialty referral and a concluding chapter on danger signs in the head and neck field.

In summary, this type of work is especially useful for practicing family physicians for the conciseness of its symptom-based approach and has added value in teaching situations for medical students, residents, and allied health professionals. It would be a welcome addition to the family physician's reference library.

Kathryn M. Larsen, MD
Health Science Clinical Professor and Chair
University of California at Irvine

Preface

This book was written by the faculty at the University of California, Irvine as a guide for the primary care and emergency medicine physicians, residents, and medical students to diagnose and treat conditions affecting the ear, nose, throat, and the head and neck. Contrary to standard texts that discuss diseases one at a time, this text was organized in a symptom-based fashion. This allows the clinician to look at a symptom and, based on the algorithm and the description of the disease, come to a diagnosis. For each problem, we tried to create a guide for diagnosis, what tests to order, how to treat, and when to refer. Two chapters at the end outline the most common danger signs in the head and neck of which the primary care physician should be aware and common procedures in otolaryngology-head and neck surgery. We hope that this book will allow the primary care physician to come to a diagnosis for a complaint in the head and neck in less than 10 minutes.

Sixty years ago, the field of otolaryngology-head and neck surgery was still combined with ophthalmology. Now each field has seven subspecialties. The subspecialization in the field of otolaryngology-head and neck surgery has allowed for better patient care in some areas of the field. Although most problems in the head and neck can be cared for by the general otolaryngologist, some patients will need subspecialty care. The current subspecialties in otolaryngology include:

- Otology, Neurotology, and Skull Base Surgery: This specialty treats the diseases of the temporal bone. These include, ear disease, hearing problems, vertigo and balance issues, facial nerve disorders, and posterior and lateral skull base tumors (eg, acoustic neuromas, etc), and stereotactic radiation (radiosurgery/GammaKnife/CyberKnife) for skull base tumors.
- Head and Neck Surgery: This subspecialty cares for the patients with benign and malignant tumors of the head and neck, including upper aerodigestive tumors, salivary gland, thyroid, and parathyroid tumors.
- Rhinology, Nasal Allergy, and Endoscopic Sinus and Anterior Skull Base Surgery: This subspecialty treats diseases of the nose and sinuses as well as tumors of the anterior skull base, including pituitary tumors, and so forth. These clinicians also diagnose and treat allergies using immunotherapy.
- Facial Plastic and Reconstructive Surgery: Specialists in this field are aesthetic and reconstructive specialists of the head and neck.
- Laryngology: This subspecialty treats diseases of the larynx including voice and swallowing disorders.
- Microvascular Reconstructive Surgery: These surgeons work in conjunction with head and neck surgeons for reconstruction of complex defects of the head and neck using free flaps. These flaps are brought to the head and neck from other areas of the body and their

vasculature is anastamosed to the head and neck vessels allowing for more functional outcomes after cancer surgery.

- Pediatric Otolaryngology: This field is dedicated to the treatment of pediatric patients, especially treatment of the pediatric airway problems.

This book would not be possible without the inspiration from my father, Dr. Mohsen Djalilian, who taught me the basics of otolaryngology and how to be a great physician and teacher, my brother, Dr. Ali Djalilian, who always pushed me to be the best I can be, my mentor, the late Dr. George L. Adams, chairman of Otolaryngology-Head and Neck Surgery at the University of Minnesota, and all the faculty at the University of Minnesota, who were my guiding light in my residency training and beyond, and Dr. Victor Passy at the University of California, Irvine who encouraged me to undertake this project.

Hamid R. Djalilian, MD

Contributors

Gurpreet S. Ahuja, MD
Associate Clinical Professor
Department of Otolaryngology-Head and Neck
  Surgery
Division of Pediatric Otolaryngology
University of California, Irvine
Irvine, California
Chapters 21 and 27

William B. Armstrong, MD, FACS
Associate Professor and Interim Chair
Department of Otolaryngology-Head and Neck
  Surgery
University of California, Irvine
Irvine, California
Chapter 23

Roberto L. Barretto, MD
Clinical Assistant Professor
Department of Otolaryngology-Head and Neck
  Surgery
University of California, Irvine
Irvine, California
Chapters 22 and 27

Aaron G. Benson, MD
Clinical Adjunct Professor

Department of Otolaryngology-Head and Neck
   Surgery
University of Michigan
Otology-Neurotology
Ann Arbor, Michigan
Chapter 17

Roger L. Crumley, MD, MBA
Professor, Department of Otolaryngology-Head and
   Neck Surgery
University of California, Irvine
Irvine, California
Chapter 19

Amir Deylamipour, MD
Research Fellow
Department of Otolaryngology-Head and Neck
   Surgery
University of California, Irvine
Irvine, California
Chapter 8

Hamid R. Djalilian, MD
Associate Professor
Director of Otology, Neurotology, and Skull Base
   Surgery
University of California Irvine Medical Center
Orange, California
Chapters 1-18, 20-22, 25-28

Esther L. Fine, MD
Resident Physician
University of California, Irvine
Irvine, California
Chapters 19 and 20

Rohit Garg, MD, MBA
Resident Physician
Department of Otolaryngology-Head and Neck
 Surgery
University of California, Irvine
Irvine, California
Chapter 12

Sanaz Hamidi, MD
Research Fellow
Department of Otolaryngology-Head and Neck
 Surgery
University of California, Irvine
Irvine, California
Chapters 2, 5, and 8

Paul K. Holden, MD, MS
Resident Physician
Department of Otolaryngology-Head and Neck
 Surgery
University of California, Irvine
Irvine, California
Chapter 15

Jason H. Kim, MD
Assistant Professor
Director of Endocrine Surgery
Department of Otolaryngology-Head and Neck
 Surgery
University of California, Irvine
Irvine, California
Chapter 24

Kathryn M. Larsen, MD
Health Science Clinical Professor and Chair
Gerald B. Sinykin, M.D., Endowed Chair in Family
 Medicine
Department of Family Medicine

University of California at Irvine
Irvine, California
Foreword

Alice D. Lee, MD
Fellow, Neurotology and Skull Base Surgery
Wayne State University/Michigan Ear Institute
Farmington Hills, Michigan
Chapter 3

Ryan Leonard, DO
Resident Physician
Department of Otolaryngology-Head and Neck
    Surgery
Michigan State University
Detroit, Michigan
Chapter 17

John F. McGuire, MD, MBA
General Otolaryngology
Fallbrook, California
Chapter 26

Quoc A. Nguyen, MD
Clinical Associate Professor of Otolaryngology
Department of Otolaryngology-Head and Neck
    Surgery
University of California, Irvine
Irvine, California
Chapter 13

Victor Passy, MD
Professor and Emeritus Chair
Department of Otolaryngology-Head and Neck
    Surgery
University of California, Irvine
Irvine, California
Chapter 18

James M. Ridgway, MD
Resident Physician
Department of Otolaryngology-Head and Neck
  Surgery
University of California, Irvine
Irvine, California
Chapter 7

Vanessa S. Rothholtz, MD, MSc
Resident Physician
Department of Otolaryngology-Head and Neck
  Surgery
University of California, Irvine
Irvine, California
Chapters 1, 4, 5, 10, and 16

Paul Schalch, MD
Resident Physician
Department of Otolaryngology-Head and Neck
  Surgery
University of California, Irvine Medical Center
Irvine, California
Chapters 11, 13, and 18

Ali Sepehr, MD
Resident Physician
Department of Otolaryngology-Head and Neck
  Surgery
University of California, Irvine School of Medicine
Irvine, California
Chapters 1 and 6

Mehdi Sina-Khadiv, BA
MD/MBA Candidiate
University of California, Irvine
Irvine, California
Chapter 18

David M. Stone, MD, FACS
Associate Professor
Department of Otolaryngology-Head and Neck
    Surgery
Aesthetic Facial Plastic Surgery
University of California, Irvine
Irvine, California
Chapter 27

Brian J. F. Wong, MD, PhD
Professor of Otolaryngology-Head and Neck Surgery
Director of Facial Plastics and Reconstructive Surgery
University of California, Irvine
Irvine, California
Chapter 15

Hau Sin Wong, MD
Clinical Assistant Professor
Department of Otolaryngology-Head and Neck
    Surgery
Pediatric Otolaryngology
University of California, Irvine
Irvine, California
Chapters 24 and 27

Edward C. Wu, BA, BS
MD/MBA Candidate
University of California, Irvine School of Medicine
Irvine, California
Chapters 10 and 16

*To my wife who has been especially patient
and supportive throughout.*

*To my family who gave me every opportunity,
and to all my teachers for their dedication
and patience.*

PART I

Diseases of the Ear, Dizziness, and Facial Paralysis

CHAPTER 1

History and Examination of the Ear

ALI SEPEHR
VANESSA S. ROTHHOLTZ
HAMID R. DJALILIAN

HISTORY

Taking a history for ear problems depends on the age of the patient and the presenting problem. The patients who present with ear pain or drainage must be asked the usual questions regarding chronology, location, severity, radiation, character, related symptoms, and modifying symptoms. Patients with hearing loss also need to have questions on chronology, location, severity, situations in which they have difficulty, and related symptoms (eg, tinnitus, vertigo, ear drainage), and previous otologic surgery.

In neonates who present with hearing loss upon screening, a detailed birth history is required. This includes any complications during the mother's pregnancy such as illnesses, drug use, or trauma. Any genetic abnormalities noted in the family history, siblings, or

3

parents should also be discussed. A history of intubation, a stay in the neonatal intensive care unit, or medications administered to the neonate postpartum must be documented. Hyperbilirubinemia at birth and the need for exchange transfusion increases the risk of hearing loss. All parents must be questioned about activity, babbling, if certain developmental milestones have been achieved and the infant's response to startling sounds. Children may present to the pediatrician having failed a hearing screening at school. Hearing loss in a child who is in elementary school may divulge itself through adverse behavior, inattention, poor grades, and social isolation. Parents may note a failure for their child to respond to requests or listening to the television at an unusually high sound level.

In adults and the elderly, a history of hearing loss may originate with the patient, from a spouse, caretaker, or loved one. Patients may complain of having difficulty hearing an individual in a crowded room or at a restaurant. The patient may also describe the sensation of hearing well, but not understanding the speaker. These may be signs of high-frequency hearing loss. History of noise exposure, including that in the military or occupational exposure, should be acquired. Age of onset, sidedness, exacerbating and alleviating factors, and prior episodes of the condition should be elicited. Additionally, the presence of any associated symptoms including ear pain, fullness, discharge, tinnitus, vertigo, trauma, facial weakness, numbness, and other neurologic manifestations must be communicated.

At any age, the physician should ask the patient about current medication use, past surgical history, past medical history, social habits, and family otologic history. Any past or present history of ototoxic medication use should be noted as a probable etiology. A history of trauma may indicate a fracture of the temporal bone or ossicular chain disruption.

Physical Exam

After a thorough history is acquired, the physician should next perform a physical exam. The patient's anterior and posterior nasal cavity should be examined for masses or lesions that may manifest as a chronic unilateral ear effusion. The patient's oral cavity should be examined for any congenital malformations such as a cleft palate. Any masses or enlarged lymph nodes should be noted in the neck and a complete cranial nerve examination should be performed.

The complete ear exam is imperative when evaluating the patient for hearing loss. The external ear should be evaluated for any signs of inflammation, infection, or malformation. Any masses or lesions in, on, or around the ear should be noted. An edematous and erythematous external auditory canal without visualization of the tympanic membrane (TM) is likely otitis externa. An atresia (complete closure) of the external canal may also be present. Patients with an atresia of the ear canal need to be evaluated by an audiologist and an otologist/neuro-otologist for hearing rehabilitation/reconstruction.

For the otoscopic exam, the physician should choose the largest available otoscope tip (typically 5 mm) for all patients over the age of 5 years. The 4-mm tip should be used for children 2 to 5 years, and the 2.5-mm tip should be used for those under the age of 2 years. If the otoscope tip is too large, it can be downsized although that is uncommonly needed. The larger tip gives the examiner a better view of the TM and the ability to seal the ear canal for pneumatic otoscopy. The otoscope should be held close to the lighted end so as to give better control over the movement of the otoscope. The senior author (HD) prefers holding the otoscope like a handgun, which provides superior control over the otoscope, especially in an otoscope that is tethered by a power cord which could pull on the otoscope (Fig 1-1). One of the fingers should be extended to brace the otoscope against the patient's head (generally second or third finger). This will prevent a sudden insertion of the otoscope into the canal with head movement. The otoscope should be inserted after pulling the auricle back to align the cartilaginous canal with the bony canal. The otoscope should only be inserted for a short distance in the cartilaginous canal. Deep insertion should be avoided as touching the bony canal causes significant pain. If the ear canal is pulled back properly, only 2 to 3 mm of insertion is needed for an adequate exam. After placing the otoscope in the ear canal, the examiner should aim the otoscope anteriorly as the ear canal in most patients turns anteriorly.

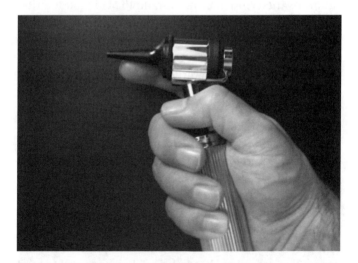

Fig 1-1. The proper method of holding the otoscope. This way, the otoscope is secure and can be held tightly. The second finger will sit in the concha preventing a sudden deep insertion of the otoscope into the canal, which can cause injury.

In a child, the otoscope tip should be shown to the child and placed against his or her finger, arm, leg, and so on. to show that it will not cause pain. If an older sibling is available, looking into his or her ear will place the patient at ease. Otherwise, an ear exam of the parent can be demonstrated to lessen anxiety. The senior author (HD) will always hold the otoscope a few centimeters away from his own ear and have the child peer into his ear to demonstrate its harmlessness. Finally, the child should be asked, "Which ear should I look at?" while the examiner points to each ear separately. The child should not be asked, "Can I look in your ears?" as the answer will always be a resounding "No!" If the child is not cooperative (which occurs rarely with the above techniques), the parent should be instructed to hold the child in his or her lap with the child's legs between their legs, one arm to control the two arms of the child, and one hand holding the forehead.

Obstruction of the external auditory canal by cerumen, a foreign body, or blood may be the cause of a conductive hearing loss. If the physician feels comfortable and has experience in removing the cerumen with a small curette under direct visualization, it should be done. Alternatively, cerumen may be removed with an alligator or Frasier tip suction (Fig 1–2). When an instrument is used through the otoscope, the hand holding the instrument should be braced against the otoscope to prevent a deep insertion of the instrument if there is a sudden head motion.

Ear-irrigating devices should be used with caution as they can increase the risk of otitis externa. Also, when vigorous irrigation is used in the presence of a thinned tympanic membrane (TM) or a TM perforation, a middle ear infection may occur. If a patient has had a previously documented normal TM, then irrigation may be used. Body-temperature water should

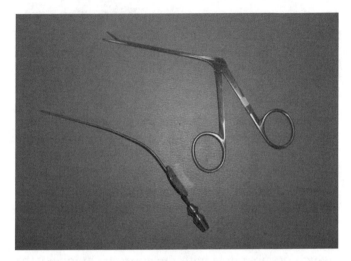

Fig 1–2. Alligator forceps and Frasier tip suction used for cerumen removal. Generally, a size 5 or 7 French suction tip is used for cerumen removal. Close to the tympanic membrane, a size 3 is used. A metal curette generally works better for cerumen removal than a plastic one due to its finer tip.

be used for irrigation. After irrigation, 3 to 4 drops of a 50:50 solution of isopropyl alcohol and white vinegar can be placed in the ear for prevention of an otitis externa. For impacted, hardened cerumen in an ear without prior history of trauma, otologic surgery, or tympanic membrane perforation, the physician can prescribe otic drops, such as Debrox or hydrogen peroxide drops, to soften the wax for removal at the next visit. If the cerumen cannot be removed easily under visualization or is causing the patient discomfort, the patient should be referred to an otolaryngologist for removal and evaluation.

Once the external canal is clear, the physician should obtain a complete view of the patient's tympanic membrane and note the integrity of the membrane. A perforation may lead to a conductive hearing loss. The eardrum should be evaluated for tympanosclerosis, or white thickening of the middle fibrous layer of the TM, and dimeric TM, thinned sections of the TM. The physician should always be able to see the malleus in the TM as the malleus is embedded within the TM. The cone of light (reflection of the light from the TM) seen anteroinferiorly will always indicate the visualization of the TM. The cone of light should not be used as a marker of a normal TM, as a cone of light will be seen in many disease states. It is critical for the physician to visualize the pars flaccida, area of the TM above the lateral process of the malleus (Fig 1–3).

Pneumatic otoscopy will determine the mobility of the tympanic membrane and assist the physician in knowing if a middle ear effusion exists. The examiner should use the largest available otoscope tip or use a

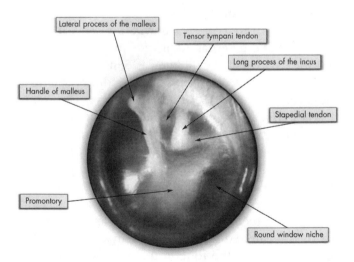

Fig 1–3. Normal left tympanic membrane. (From: Touma, J. B. and Touma, B. J., 2006. *Atlas of Otoscopy.* Copyright 2006, San Diego: Plural Publishing. Printed with permission.)

Siegel tip for better seal of the canal. Sealing of the canal for pneumatic otoscopy should be done at the cartilaginous canal level and not in the bony canal, which will cause great discomfort. Using a finger to push the tragus onto the otoscope may help in obtaining a seal. The pneumatic bulb should be held in the hand opposite the one holding the otoscope. This allows pumping of the bulb without motion of the otoscope. If a seal is not properly obtained, the TM will not move and create a false positive test. Pneumatic otoscopy is done with very slight pressure on the bulb (depressing it 5 to 6 mm). If the bulb is squeezed entirely to the point of flattening it and a seal of the ear canal is present, it will cause significant pain from the pressure generated in the ear canal. If the air pressure is not causing some mild discomfort, no seal is present.

Tuning fork tests can assist the physician in differentiating between conductive hearing loss and sensorineural hearing loss. Conductive hearing loss (CHL) is the disruption of sound along its transduction from the external ear to the oval window. This includes defects in the external auditory canal, the eardrum, and the ossicles of the middle ear. Sensorineural hearing loss (SNHL) is disruption of the auditory system at the level of the cochlea or auditory nerve. The Weber test is performed with a 512-hertz tuning fork. After striking the tuning fork to elicit a vibration, the physician should place the base of the tuning fork in the midline of the patient's forehead. If the patient is unable to hear the transmitted sound, the physician may place the clean tuning fork on the patient's maxillary incisor teeth. The patient is then asked in which ear the transmitted sound is heard. In a normal exam, the patient hears the tone in the midline. In a unilateral conductive loss, the tone is louder in the affected poorer hearing ear. In a unilateral sensorineural loss, the tone is louder in the unaffected better hearing ear.

The Rinne test is also performed with a 512-hertz tuning fork. After striking the tuning fork, the physician will initially place its base on the patient's mastoid bone behind his or her ear. This is known as bone conduction. The fork will then be moved to a location 1 inch lateral to the ear canal on the same side (air conduction) and the patient is then asked which position was perceived as louder. The normal exam will result in air conduction being louder than bone conduction. This is also observed in patients with sensorineural hearing loss. Patients with a conductive loss will perceive the bone conduction condition as being louder than the air conduction in the affected ear. This signifies a conductive hearing loss of at least 30 dB. Although the tuning fork test is useful for the frequency in which it is tested (generally 512 Hz), its usefulness is limited. Therefore, all patients with a suspected hearing loss should be evaluated using an audiogram. Tympnanometry, otoacoustic emissions, and an auditory brainstem response (ABR) can complement the testing.

AUDIOLOGY

Although a complete description of audiologic measuring systems is beyond the scope of this text, key terminology and basic methods incorporated into an examination to evaluate a patient for hearing loss are presented.

The Audiogram

The audiogram illustrates the relative measure of a patient's hearing by depicting the softest intensity level that the patient can hear (threshold in decibels) as it relates to frequency along a scale from 250 Hz to

8000 Hz. Hearing threshold levels are grouped in ranges of 20 dB HL to identify patients who have normal hearing from those who have a mild, moderate, severe or profound hearing loss (Table 1-1). Air conduction testing is performed by sending the sound signal through the ear canal. This tests the integrity of the middle ear and inner ear together. The bone conduction testing is performed by sending the sound signal through the bone, which will directly stimulate the cochlea. The thresholds at various frequencies are obtained by finding the quietest sound that the patient can hear at that frequency. In normal situations, both the air and bone thresholds should be equal and better than the 20 dB level (less than or equal to 20).

The audiologist often tests the pediatric patient utilizing sound fields and the adult patient with both masked and unmasked air conduction as well as bone conduction if indicated. The pediatric audiogram is done differently in various age ranges depending on the ability of the child to cooperate. Masking is the administration of sound to the ear that is not being tested to prevent that ear from interfering with the sound perception of the ear that is being tested. An air-bone gap is the difference between air conduction and bone conduction in each frequency and is abnor-

Table 1–1. Hearing Loss Standards

Decibel	Clinical Correlation
<20 dB	Normal Hearing
21–40 dB	Mild Hearing Loss
41–60 dB	Moderate Hearing Loss
61–80 dB	Moderately Severe Hearing Loss
81–100 dB	Severe Hearing Loss
>101 dB	Profound Hearing Loss

mal at greater than 15 dB HL, signifying a conductive hearing loss. Averaging the air conduction thresholds at 500, 1000, and 2000 hertz, which are the frequencies located in the speech range, calculate the pure-tone average (PTA). The speech reception threshold (SRT) is the lowest intensity that a patient can identify 50% of a set of double-syllabic words. This threshold should be within ±6 dB of the PTA. Speech discrimination values, or word recognition testing, of more than 90% correct are considered normal when single-syllable words are presented at 30 to 40 dB above the speech reception threshold. Figure 1–4 demonstrates an audiogram in a patient with normal hearing, a conductive hearing loss, and a sensorineural hearing loss.

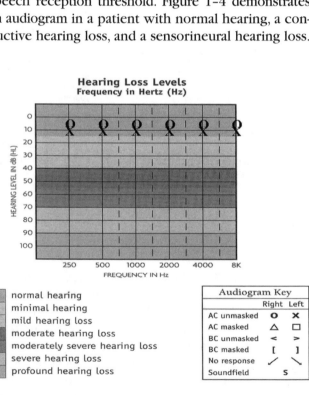

A

Figure 1–4. The audiogram. In normal hearing (**A**), all thresholds are better than 20 dB. *continues*

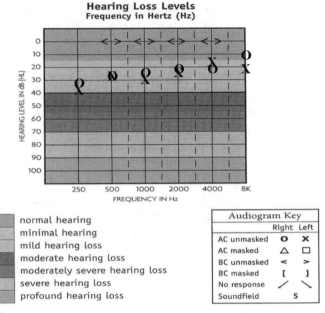

Figure 1–4. *continued* In conductive hearing loss (**B**), the bone conduction thresholds are better than the air conduction thresholds. *continues*

Tympanometry and Acoustic Immittance

Acoustic immittance testing is a group of tests that ascertain the integrity of the tympanic membrane and middle ear. These tests include tympanometry, acoustic reflexes, and static compliance. Tympanometry is an indirect determination of middle ear function by the measurement of the degree of reflection of the eardrum when an 85 dB SPL low-frequency tone is introduced into the ear canal under varying pressure. Three types of compliance plots can result from tym-

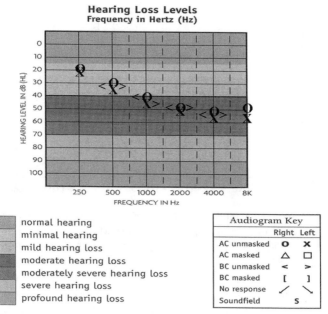

C

Figure 1–4. *continued* In sensorineural hearing loss (**C**), both the bone and air conduction thresholds are worse than 20 dB.

panometric testing (Fig 1-5). A type "A" tympanogram signifies a normal peak between −100 and +100 daPa. A shallow peak in a type A tympanogram indicates a TM that has reduced compliance. This stiffness may indicate otosclerosis or tympanosclerosis. A deep peak in the tympanogram indicates a hypercompliant eardrum that may lead to the diagnosis of ossicular chain disruption or a very thin atelectatic tympanic membrane. A flat tympanogram that indicates an immobile eardrum is a type "B" tympanogram. This may suggest the presence of middle ear effusion, tympanic membrane

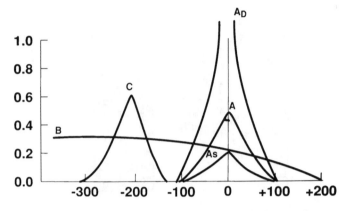

Fig 1–5. The tympanograms in normal and diseased ears. The normal tympanogram peak should fall between −100 and +100 daPa (type A). A flat tympanogram (type B) indicates a hole in the TM or a middle ear effusion. A type C tympanogram will have a peak that is less than −100 daPa. Type A_S (a shallow curve) tympanogram indicates a hypomobile TM due to ossicular fixation or tympanosclerosis (thickening of the TM). Type A_D (deep curve) tympanogram indicates hypermobility of the TM due to ossicular discontinuity or a very thin TM.

perforation, or the presence of a patent pressure equalization tube. A perforation or PE tube is distinguished from middle-ear fluid by the ear canal volume reading. A volume reading of less than one milliliter (mL) indicates an intact TM (measuring ear canal volume indicating a middle ear effusion), and a volume of greater than one mL indicates a hole in the TM (including the middle ear volume and ear canal volume). Finally, a type "C" tympanogram is one in which the peak is shifted to a more negative pressure thereby indicating the presence of a retracted TM from negative middle ear pressure or eustachian tube dysfunction. Tympanograms are inaccurate in children under the age of

6 months and should not be relied upon for diagnosis in this age group.

Acoustic reflex testing measures the contraction of the stapedial muscle in response to a loud controlled sound. The thresholds measured are the least intense stimulation that can be administered with a response, and the presence of the response measures the function of cochlea, ventral cochlear nucleus, the auditory nerve, the facial nerve, and the stapedius muscle itself. Absent ipsilateral and/or contralateral responses may indicate a middle ear disorder, a conductive hearing loss, a sensorineural hearing loss, dysfunction at the level of the brainstem, or an acoustic neuroma.

Otoacoustic Emissions (OAE)

OAE is a screening test to quickly check between a normal and an abnormal hearing ear. It is rapid and does not require patient cooperation. A normal result indicates a threshold of 35 dB or better. An abnormal test may occur from a conductive or sensorineural hearing loss of greater than 35 dB or in the case of a middle ear effusion.

Auditory Brainstem Response

The auditory brainstem response (ABR) is the recording of the response of the central nervous system and cochlear nerve when stimulated with an acoustic signal. This test is frequently used in patients who are suspected of having a unilateral eighth nerve dysfunction due to an acoustic neuroma, intraoperatively to evaluate stimulation of the cochlear nerve, or as a screening tool in neonates. The ABR is recorded from surface electrodes placed on the vertex, forehead, mastoid, and ear lobule. Active electrodes distribute rapid clicks up to 50 pulses per second, and response electrodes average the output to record an ABR waveform. Disruption in the peaks of the waveform may lead to the discovery of dysfunction in the eighth nerve or the brainstem (cochlear nuclei, superior olive, lateral lemniscus, or inferior colliculus).

Universal newborn hearing screening is now the standard in the United States. Neonates who fail two hearing screenings at birth will need to be retested within a month. If the patient fails the outpatient test, then a definitive sedated ABR test is done. Abnormalities in the ABR include a delayed wave I—indicating a conductive or mixed hearing loss, small wave I—high-frequency sensorineural hearing loss, prolonged interwave latency: I to V—lesion involving CN VIII.

BALANCE TESTS

Balance depends on vestibular, visual, and somatosensory information that is integrated in the brainstem to produce a motor response to recover from the perturbation. The goal of testing is to localize the lesion and determine severity.

Videonystagmography (VNG) (aka Electronystagmography [ENG])

The VNG test is performed using infrared or electrodes to track eye movement to characterize abnormalities of the vestibular organ and the brainstem and cerebellar coordination of eye movement. The two subsets of the test check for central or peripheral balance problems. It is useful for understanding whether the patient's problem is from the vestibular organ/nerve or from the brainstem/cerebellum. It is the first test that is obtained if the patient has vertigo.

Posturography

Computerized dynamic posturography (CDP) is performed to detect the etiology and extent of imbalance. It can characterize the etiology of imbalance as being musculoskeletal, vestibular, or central.

IMAGING

Imaging of the ear, temporal bone, or the neural structures in and around the temporal bone depends on the pathology that is being evaluated. A plain x-ray is of no value in the work up of an otologic condition. A high-resolution computed tomography (CT) without contrast is often used to evaluate the temporal bones for abnormal processes especially in cases of an abnormal ear examination or conductive hearing loss. The CT scan may demonstrate congenital malformations, complications of chronic infection with erosion of the bones of the middle ear, neoplasms, cholesteatoma, mastoiditis, and temporal bone fractures.

If abnormalities of the neural structures are suspected, a magnetic resonance imaging (MRI) of the temporal bone (internal auditory canal sequence) with gadolinium is needed. For cases of unilateral hearing loss or tinnitus in which an acoustic neuroma is suspected or in patients who are suspected of having multiple sclerosis, MRI is the test of choice. Conventional angiography is rarely needed, but magnetic resonance angiography (MRA) is beneficial in evaluating a pulsatile tinnitus.

CHAPTER 2

Ear Pain

HAMID R. DJALILIAN
SANAZ HAMIDI

GENERAL APPROACH TO EAR PAIN

It is not uncommon for a physician to not find any pathology on ear exam of patients with otalgia (Fig 2-1). This is usually due to the complex anatomy and innervation of the ear. Cranial nerves V, VII, IX, X, and the cervical plexus all have branches in the ear that cause referred pain from any pathology in their pathways. It is not unusual that pathology in the teeth, larynx, tonsils, thyroid, parotid, or even GERD can cause ear pain in the patient.

Patients who present with ear pain should be asked about location of pain, what makes the pain better or worse (eg, chewing, swallowing), radiation of pain, and associated symptoms such as sore throat or hearing loss.

Physical examination usually starts with the ear looking for an intact tympanic membrane and a normal external canal. If ear examination is completely normal, then the physician must proceed with examining

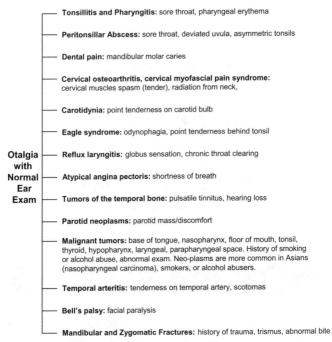

Tonsillitis and Pharyngitis: sore throat, pharyngeal erythema

Peritonsillar Abscess: sore throat, deviated uvula, asymmetric tonsils

Dental pain: mandibular molar caries

Cervical osteoarthritis, cervical myofascial pain syndrome: cervical muscles spasm (tender), radiation from neck,

Carotidynia: point tenderness on carotid bulb

Eagle syndrome: odynophagia, point tenderness behind tonsil

Reflux laryngitis: globus sensation, chronic throat clearing

Atypical angina pectoris: shortness of breath

Tumors of the temporal bone: pulsatile tinnitus, hearing loss

Parotid neoplasms: parotid mass/discomfort

Malignant tumors: base of tongue, nasopharynx, floor of mouth, tonsil, thyroid, hypopharynx, laryngeal, parapharyngeal space. History of smoking or alcohol abuse, abnormal exam. Neo-plasms are more common in Asians (nasopharyngeal carcinoma), smokers, or alcohol abusers.

Temporal arteritis: tenderness on temporal artery, scotomas

Bell's palsy: facial paralysis

Mandibular and Zygomatic Fractures: history of trauma, trismus, abnormal bite

Otalgia with Normal Ear Exam

Fig 2–1. The most common causes of ear pain with a normal ear exam.

the oral cavity, pharynx, neck, parotid, and the facial nerve. On oral cavity/pharynx exam, each tonsil and base of tongue must be palpated for tumors. Also, dental abnormalities (eg, dental caries, evidence of grinding of teeth) must be looked for and a tongue depressor must be used to percuss the mandibular teeth. The temporomandibular joint (TMJ), which is located in front of the ear, should be palpated and the patient is asked to open and close the mouth and elicit tenderness while the physician feels and listens for clicking, and tries to recognize movement of the condyle of the mandible out of the joint (anteriorly or laterally).

When to Refer

Persistent ear pain (beyond 3 weeks) despite conservative therapy or inability to examine the nasopharynx or larynx mandates referral to an otolaryngologist for nasal endoscopy and laryngoscopy. Pain that wakes patient at night despite therapy requires referral as well. Post-trauma patients especially those with abnormal bite after trauma (could indicate mandible fracture), patients with a long history of smoking or heavy alcohol use, or patients with neck mass must also be referred to an otolaryngologist. TMJ problems are referred to a dentist or oral surgeon.

OTALGIA WITH A NORMAL EAR EXAM

TEMPOROMANDIBULAR JOINT DISORDERS

Developmental and congenital anomalies, traumatic injuries, dislocations, ankylosis, arthritis, and neoplasm of temporomandibular joint all can cause referral of pain to the ear and otalgia.

Symptoms and Signs

Trauma to the temporomandibular joint causes difficulty and asymmetry in opening the mouth, periauricular pain, and tenderness over the mandibular condyle. Dislocation of the mandible causes the mouth to remain open. Myofascial pain dysfunction (MPD) syndrome is a disorder that presents with dull pain or acute pain with jaw movement and limitation of mouth opening. The patient will have radiation of the pain on all parts of the face, ear, and neck where the fascial planes are contiguous. The MPD patients will have tenderness upon palpation of all the facial muscles and the sternocleidomastoid muscle.

Diagnosis and What Tests to Order

The diagnosis of TMJ disorders is based on the tenderness or clicking of the TMJ on movement. A panoramic x-ray of the TMJ can be obtained to look for erosion or arthritis of the TMJ. An oral surgeon may obtain an MRI of the TMJ for a better view of the joint. The diagnosis of MPD is dependent on the tenderness of all facial muscles and their contiguous fascial planes (eg, sternocleidomastoid).

Treatment and When to Refer

Arthritis of the TMJ is treated with heat application on the muscles of mastication (temporalis and masseter) and nonsteroidal anti-inflammatory drugs (NSAIDs) (eg, ibuprophen 600 mg po TID × 7–14 days). Muscle relaxants (eg, cyclobenzaprine 10 mg TID × 7–14 days) will also help in symptom relief. The patient must be counseled about home therapy and avoidance of clenching and grinding of the teeth, and a soft diet. Acute dislocation of TMJ should be referred to an oral surgeon or emergency department with access to an oral surgeon. MPD syndrome is treated in the same way as TMJ disorder. If symptoms persist despite all described measures, a referral to a dentist or oral surgeon for a bite appliance is recommended.

TONSILLITIS, PHARYNGITIS, OR ANY IRRITATION IN PHARYNX

Tonsillitis, pharyngitis, or any irritation in the pharynx can cause ear pain by irritating cranial nerve IX (see Chapter 18).

CANCERS OF THE SKULL BASE, PHARYNX, OR LARYNX

Any cancer in the skull base, pharynx, or larynx can cause ear pain due to the irritation of cranial nerve V, IX, or X. If otalgia continues beyond 2 months despite maximal medical therapy for other presumed causes, a referral to an otolaryngologist is warranted for examination and possible CT of the skull base with contrast.

FACIAL PARALYSIS

Paralysis can cause ear pain by irritation of cranial nerve VII and its branch to the ear canal.

CAROTIDYNIA

These patients most commonly present with pain on the side of the face, neck, and the ear. See Chapter 25 on Neck Pain for carotidynia.

EAGLE SYNDROME

This syndrome usually presents with a chronic sore throat, but otalgia is also common in these patients. See Chapter 20 on Swallowing Problems.

LARYNGOPHARYNGEAL REFLUX

See Chapter 18.

OTALGIA WITH AN ABNORMAL EAR EXAM

The ear is a highly sensitive organ that derives its sensory input from the cervical spine as well as contributing branches from cranial nerves V, VII, IX, and X. This pattern of innervation results in the symptom of otalgia occurring when pathology affects other areas of distribution of the affected nerves. Although ear pain in adults is most commonly referred, many diseases of the ear can cause otalgia. The key to the diagnosis is a thorough, yet directed, history and a physical examination of the ear as well as the temporomandibular joint, the pharynx, and the base of tongue. If the etiology of the otalgia is not discovered with the directed examination, a referral to an otolaryngologist for nasopharyngoscopy and laryngoscopy is required to rule out pathology in those areas. Otalgia with a normal ear examination is discussed in more detail in the previous section. This section is organized starting with abnormalities of the auricle, then proceeding to those of the external auditory canal, and finally the middle ear. Figure 2-2 shows a brief description of the most common causes of otalgia with an abnormal ear exam.

RELAPSING POLYCHONDRITIS

Relapsing polychondritis (RP) is a rare, autoimmune condition that is characterized by recurrent inflammation and subsequent destruction of cartilage in the ear, nose, Eustachian tube, joints, trachea, and ribs. The underlying pathology in RP is the development of antibodies that become reactive with collagen type II in various tissues. The disease also causes involvement of noncartilaginous organs such as kidneys, eyes, and peripheral or central vessels. RP is usually seen between the third and fourth decade of life.

Signs and Symptoms

The patient may present with inflammation of the ear and/or nasal cartilage and will mainly complain of redness, pain, and eventually deformity of these organs. When the ear cartilage is involved, the main complaint is ear pain. Trachea involvement manifests with throat pain, hoarseness, and breathing difficulty that may need mechanical ventilation. Hands, knees, ankles, wrists, and feet are the joints that are typically involved in a migratory fashion in the RP patients. Other tissues that may be involved are cranial nerves, cardiac vessels, ribs, and cardiac membrane. Systemic symptoms such as fever, anemia, and fatigue may occur. On examination, the auricular cartilage will be swollen, red, and tender to touch. The lobule will be characteristically normal.

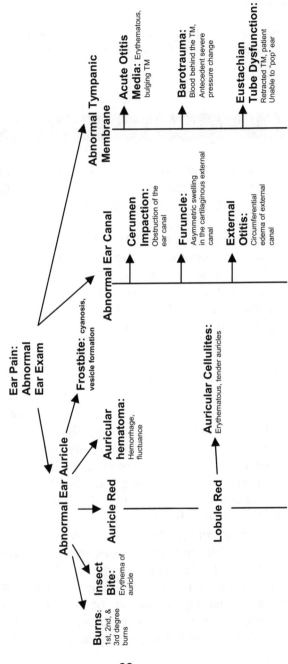

Ear Pain: Abnormal Ear Exam

Abnormal Ear Auricle

Burns: 1st, 2nd, & 3rd degree burns

Insect Bite: Erythema of auricle

Auricle Red

Auricular hematoma: Hemorrhage, fluctuance

Frostbite: cyanosis, vesicle formation

Auricular Cellulites: Erythematous, tender auricles

Lobule Red

Abnormal Ear Canal

Cerumen Impaction: Obstruction of the ear canal

Furuncle: Asymmetric swelling in the cartilaginous external canal

External Otitis: Circumferential edema of external canal

Abnormal Tympanic Membrane

Acute Otitis Media: Erythematous, bulging TM

Barotrauma: Blood behind the TM, Antecedent severe pressure change

Eustachian Tube Dysfunction: Retracted TM, patient Unable to "pop" ear

28

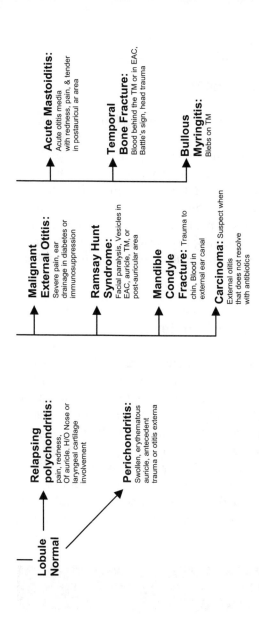

Fig 2-2. The most common causes of otalgia with an abnormal ear exam.

Lobule ——— Normal

Relapsing polychondritis: pain, redness, Of auricle. H/O Nose or laryngeal cartilage involvement

Perichondritis: Swollen, erythematous auricle, antecedent trauma or otitis externa

Malignant External Otitis: Severe pain, ear drainage in diabetes or immunosuppression

Ramsay Hunt Syndrome: Facial paralysis, Vesicles in EAC, auricle, TM, or post-auricular area

Mandible Condyle Fracture: Trauma to chin, Blood in external ear canal

Carcinoma: Suspect when External otitis that does not resolve with antibiotics

Acute Mastoiditis: Acute otitis media with redness, pain, & tender in postauricul ar area

Temporal Bone Fracture: Blood behind the TM or in EAC, Battle's sign, head trauma

Bullous Myringitis: Blebs on TM

Diagnosis and What Tests to Order

Diagnosis of the disease is entirely clinical. Inflammation in two of three of auricular, nasal, or laryngotracheal cartilages or inflammation found in one of three of the auricular, nasal, or laryngotracheal cartilages plus two other signs of the following: inflammatory arthritis, ocular inflammation, vestibular dysfunction, and hearing loss. An accurate history of previous inflammations involving the auricular cartilages, nasal cartilage, or laryngeal cartilage will help in establishing the diagnosis.

Treatment and When to Refer

Glucocorticoids are the main therapy of the disease. Prednisone 1 mg/kg/day up to 80 mg per day is the mainstay of initial therapy. Long-term maintenance with prednisone is commonly required and is generally best done under the care of a rheumatologist. A referral to a rheumatologist is needed for long-term management. If eustachian tube involvement (middle ear effusion or tympanic membrane retraction) or laryngeal/tracheal disease is suspected referral to an otolaryngologist is also warranted.

AURICULAR CELLULITIS AND ERYSIPLAS

Auricular cellulitis is a cutaneous and subcutaneous infection of the auricle and external ear usually caused by group-A Streptococcus or *Staphylococcus aureus* that usually follows a minor trauma. Erysiplas is commonly caused by streptococcal infection of the auricle and has the same symptoms and signs as cellulitis.

Signs and Symptoms

The patient will present with a few days history of pain in the ear. Inquiry should be made about recent trauma, insect bites, or even minor abrasions of the ear skin. The infection may be an extension of an otitis externa. The auricle is warm to touch, tender, erythematous, and cervical lymphadenopathy is occasionally present. The auricle and the lobule will be red and tender (unlike relapsing polychondritis where the lobule is normal on examination).

Diagnosis and What Tests to Order

The diagnosis is entirely clinical. Any purulent discharge should be sent for culture and antibiotic sensitivity studies. If facial cellulitis is present, a CBC with differential should be obtained. It is helpful to outline the edge of the erythema with a marker on the skin to monitor progress.

Treatment and When to Refer

Patients with cellulitis are best treated with penicillinase resistant penicillins which are effective against gram-positive cocci. Amoxicillin/clavulonate 875 mg po BID for 10 days (in children, amoxicillin/clavulonate 90 mg/kg/day of amoxicillin with 6.4 mg/kg/day of clavulonate) will generally cover most of the offending bacteria. Quinolones (e.g., levofloxacin 500 mg po QD × 10 days) can be used as an alternative in adults, and clindamycin 20 mg/kg/day divided Q6–8H can be used in children. If the infection appears to involve the cartilage (exquisite tenderness and blistering/blebs on skin) or systemic symptoms (fever) is present, the patient should be admitted for intravenous (IV) antibiotics with coverage of *S. aureus* and *P. aeruginosa*. A blood culture should also be obtained.

Cellulitis localized to the auricle in an immune-competent patient can be treated with oral antibiotics. Immune-suppressed or diabetic patients or those with extension of the cellulitis beyond the auricle need admission for IV antibiotics. Consultation of an otolaryngologist is recommended if the patient is admitted for IV antibiotics.

PERICHONDRITIS

Perichondritis occurs when the infection of the skin of the auricle involves the cartilage. This can occur secondary to an insect bite, cellulitis, otitis externa, infected ear piercings, trauma, or burn to the auricle.

Symptoms and Signs

The auricle will be erythematous and exquisitely tender to touch. Occasionally blisters or blebs may be present on the auricle.

Diagnosis and What Tests to Order

The diagnosis is based on the examination. A culture of the exudate from the skin and peripheral blood should be obtained.

Treatment and When to Refer

The patient should be admitted for intravenous anti-biotics with antipseudomonal and anti-*Staph aureus* coverage until culture results have been established. The need for admission is due to the tenuous blood supply of the auricular cartilage which can become compromised with the infection and lead to complete loss of the ear cartilage. This will result in a floppy ear due to the loss of structure in the auricle. An otolaryngology consultation on admission is recommended.

BURN OF THE EAR

Direct thermal injury, contact injury, and electrical burns are some common types of burns to the ear. The damage in the skin's outer layer may lead to cartilage infection and subsequent perichondritis or chondritis with final deformity of the cartilage.

Symptoms and Signs

The first degree burns manifest with minor pain and erythema whereas the second degree burns develop blistering. Third degree burns are mostly painless due to full thickness involvement and loss of neural endings. Third degree burns may appear black in color.

Diagnosis and Tests to Order

History and local signs are adequate for diagnosis and no diagnostic measure is required. A basic metabolic panel, and if signs of infection are present, a CBC with differential may be beneficial in the inpatient setting.

Treatment and When to Refer

No specific treatment is suggested in the case of first degree burns. In second and third degree burns, administration of topical antibiotics with analgesics in addition to avoiding pressure on the involved tissue is recommended. In second degree burns, draining the vesicles with a sterile needle will help prevent infection of the vesicular fluid. Skin grafts and reconstruction are used in third degree burns. Debridement of the cartilage is usually avoided. First degree burns and localized second degree burns can be managed in a primary care setting. Extensive second degree burns of the auricle and third degree burns are best managed at a burn center in conjunction with an otolaryngology consultation.

AURICULAR HEMATOMA

Auricular hematomas usually occur because of perichondrial vessel rupture in direct trauma to the ear. In some cases, the blood that accumulates between the perichondrium and cartilage deprives nutrients to the cartilage causing an organized hema-toma and the development of a "cauliflower ear." Cartilage necrosis and atrophy may also occur as a result of an auricular hematoma and can lead to a floppy auricle.

Diagnosis and What Tests to Order

The diagnosis will be clinical. The auricle will be red and ecchymotic with fluctuance.

Symptoms and Signs

The patient will present with a history of trauma and a hematoma. The cartilage may become necrotic and deformity of the ear may develop.

Treatment and When to Refer

An incision is made over the hematoma and the hematoma is completely evacuated. Cottonballs soaked in Betadine™ ointment should be placed into the crevices of the auricle (outside of the skin) to prevent reaccumulation of the hematoma. A head dressing with sponges on and behind the auricle should be used with a head wrap to keep pressure on the auricle. Alternatively, dental rolls may be placed in the concha and in the crease between the helix and the antihelix, as well as behind the ear, and sutured through and through the ear to keep pressure on the auricle. The dressing should be removed in 5 days. Ideally, the patient should be referred for evacuation of the hematoma; however, when immediate access to an otolaryngologist is not available, follow-up with an otolaryngologist is recommended in 2 to 3 days after hematoma evacuation. (See Chapter 7 on Trauma to the Ear for more details.)

FROSTBITE

Frostbite occurs when there is ice formation in the extracellular fluid. When the tissue temperature falls below 0°C, sensory input from the local neural endings is reduced causing the patient not to sense the impending frostbite.

Symptoms and Signs

The cold exposure causes cyanosis that progresses to ischemia and pallor and later vesicle formation in the case of extravasation of the fluid. On examination, the auricle is commonly edematous and occasionally has intact or ruptured bullae.

Treatment and When to Refer

Treatment is by rapid warming of the ear at the temperature of 38 to 42°C in a warm water bath and ibuprofen 600 to 800 mg po as soon as possible. Draining the vesicles with a sterile needle will help prevent infection of the vesicular fluid. Application of the topical aloe vera is suggested. Anti-*Staph. aureus* antibiotics, namely, cephalexin 500 mg po TID (children, 10 mg/kg TID) for nonpenicillin allergics, or clindamycin 150 mg po QID (in children, 15 mg/kg/day divided Q6-8H) for 1 week is suggested for prophylaxis. No debridement is performed until the necrotic tissue has completely demarcated—this may take several weeks. The use of snow or a radiating heat source for rewarming is contraindicated. Hospital admission is required in cases of hypothermia or with frostbite involving the extremities.

OTITIS EXTERNA

Infection of the external ear canal can happen in the acute or chronic forms. Swimming, humidity, maceration of the ear skin, seborrheic dermatitis, and local trauma (with the use of cotton-tipped applicators or other foreign bodies) are predisposing factors for the development of the external otitis. Acute or chronic otitis media can also secondarily cause otitis externa when the purulence drains into the ear canal and causes a local infection. The most common organisms are *Pseudomonas aeruginosa*, *Staphylococcus aureus*, *Staphylococcus epidermis*, and *Proteus vulgaris*. Fungal otitis externa may also occur and can be caused by a variety of organisms.

Symptoms and Signs

The main complaint of patients in otitis externa is ear pain. Ear discharge, external auditory canal stenosis, and hearing loss might occur as the infection progresses. Itching occurs in the setting of fungal otitis externa or in chronic otitis externa, which is also generally fungal in origin. On examination, manipulation of the tragus usually causes pain. The external auditory canal is usually erythematous and inflamed and may seem narrower than the normal side. Drainage in the ear canal is commonly present, but if early in the disease process, it may not be present. The tympanic membrane is not involved initially but may become involved in a macerated pattern if the infection persists. Examination may not be possible at the end stage when an overwhelming pain is developed or the canal has narrowed greatly. Fungal otitis externa is distinguished from bacterial disease by the much thicker and yellow character of the drainage. Occasionally, black dots or white furry appearance of the fungus can be seen in the ear canal among the pus (Fig 2–3).

Diagnosis and What Tests to Order

The diagnosis is based on the pain and edema of the ear canal and the tenderness on movement of the auricle

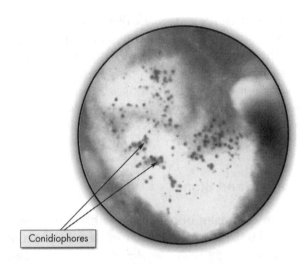

Fig 2–3. Fungal otitis externa. Yellow sludgy drainage and black dots are characteristic findings. From Touma BJ and Touma JB. (2006). *Atlas of Otoscopy.* Copyright 2006. Plural Publishing, San Diego, Calif. Reprinted with permission.

or tragus. A culture of the drainage is necessary only in patients with diabetes and those with an immuno-compromised status or in patients who have failed two courses of ear drops.

Treatment and When to Refer

Avoiding water and cleaning of the external auditory canal to remove the debris is critical for satisfactory treatment. Removal of the debris should be carried out with suction or cotton-tipped applicators, and water should not be used for cleaning. In the mild and moderate external otitis, utilization of drops that contain anti-pseudomonal agents helps. Topical antibiotics that are commonly used are polymyxin, neomycin, and hydrocortisone (Cortisporin Otic Suspension or Solution®), ciprofloxacin with dexamethasone (Ciprodex®), and ofloxacin. All otic drops can be given as 3 gtt TID for 10 days, though ciprofloxacin with dexamethasone can be given as 4 gtt BID for 7 days. To be effective, antibiotics should have contact with the skin, which requires cleansing the canal of debris. In the severe external otitis, once the edematous external canal is to the point that it is closing or closed, or if obstructed by the excessive debris, a wick soaked in the antibiotic drops is placed in the ear canal for 5 to 7 days. Commercial ear wicks are available (eg, Otowick™) or one can be made by cutting a 2 mm × 2 mm × 2 cm sliver from a nasal tampon. The wick is lubricated with a small amount of antibiotic or other lubricant and placed entirely in the ear canal. The patient should be warned of the discomfort that the wick placement will cause temporarily. Oral antibiotics are rarely necessary and can be given in cases where the canal is closed or in cases of mild otitis externa in a reliable diabetic or immunocompromised patient (see malignant otitis externa for diabetic or immune-compromised patients). If oral antibiotics are used, ciprofloxacin 500 mg BID or levofloxacin 500 mg QD is given for 10 days.

Treatment of fungal otitis externa consists of debris removal using suction and irrigation of the ear with a solution of isopropyl alcohol and white vinegar. Isopropyl alcohol and white vinegar is mixed in a 50:50 mixture and the ear is irrigated three times a day using 10 cc of the solution in an ear (bulb) syringe for 10 days. The patient is asked to point the tip of the syringe superiorly in the lateral ear canal and with gentle pressure to cleanse the ear canal. The patient should expect some mild dizziness that results from cooling of the ear canal that resembles caloric testing. The shoulder should be covered with a towel to gather the flushed debris and solution. Acetic acid drops can be given instead of irrigation as VoSol™ or VoSol HC™ (with hydrocortisone) 3 gtt TID for 10 days. The irrigation is preferred because it cleanses the ear canal of the significant debris that gathers as a result of fungal otitis externa. In cases of a tympanic membrane perforation, clotrimazole solution given with a dropper 3 gtt TID for 10 days works well.

Chronic otitis externa patients generally will have chronic itching of the ear and not as much pain. Treatment of chronic otitis externa consists of removal of debris from the external auditory canal and administration of VoSol HC™. Alternatively, nystatin and triamcinolone ointment (Mycolog™) can be given topically to be applied with a cotton-tipped applicator TID for 3 weeks. Hair care products (shampoo, conditioner, hair spray, etc) should be prevented from entering the ear by placing a cotton ball covered with an ointment or petroleum-based jelly (Vaseline™). The patient should be instructed to avoid itching the ears and warned not to use cotton-tipped applicators unless they are used for application of ointment. In resistant cases, topical calcineurin inhibitors (pimecrolimus or tacrolimus) ointments can be used TID for a 3-week period.

Patients with an external auditory canal mass, chronic otitis media, or if the infection is refractory to two different topical antibiotic drops should be referred to an otolaryngologist. Diabetic or immune-compromised patients who have severe pain or edema of the ear canal should be admitted to the hospital for IV antibiotic therapy and otolaryngology consultation.

MALIGNANT (NECROTIZING) EXTERNAL OTITIS (SKULL BASE OSTEOMYELITIS)

Malignant otitis externa (now called skull base osteo-myelitis) occurs when external otitis extends beyond the skin of the external ear canal and invades the tem-poral bone. This phenomenon is usually caused by *P. aeruginosa* in diabetics or immunesuppressed patients. The infection can spread along the skull base, involve the meninges, and cause death.

Symptoms and Signs

The patient will complain of excruciating pain that gets worse at nights in addition to ear discharge. On exam-ination, the skin of the external auditory canal is ede-matous and pus and debris generally are present. In some of the cases, granulation tissue may be visualized at the bony cartilaginous junction (in the midcanal).

Diagnosis and What Tests to Order

In an outpatient setting, a culture of the external ear should be obtained. Admission to the hospital for IV antibiotics must be arranged. A technetium-99 bone scan and otolaryngology consultation should be obtained. Gallium-67 scan should be obtained if the technetium scan is positive. The gallium scan should be repeated after 6 weeks of IV antibiotic ther-apy to monitor resolution of the infection. An erythro-cyte sedimentation rate should be obtained daily in the hospital.

Treatment and When to Refer

Treatment is by removal of debris in addition to the use of intravenous antibiotics. Until culture and sensitivity is obtained, two antipseudomonal antibiotics must be given intravenously. When culture is negative but the technetium scan is positive, intravenous ceftazidime in combination with oral ciprofloxacin should be given. The patient should be discharged with a PICC line when the pain has substantially improved or if the erythrocyte sedimentation rate drops significantly. The treatment must be continued for at least 6 weeks or until the gallium scan is normalized. The technetium scan will remain positive for an extended time period even after resolution of the infection. Upon diagnosis the patient should be admitted to the hospital and otolaryngology consultation should be obtained.

CERUMEN IMPACTION

Cerumen, or earwax, is produced by cerumenous glands in the outside part (cartilaginous) of the ear canal. The function of cerumen is in its oily, acidic nature and its antibacterial enzyme content. The epithelium of the external auditory canal naturally migrates toward the outside of the ear canal and carries the cerumen with it. As one ages (>60 years), the migration slows and the cerumen becomes harder, which leads to a higher incidence of cerumen impaction in the elderly. Occasionally, chronic obstruction of the ear canal by cerumen leads to a mild otitis externa which causes edema of the canal tightening the canal around the cerumen. Use of cotton-tipped applicators worsens the problem of cerumen impaction by pushing cerumen more medially.

Signs and Symptoms

Cerumen impaction most commonly causes hearing loss and occasionally can cause otalgia. The examination shows a cerumen plug in the ear canal. Diagnosis made by examination. No tests need to be ordered.

Treatment and When to Refer

Treatment of cerumen impaction consists of manually removing the cerumen. This can be achieved using loops, suction, or an alligator forceps. If the tympanic membrane has been visualized previously, then irrigation with warm water can help. If the ear canal appears edematous, it is best that irrigation is not used. In these cases, polymyxin, neomycin, hydrocortisone drops (Cortisporin otic suspension® 3 gtt TID in affected ear for 12 days) can be used. In noninfected ears, docusate drops can be used using the same regimen. If the patient is diabetic or immune-compromised and the cerumen cannot be removed atraumatically and without irrigation, then the patient can be referred to an otolaryngologist for removal. Irrigation of the ear increases the risk of otitis externa, which can become severe in diabetic and immune-compromised patients.

RAMSAY HUNT SYNDROME

When facial paralysis is caused by varicella zoster virus, it is termed Ramsay Hunt syndrome. It is distinguished from Bell's palsy by the presence of multiple vesicles present in the external auditory canal, the tympanic membrane, the auricle, or the postauricular areas.

Symptoms and Signs

These patients generally have a severe, excruciating pain in addition to vesicles along the sensory fibers of the facial nerve as described above. The unilateral facial paralysis is more severe and the prognosis is poorer than Bell's palsy with approximately 50 to 60% recovery back to normal (vs 85% in Bell's palsy). Hearing loss and vertigo may also occur due to the cochlear or vestibular nerve involvement. Hyperacusis (sensitivity to sound) may occur due to stapedius muscle paralysis. On examination, CN VII is peripherally involved, which leads to facial asymmetry, eyebrow droop, droop in corner of the mouth, inability to close the eye, lips that cannot be held tightly together, and difficulty keeping food in mouth. Vesicles may be seen in the EAC, TM, auricle, and/or postauricular area.

Diagnosis and What Tests to Order

The diagnosis is by history and examination findings. An MRI of the temporal bone and parotid gland with gadolinium must be ordered to rule out a tumor if the facial paralysis lasts more than 6 months, if there is a slow onset of paralysis (>7 days), recurrent paralysis on the same side, or in a patient with a history of a cutaneous malignancy of the face.

Treatment and When to Refer

Oral corticosteroids and antivirals are the treatment of choice for patients. Prednisone is usually given at a dose of 1 mg/kg (up to 80 mg) per day for 7 days with an 8-day taper. Acyclovir (800 mg po 5 times a day), valacyclovir (1000 mg po q8h), or famcyclovir (500 mg po q8h) should be given for 7 days. Patient should be referred to an otolaryngologist if complete paralysis is present for electrical testing.

CARCINOMA OF THE EAR CANAL

Carcinoma of the ear canal occurs rarely. It is most commonly found in the setting of chronic otitis externa. Similar to cancer in other areas of the head and neck, nonhealing lesions, persistent drainage, a visible mass with pain, or cranial nerve palsies should raise the suspicion for carcinoma.

Symptoms and Signs

The patients most commonly present with chronic drainage from the ear and pain. On examination, the skin of the ear canal can vary from edema of the skin to a fleshy or polypoid mass in the ear canal.

Diagnosis and Treatment

The diagnosis depends on tissue diagnosis upon biopsy. The patient should be referred to an otolaryngologist for biopsy and treatment.

FURUNCLE

A furuncle is an infection of a hair follicle in the external ear canal, which is generally caused by *S. aureus*.

Symptoms and Signs

A red, warm, indurated lesion usually in the orifice of the external auditory canal can be seen and may cause stenosis of the ear canal. The edema of the external canal will be only on one side (vs otitis externa where the canal will be circumferentially edematous).

Diagnosis and Tests to Order

The diagnosis is by the asymmetric edema of the ear canal (Fig 2-4). If purulence is seen, a culture should be obtained.

Treatment and When to Refer

Treatment is with systemic antibiotics (cephalexin 500 mg po TID, in children, 10 mg/kg TID) for 10 days. For penicillin allergics, clindamycin 300 mg po QID (in children, 20 mg po/kg/d divided Q6-8hrs). Warm compresses may help in the early stages, but incision and drainage generally needs to be performed with an 11 blade or an 18-g needle after lidocaine injection if there is no spontaneous drainage or if there is fluctuation in the furuncle that can be palpated. A culture of the abscess contents should be obtained. If the pain and swelling do not subside after antibiotic therapy, a CT scan with and without contrast of the temporal bone may be obtained to rule out the presence of a mass lesion, after a week of treatment.

If the furuncle does not resolve with 3 days of oral antibiotics and the physician is not comfortable with the incision and drainage, referral to an otolaryngologist is warranted.

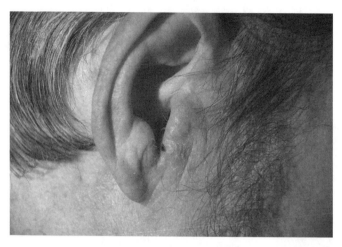

Fig 2–4. Furuncle of the ear canal. Note the edema of tragus and the normal posterior aspect of the ear canal.

MANDIBLE CONDYLE FRACTURE

The mandibular condyle is located a few millimeters anterior to the external auditory canal. Trauma to the chin such as a fall or other external trauma can cause pressure on bilateral mandibular condyles and lead to fracture of the condyle(s). The condyle can sometimes fracture the anterior wall of the external canal and the patient may present with bloody drainage and otalgia after a fall or a strike on the chin.

Symptoms and Signs

In addition to otalgia and occasionally bloody otorrhea, the patient will complain of a difficulty in opening or closing his or her mouth as well as feeling like the teeth do not fit together properly. On examination, occasionally bloody drainage from the ear may be observed. If the patient has an additional fracture of the mandibular symphysis (chin area), a sublingual hematoma may be observed. Palpation of the affected condyle(s) will cause great discomfort.

Diagnosis and What Tests to Order

A panorex of the mandible with a separate panorex of the condyles will help in establishing the diagnosis.

Treatment and When to Refer

If a mandible fracture is suspected or diagnosed, referral to an otolaryngologist is warranted.

TEMPORAL BONE FRACTURE

Temporal bone fractures occur as a result of a severe head trauma. Cochlea, vestibulae, and facial nerves are located within the temporal bones. Temporal bone fractures may involve the tympanic membrane, dislocate the ossicles of the middle ear causing conductive hearing loss, disrupt the facial nerve, or fracture or cause concussive effects on the cochlea leading to sensorineural hearing loss.

Symptoms and Signs

The symptoms include pain in the ear, hearing loss, vertigo, facial paralysis, and bloody ear discharge. Otoscopy may reveal the blood in the external auditory canal, hemotympanum, or otorrhea. A Battle's sign (ecchymosis of the mastoid area) may also be seen. Fracture of the external auditory canal, laceration, or stenosis of the canal also may occur. Rinne and Weber test may demonstrate conductive or sensorineural hearing loss. Neurologic examination may show peripheral facial nerve paralysis or nystagmus.

Diagnosis and What Tests to Order

High-resolution CT of the temporal bone is suggested to evaluate the line and extent of the fracture. If fracture of the temporal bone is suspected, a CT of the brain should also be obtained to rule out an intracranial hemorrhage. An audiogram should be performed after stabilization of the patient looking for potential hearing loss. Facial nerve studies (Electroneuronography [evoked-EMG]) will help in determining prognosis and the need for decompression when facial paralysis is present.

Treatment and When to Refer

If temporal bone fracture passes the external auditory canal, a pack should be inserted to avoid possible stenosis of EAC. This would be best done by an otolaryngologist. In the presence of tympanic membrane perforation, no antibiotic drops should be instilled into the ear and spontaneous healing of the membrane is expected. Ossicular dislocation usually is repaired several months after the fracture. If a temporal bone fracture is suspected, the patient should be sent to an emergency department for CT imaging of the temporal bone and brain. Otolaryngology consultation should be obtained if the diagnosis is made by CT imaging.

ACUTE OTITIS MEDIA

Acute otitis media (AOM) presents with the acute signs of infection such as otalgia and fever. The most common organisms involved in the development of AOM are *Streptococcus pneumoniae*, *Haemophilus influenzae*, and *Moraxella catarrhalis*.

Symptoms and Signs

Young children and adults may present with fever, earache, sensation of fullness in the ear. Less frequently otorrhea, hearing loss, and vertigo may occur. Infants may present with poor sleep, poor feeding, tugging on the ear, and restlessness due to otitis media.

Diagnosis and What Tests to Order

The diagnosis of AOM requires (1) a history of acute onset of signs and symptoms, (2) the presence of middle ear effusion (MEE) (bulging of TM, limited or no mobility of the TM, air-fluid level behind the TM, or otorrhea), and (3) signs and symptoms of middle-ear inflammation (erythema of the TM, otalgia). An audiogram may be warranted if there are signs of speech delay or persistent effusions.

Treatment and When to Refer

For children under the age of 6 months, antibiotic therapy should be used in all patients with certain or uncertain diagnosis. For patients between 6 mo and 2 yrs, antibiotic therapy should be given if the diagnosis is certain. If the diagnosis is uncertain in this age group, antibiotic therapy should be given in patients with severe illness (defined as moderate to severe otalgia or fever of 39°C or higher). For patients over the age of 2 years, antibiotic therapy should be given if the diagnosis is certain and the patient has severe illness. If there is no severe illness or the diagnosis is uncertain, there is an option of observation in children over the age of 2 years. If the observation option is chosen, an antibiotic prescription must be given to the patient to be filled if the symptoms do not significantly improve within 2 days. The patient should follow-up in 2 to 3 days for a recheck. The observation option should not be chosen in a patient who would not be available for a follow-up in 2 to 3 days or in a nonreliable patient.

Antibiotic therapy at diagnosis or at 48 to 72 hours after initial observation (if symptoms do not resolve) is amoxicillin (90 mg/kg/day) in three divided doses for patients without severe illness. For penicillin allergics, cefuroxime or cefpodoxime should be given in non-type-1 reactions and azithromycin or clarithromycin in type 1 allergic reactions to penicillin. In cases of severe illness amoxicillin-clavulonate (90 mg/kg/day of amoxicillin with 6.4 mg/kg/day of clavulonate) should be given. Ceftriaxone 50 mg/kg/d intramuscularly for 1 to 3 days may be given in penicillin allergics with severe illness. In patients with treatment failure at 2 to 3 days after initial management with antibiotic therapy, amoxicillin-clavulonate (in nonsevere illness) or ceftriaxone (severe illness) should be given. For penicillin allergics in treatment failure, ceftriaxone (nontype-1 allergy) or clindamycin (type 1 allergy) should be prescribed. Tympanocentesis or clindamycin should be considered for amoxicillin-clavulonate failures with severe illness.

Refer the patient in case of severe pain/infection that does not resolve with antibiotics, or acute otitis media in the presence of mastoiditis, facial paralysis, meningitis, or vertigo. If pain or tenderness of the mastoid area is noticed or mental status or neurologic changes are seen, the patient should be referred to an emergency department for evaluation and otolaryngology consultation. Recurrent acute otitis media (6 per year), persistent effusion after 4 months, persistent hearing loss, speech delay, or otorrhea warrant outpatient referral to an otolaryngologist for myringotomy and tube placement.

BULLOUS MYRINGITIS

Bullous myringitis manifests with ear pain and blebs that usually appear on the tympanic membrane. The most common organisms responsible for bullous myringitis are *Mycoplasma pneumoniae* and other bacteria that cause otitis media. The blebs usually resolve after a few days of treatment.

Symptoms and Signs

Otalgia is the most common symptom. The examination finding of blebs on the tympanic membrane is diagnostic. No tests need to be ordered.

Treatment and When to Refer

Azithromycin (500 mg po QD × 3 days, children 10 mg/kg QD for 3 days) can be given to cover otitis media and *Mycoplasma spp.* Analgesics for ear pain is recommended. Referral should be considered in cases of excruciating pain. An otolaryngologist can perform a myringotomy and open the blebs and also drain the middle ear of the acute otitis.

ACUTE MASTOIDITIS

Infection of mastoid air cells or mastoiditis as a complication of acute otitis media was more common in the preantibiotic era. The most common organisms responsible in acute mastoiditis are the same organisms that cause acute otitis media.

Symptoms and Signs

The symptoms usually start 1 week after acute otitis media. The patients are usually acutely ill, presenting with fever, otalgia, and sometimes otorrhea.

Signs and Symptoms

The postauricular area will be red, tender, and edematous. Fluctuation of the postauricular area points to a subperiosteal abscess.

Diagnosis and What Tests to Order

The diagnosis is based on the history and exam findings. CT scan is warranted to evaluate for a coalescent mastoiditis or a subperiosteal abscess.

Treatment and When to Refer

Intravenous antibiotic administration is the mainstay of therapy. Surgery is recommended when the patient has otorrhea for more than 2 weeks despite antibiotic therapy, complications of mastoiditis (eg, intracranial complications, sigmoid sinus thrombosis, facial nerve paralysis, and labyrinthitis), or in cases of coalescent mastoiditis (when all the bony septa in the mastoid have been destroyed by the infection as seen on CT imaging). If the patient with acute otitis media has postauricular tenderness or redness, the patient should be admitted with an otolaryngology consultation.

BAROTRAUMA

Barotrauma occurs when there is sudden external pressure change and the patient is not able to equalize their middle ear pressure through Valsalva or other means. This most commonly occurs on descent of a plane and during SCUBA diving. Most commonly, it occurs when the patient's eustachian tube function is poor (eg, upper respiratory infection (URI), allergic rhinitis, nasal congestion, etc) and does not allow equalization of the middle ear pressure using Valsalva, swallowing, and yawning.

Symptoms and Signs

If the middle ear pressure does not normalize with the environment, an excruciating pain, sense of ear fullness, and a mild conductive hearing loss may occur. Occasionally, the patient may develop concomitant vertigo. On otoscopic examination of the ear, red or blue discoloration of the tympanic membrane and blood or fluid in the middle ear may be visualized. The tympanic membrane may rupture and bleeding may occur in to the ear canal.

Diagnosis and What Tests to Order

The diagnosis is based on the history and examination findings. An audiogram must be obtained to evaluate for sensorineural hearing loss, indicating an inner ear loss of function.

Treatment and When to Refer

Generally, no instrument is necessary as the blood or middle ear fluid will resolve. If a TM perforation is seen, the patient should avoid blowing of the nose and prevent water from getting in to the ear by using an ear plug while bathing. Referral to an otologist/ neuro-otologist is required if sensorineural hearing loss or vertigo occurs. This may represent a rupture of the round window membrane, which requires surgical repair.

EUSTACHIAN TUBE DYSFUNCTION (ETD)

ETD can cause pain in the ear. For more detail on the diagnosis or treatment please see Chapter 6 on Ear Plugging.

CHAPTER 3

Ear Drainage

ALICE D. LEE
HAMID R. DJALILIAN

BACKGROUND

Ear drainage can be caused by a variety of pathology in the external ear and the middle ear. This chapter discusses the various disorders based on presentation with or without pain. Figure 3–1 shows the most frequent causes of ear drainage.

EAR DRAINAGE WITH EAR PAIN

Ear drainage, or otorrhea, can be caused by cerumen, exudative or purulent material, fungal debris, carcinoma, or blood or cerebrospinal fluid. Infectious causes are the most common etiologies of otorrhea, but high clinical suspicion for less common causes must be maintained for otorrhea that does not resolve despite reasonable treatment.

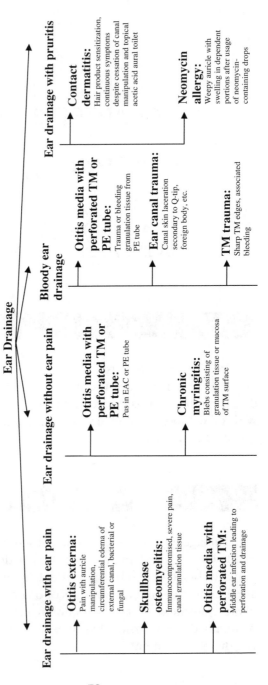

Ear Drainage

Ear drainage with ear pain

Otitis externa:
Pain with auricle manipulation, circumferential edema of external canal, bacterial or fungal

Skullbase osteomyelitis:
Immunocompromised, severe pain, canal granulation tissue

Otitis media with perforated TM:
Middle ear infection leading to perforation and drainage

Ear drainage without ear pain

Otitis media with perforated TM or PE tube:
Pus in EAC or PE tube

Chronic myringitis:
Blebs consisting of granulation tissue or mucosa of TM surface

Bloody ear drainage

Otitis media with perforated TM or PE tube:
Trauma or bleeding granulation tissue from PE tube

Ear canal trauma:
Canal skin laceration secondary to Q-tip, foreign body, etc.

TM trauma:
Sharp TM edges, associated bleeding

Ear drainage with pruritis

Contact dermatitis:
Hair product sensitization, continuous symptoms despite cessation of canal manipulation and topical acetic acid aural toilet

Neomycin allergy:
Weepy auricle with swelling in dependent portions after usage of neomycin-containing drops

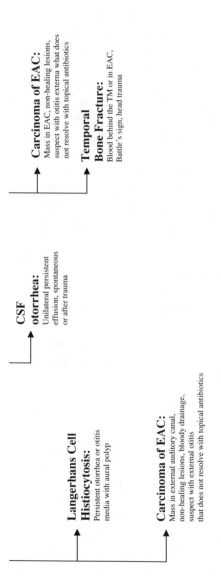

Langerhans Cell Histiocytosis:
Persistent otorrhea or otitis media with aural polyp

Carcinoma of EAC:
Mass in external auditory canal, non-healing lesions, bloody drainage, suspect with external otitis that does not resolve with topical antibiotics

CSF otorrhea:
Unilateral persistent effusion, spontaneous or after trauma

Carcinoma of EAC:
Mass in EAC, non-healing lesions, suspect with otitis externa what does not resolve with topical antibiotics

Temporal Bone Fracture:
Blood behind the TM or in EAC, Battle's sign, head trauma

Fig 3–1. The most common causes of ear drainage.

Otitis Externa

Otitis externa (OE) will most commonly present with severe pain with or without ear drainage. A moist obstructed environment (eg, from ear plugs or hearing aids) or a history of microtrauma (eg, from Q-tip or fingernail manipulation) will cause removal of the normal external auditory canal (EAC) oils and cerumen and can allow bacterial invasion of the skin of the EAC. This leads to an infection, or otitis externa. Swelling of the external auditory canal, canal debris, and pain with tragal pressure and auricular manipulation are classic signs of OE. Patients will often report hearing loss secondary to canal obstruction. The infection is bacterial or fungal in origin. The most common bacterial causes in acute OE are *Pseudomonas aeruginosa* and *Staphylococcus aureus*. Fungal infections usually occur in the setting of immunocompromise (eg, diabetes) or after use of antibacterial ear drops. However, primary fungal OE may occur as well especially in moist environments such as hearing aid use. Fungal OE is characterized by the visualization of fungal debris in the ear canal. This debris may appear as black dots, furry white debris, or a thick sludgy yellow drainage (see Fig 2–1 in Chapter 2).

Treatment and What Tests to Order

The treatment of bacterial OE consists of removal of the debris (with suction), otic drops (eg, ciprofloxacin/dexamethasone (Ciprodex®), polymyxin/neomycin/hydrocortisone (Cortisporin Otic Suspension®), or ofloxacin (Floxin®) 3 drops TID in the affected ear for 10 days) and the avoidance of water or any manipulations of the ear by the patient. Ciprofloxacin/dexamethasone can be given as 4 gtt BID for 7 days. The addition of oral antibiotics with *Pseudomonas* coverage (ciprofloxacin 750 mg po BID × 10 days) is necessary in early infections in diabetics or immunocompromised patients. Patients with near total or total blockage of the external canal from edema must have a wick placed in the ear to allow delivery of the drops to the skin surface. The wick can be obtained commercially (eg, Microwick or Otowick) or can be made with cotton or using a sliver (2 mm × 2 cm) of a nasal tampon. The wick will need to be lubricated and placed in the ear canal with forceps. The wick must be removed in 5 to 7 days. In severe obstruction and in the absence of a wick, oral ciprofloxacin will help in faster alleviation of the patient's symptoms. In cases of MRSA, sulfacetamide drops (3 gtt TID × 2 wks) is generally curative if sensitivity to sulfamethoxazole is found. Generally, all ophthalmic antibiotic drops can be used in the ear if there is no tympanic membrane perforation present.

Patients with fungal otitis externa should be treated with clotrimazole solution applied topically using a dropper (3 gtt TID × 10 days). Alternatively, the patient can be treated with a 9:1 mixture of isopropyl alcohol and white vinegar applied using a bulb syringe or a 10-cc syringe in a flushing manner 3 times a day for 10 days. Patients with tympanic membrane perforations should be treated with clotrimazole and not the alcohol/vinegar combination.

What Tests to Order

Gram stains and cultures can direct antibiotic coverage but are only necessary after failure of a course of otic drop or in the setting of a suspicion for malignant otitis externa (in diabetics or immune-compromised patients). The emergence of methicillin-resistant *Staph aureus* (MRSA) cultured from the EAC must also be considered in refractory cases. Fluoroquinolone otic drops generally do not provide coverage for MRSA and if not recognized, can lead to repeated usage of ineffective medications.

When to Refer

Debridement of the canal using suction is ideal but may be limited in a primary care setting and require otolaryngology referral if these initial steps do not lead to improvement. Flushing of the ear canal should be avoided in otitis externa patients. Granulation (friable polypoid appearing) tissue in the external auditory canal, cranial nerve palsies, extensive otologic pain (especially that which wakes the patient at night), and an immunnocompromised status are warning signs for malignant otitis externa, now referred to as skull base osteomyelitis. These patients require urgent hospitalization with otolaryngology consultation and intravenous antibiotics.

Skullbase Osteomyelitis (aka Malignant Otitis Externa, Necrotizing Otitis Externa)

As mentioned in the prior section, otitis externa that has extended into the temporal bone is termed skullbase osteomyelitis.

Symptoms and Signs

The patients will present with a history of severe otologic pain combined with otorrhea granulation tissue (friable beefy red tissue) in the ear canal on exam. This condition almost exclusively occurs in immune-compromised or diabetic patients and is most commonly caused by *P. aeruginosa*.

Diagnosis and What Tests to Order

The diagnosis depends on the history, examination, and increased uptake on the technetium-99 bone scan. The white blood cell count is often normal but the erythrocyte sedimentation rate (ESR) is elevated. The patient suspected of having skull base osteomyelitis should be admitted to the hospital and a technetium-99 bone scan for diagnosis and gallium-67 scan to follow the progression of the disease should be obtained. A culture of the ear canal should be obtained. The ESR level, gallium scan, improvement of pain, and diminishing granulation tissue are markers of resolution. Treatment consists of an initial 6 week course of culture-directed IV antibiotics, placement of an Otowick, the use of otic ear drops, supportive care for cranial nerve palsies, and pain management. A gallium-67 scan is repeated every 3 weeks after the initial 6 weeks of IV antibiotics to monitor for resolution of inflammation. A normal scan marks the end of antibiotic usage. Clinical suspicion must remain high for a malignancy in this scenario and a biopsy of the granulation tissue should be performed if there is no resolution within 1 to 2 weeks.

Treatment and When to Refer

Initial treatment consists of double coverage IV antibiotics against *Pseudomonas spp*. The antibiotics should be changed once culture has been obtained. The patient should be hospitalized immediately if there is suspicion for skull base osteomyelitis and otolaryngology consultation should be obtained.

Otitis Media with Perforated Tympanic Membrane

In the setting of a draining ear without evidence of otitis externa, a perforated tympanic membrane or a pressure equalizing tube (PE tube) causing drainage of the middle ear infection into the ear canal is a common scenario. Purulent drainage or debris in the external auditory canal (EAC) is often mistaken for isolated otitis externa until the EAC is cleaned out and the tympanic membrane (TM) is examined. The patient with acute otitis media with TM perforation generally will present with a history of otalgia which resolved after the ear drainage started. This is in contrast to the otitis externa patient who will present with ear pain and drainage together. Occasionally, purulence from the middle ear that drains into the EAC can cause a secondary otitis externa. These patients will have a perforation of the TM and edematous and inflamed EAC skin.

Diagnosis and What Tests to Order

The diagnosis depends on visualization of the perforation or tube in the TM. A known history of a PE tube placement and ear drainage should alert the physician of a middle ear infection. Fluoroquinolone otic drops (ofloxacin or ciprofloxacin/dexamethasone 3 gtt TID × 10 days) are the treatment of choice. Gram stain and cultures may direct refractory cases.

Treatment and When to Refer

Depending on the size and location, the majority of TM perforations that occur after acute otitis media will heal spontaneously. A history of repeated infections, subjective or objective hearing loss, and speech delay require otolaryngology referral for formal audiologic assessment and the potential need for surgery for repair of the perforation and treatment of the possible underlying mastoid disease

Cholesteatoma

Cholesteatoma is the presence of squamous epithelium in the middle ear or mastoid that is formed when epithelium is trapped in a retraction pocket, trapped from a tympanic membrane perforation, chronic infection, head trauma, prior surgery, or from congenital presence. It is locally destructive and may be primarily or secondarily acquired or congenital in origin. Diagnosis can be made from physical examination of the ear. A white glistening or yellow mass may be seen in the middle ear and may be accompanied by chronic otorrhea. Immobile cerumen near the tympanic membrane that causes dizziness or severe pain with manipulation may also indicate the presence of cholesteatoma (Fig 3–2). A patient may also present with the chief complaint of hearing loss or plugging sensation of the ear. Treatment is by surgical removal of the epithelium in the middle ear, a mastoidectomy and possible ossicular chain reconstruction if necessary. The patient should be referred to an otologist-neurotologist for evaluation and treatment.

Langerhans Cell Histiocytosis (LCH)

Persistent otorrhea and otitis media in a child despite adequate antibiotic treatment and a polyp on exam with or without other systemic symptoms (eg, fever) is concerning for LCH. LCH is a proliferation of histiocytes in the serum, lymph nodes, and junctional areas in the body (endothelial and epithelial surfaces) of

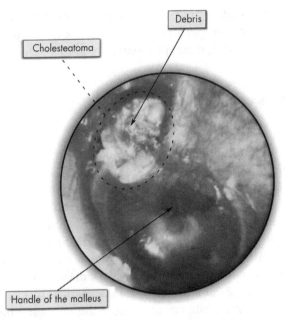

Fig 3–2. Cholesteatoma of the ear. The area most commonly involved is the pars flaccida (superior to the malleus). The cholesteatoma will appear similar to cerumen on the tympanic membrane. From: Touma BJ, Touma JB. (2006). *Atlas of Otoscopy.* Copyright 2006. San Diego, Calif: Plural Publishing. Reprinted with permission.

unclear etiology. Immune dysfunction, lymphoma, and an aberrant immunologic reaction to infection have all been suggested as theories. Twenty percent of patients with LCH present with otorrhea. Clinical suspicion should be high in a child with persistent otorrhea, otitis media, or mastoiditis, with granulation tissue or polyp in the ear canal. Other nonotologic manifestations include lytic skull lesions on x-ray and CT, CNS lesions especially of the pituitary stalk along with presentation of diabetes insipidus, cervical adenopathy, and other signs of bone marrow, lung, liver, and other organ involvement depending on the extent of the disease. Both chemotherapy and low-dose radiation are the mainstays of treatment.

Carcinoma of the External Auditory Canal

Primary squamous cell carcinoma is the most common type of cancer of the external auditory canal. The temporal bone is also a frequent site for metastatic disease. These patients are generally older than 65 years of age and will most commonly present with a history of ear drainage that does not respond to topical antibiotic drops. Patients with a history of smoking or irradiation in the past or those with a history of recurrent otitis externa are at highest risk for developing carcinoma of the external auditory canal. Abnormal tissue in the external auditory canal can be difficult to distinguish from granulation tissue, polyps, infectious debris, and so forth. especially in the setting of infection and limited equipment to examine the ear. Similar to cancer in other areas of the head and neck, nonhealing lesions, persistent drainage, a visible mass with pain, or cranial nerve palsies, should raise the suspicion for carcinoma. These patients should be referred to an otolaryngologist for evaluation and biopsy.

EAR DRAINAGE WITHOUT EAR PAIN

Otitis Media with Perforated Tympanic Membrane or Pressure Equalization (PE) Tube

The patient with a tympanic membrane perforation or PE tube and otitis media will generally present with otorrhea without pain. Examination will show pus in the ear canal or drainage from the tube which may be accompanied by granulation tissue surrounding or filling the tube. Occasionally, a patient with a history of a PE tube will present with blood draining from the ear which can alarm the parents. This is most commonly due to inflamed middle ear mucosa and granulation coming through or around the PE tube and causing some bleeding and indicative of an acute otitis media.

Treatment, What Tests to Order, and When to Refer

Treatment consists of topical quinolone antibiotics (ofloxacin or ciprofloxacin/dexamethasone gtt 3 gtt TID × 10 day). The patient/parent should be instructed to "pump" the tragus after placement of the ear drops to push the drops through the tube into the middle ear. Topical antibiotic drops can achieve concentrations that are significantly higher than oral antibiotics. Bacterial cultures are necessary when topical antibiotic drops are unsuccessful in stopping the drainage. The patient should be referred to an otolaryngologist if an abnormal tympanic membrane (eg, perforation, cholesteatoma) is found or in the setting of recurrent otorrhea (>6 times a year) in a child with a PE tube.

Chronic Myringitis

Chronic myringitis is a chronic inflammation involving the tympanic membrane (TM). It most commonly occurs as a result of trapped mucosal epithelium from the middle ear on the outside surface of the TM. The patient will have a distant history of a TM perforation or PE tube which allowed mucosa to escape the middle ear and settle on the outside surface of the TM. The patient will present with chronic otorrhea and the examination reveals granulation tissue or mucosal surface on the TM. The diagnosis is made after CT scanning which confirms the absence of middle ear and mastoid disease. Treatment is best performed by an otolaryngologist under microscopy in the clinic. It consists of repeated ablation of the mucosa/granulation tissue with silver nitrate with steroid ointment application onto the surface of the TM and antibiotic/steroid ear drops.

Cerebrospinal Fluid (CSF) Otorrhea

CSF otorrhea is most commonly seen after temporal bone trauma and following skull base surgery, but can also occur spontaneously in children with congenital temporal bone defects and a PE tube or spontaneously in adults, most often in middle-aged obese females. Children will often present with meningitis along with pre-existing sensorineural hearing loss and other congenital abnormalities of the temporal bone on CT scan. Adults will present with persistent serous middle ear effusion, aural fullness, persistent watery otorrhea either through a spontaneous TM perforation or after PE tube placement, and a skull base defect on CT scan. It is thought that congenital arachnoid granulations cause erosion of the thin bone of the middle fossa secondary to chronic pulsations and pressure. Suspicion for CSF otorrhea warrants high resolution CT scan of the temporal bone and a referral to an otologist/neuro-otologist for treatment.

BLOODY EAR DRAINAGE

Bloody Ear Drainage in a Patient with a PE Tube or a TM Perforation

Though alarming to patients, bloody ear drainage in the absence of trauma most commonly occurs in a patient with a PE tube and granulation tissue surrounding or through the tube. It can also occur in the setting of TM perforation. The patient who has a tube and develops middle ear inflammation will have the inflamed middle ear mucosa or granulation penetrate through or around the tube to be exposed to the external ear canal. The granulation has fragile blood vessels which will lead to bleeding from the ear. The treatment consists of topical quinolone antibiotics (ofloxacin or ciprofloxacin/dexamethasone gtt 3 gtt TID × 10 day). Ciprofloxacin/dexamethasone will achieve a faster resolution of the granulation tissue. The patient/parent should be instructed to "pump" the tragus after placement of the ear drops to push the drops through the tube into the middle ear.

BLOODY EAR DRAINAGE IN A PATIENT WITH A HISTORY OF TRAUMA

Ear Canal Trauma

The skin of the bony EAC is the thinnest skin in the body. It is easily traumatized by manipulation (eg, Q-tips, fingernail, etc), which will cause bleeding. The bleeding will be more significant in patients on NSAIDs or other anticoagulants.

Symptoms and Signs

The patient will present with bleeding from the ear after apparently minor trauma. Examination may show the source of the bleeding or there may be dried coagulated blood in the ear canal. No tests are required.

Treatment and When to Refer

The patient should make sure that water does not enter the ear by using an ear plug or a cotton ball covered with Vaseline to cover the outside of the ear for one week. This will ensure that water, carrying bacteria, does not cause an otitis externa. If there is a great amount of blood in the canal, topical otic drops (eg, neomycin, polymixin and hydrocortisone (Cortisporin®), ofloxacin, or ciprofloxacin/dexamethasone gtt 3 gtt TID × 5 days). The drops will help dissolve the clot and prevent an otitis externa. The patient should be referred if there is copious blood, if there appears to be tympanic membrane trauma, or if the patient has vertigo (indicating tympanic membrane and ossicular disruption).

Tympanic Membrane Trauma

Trauma to the tympanic membrane (TM) can occur from direct penetrating injury (eg, Q-tip) or indirectly from blast or thermal injury, such as from a slap to the ear or a hot slag. The history is obviously indicative of the mechanism of trauma, and the patient may have bloody otorrhea, partial to total hearing loss, pain and dizziness. Microscopic examination of the external auditory canal, the tympanic membrane and the middle ear after clearing the blood or foreign body is necessary to determine where the trauma has occurred and if there is a need for surgical exploration. Trauma to the posterior superior quadrant has a higher likelihood of ossicular injury and resultant conductive or sensorineural hearing loss. Ossicular injury will require surgical intervention to reconstruct the ossicular chain. Referral to an otolaryngologist is warranted for examination, audiologic evaluation, and evaluation for surgery. Urgent (same day) referral is needed if the patient has vertigo or if tuning fork testing shows a sensorineural hearing loss. Prednisone 1 mg/kg should be started for 7 days if the patient is not diabetic. Normally, a simple TM disruption should cause a conductive hearing loss. Therefore, a Weber test (tuning fork on the forehead) will be lateralized to the side of the injury. If the Weber test lateralizes to the side away from the injury, it may indicate a sensorineural hearing loss in the traumatized ear.

Temporal Bone Trauma

Fractures of the petrous temporal bone occur after forceful blunt trauma to the skull. The patients will generally present to an emergency department but may occasionally present to the primary care setting. The patient may not be aware of the injury due to the loss of consciousness that may have occurred from the injury. The most common sign on examination is bleeding in the ear canal or blood in the middle ear. The patient may also have a Battle's sign—ecchymosis of the mastoid area. Computed tomography of the head and preferably of the temporal bone make the diagnosis. Fractures of the temporal bone may be associated with facial nerve injury, CSF leak, other intracranial complications, and hearing loss. An otologic exam along with careful documentation of facial nerve function should always be performed soon after the injury. If the facial nerve function is normal initially after injury and then becomes weak, then the facial nerve function will spontaneously return. If the facial nerve becomes paralytic immediately following the trauma, the patient will need surgical repair of the nerve. Temporal bone fracture will generally occur from a severe head trauma. Therefore, if it is suspected, the patients should be sent to an emergency department for a head CT to rule out an intracranial bleed. A referral to an otolaryngologist during hospitalization should be made to manage the potential complications. An audiogram will need to be obtained on an outpatient basis.

Carcinoma of the External Auditory Canal

Carcinoma of the external ear canal can present with bloody drainage. It is most common in the older adult (>65 yr). See above for greater detail on this disorder.

Pruritic (Itchy) Ears

Isolated pruritic external auditory canals are a common problem that most often represent an allergic contact dermatitis. However, patients with this presenting complaint must also be ruled out for carcinoma of the EAC, foreign body, psoriasis, fungal otitis externa, dermatophytid reaction, and other entities. Given an ear exam that is otherwise normal with the exception of inflamed EAC skin, the majority of patients will have return of normal cerumen and oil production after treatment with topical acetic acid 2% with or without hydrocortisone. For patients who fail this treatment, chronic use of topical steroids is not ideal. The already thin skin of the EAC may thin further with chronic topical steroid use and undergoes changes that do not restore normal function. The topical immune modulators tacrolimus and picrolimus have been found to be efficacious for these stubborn cases. Application with a cotton-tipped applicator twice daily for 3 weeks to 3 months along with keeping the ears plugged when washing hair to prevent shampoo and conditioners from entering the ear canals is very effective. Referral to an otolaryngologist is warranted if the patient fails a short course of topical steroids or calcineurin inhibitors.

Neomycin allergy is the most common allergy seen with the use of otic drops. Cortisporin® otic drops consist of neomycin, polymixin, and hydrocortisone. Cortisporin® otic solution is more acidic than Cortisporin® otic suspension. A dependent distribution of skin irritation is a telltale sign of this allergy. Treatment consists of stopping the drops and a short course of topical steroids. The patient should be switched to either ciprofloxacin/dexamethasone or ofloxacin drops to treat the infection.

FURTHER READING

Djalilian HR, Memar O. Topical pimecrorlimus 1% for the treatment of pruritic external auditory canals. *Laryngoscope.* 2006;116:1809–1812.

Djalilian HR, Shamloo B, Thakker KH, Najme-Rahim M. Treatment of culture-negative skull base osteomyelitis. *Otol Neurotol.* 2006;27:250–255.

Lasak JM, Van Ess M, Kryzer TC, Cummings RJ. Middle ear injury through the external auditory canal: a review of 44 cases. *Ear, Nose, Throat J.* 2006;85:722,724–728.

Rao AK, Merenda DM, Wetmore SJ. Diagnosis and management of spontaneous cerebrospinal fluid otorrhea. *Otol Neurotol.* 2005;26:1171–1175.

Surico GS, Muggeo P, Muggeo V, Conti V, Novielli C, Romano A, et al. Ear involvement in childhood Langerhans' cell histiocytosis. *Head Neck.* 2000;22:42–47.

CHAPTER 4

Hearing Loss

VANESSA S. ROTHHOLTZ
HAMID R. DJALILIAN

BACKGROUND

Hearing impairment may present itself at any time and at any age. It may exist as a single entity or may be a part of a syndrome or larger disease process. Hearing loss exists in approximately 28 million Americans, affecting 2 to 3 in 1,000 newborns and 314 in 1,000 adults over the age of 65. Undetected and untreated hearing impairment in early childhood may result in lifelong deficits in language skills and cognitive learning, whereas even mild hearing difficulties that are undiagnosed and not addressed in the elderly may cause decreased interactions among peers and family that could diminish mental and physical health.

A detailed history and examination is fundamental in identifying hearing loss and its etiology. Some patients may complain of hearing loss as their primary concern; however, the impairment may be discovered on routine screening or mentioned incidentally by a family member. See Chapter 1 for the history and examination of the ear.

CONGENITAL HEARING LOSS

Congenital hearing loss can be genetic or nongenetic and syndromic or nonsyndromic. It can be sensorineural in etiology or conductive. It is important to note the presence of congenital hearing loss whether it is discovered upon screening or by strategic questioning of the parents with respect to developmental milestones in order to create a prompt treatment plan. When evaluating hearing loss of congenital origin, it is important to examine the patient for syndromic characteristics that will affect the overall health. As stated previously, a thorough family and maternal birth history, including gestational diabetes, infections, and medications, should be discussed. Immediate postpartum history of the neonate should also be acquired, including low Apgar scores, meconium aspiration, intubation with prolonged ventilation, or hyperbilirubinemia. It is important to recognize hearing loss early in childhood and to treat it. The critical period to learn speech and language is between 1 and 4 years of age and if the child passes that time and does not obtain language skills, she or he may never gain the ability to speak normally for his/her age. However, if a child is diagnosed with deafness at birth and receives a cochlear implantation before the age of 2 years, she or he has a 90% chance of enrolling in school with normal hearing children by the age of 6 years. Recognition of hearing loss at a young age depends on specifically asking the patient's parents about the language milestones (Table 4–1).

Table 4–1. Language Milestones

3 months	Infants respond to parents' voices by being quiet or are startled with loud sounds such as telephone ringing
6 months	Babble with sounds like mama or dada
12 months	Say their first word
2 years	2-word sentences, 100–300 words
3 years	3-word sentences

Workup of Congenital Hearing Loss

Once the newborn hearing screening is found to indicate a hearing loss, a second auditory brainstem response (ABR) test should be scheduled as an outpatient. If the second ABR indicates a hearing loss, a more detailed ABR, possibly under sedation will be obtained. If the third ABR indicates a hearing loss, the patient will be fitted with hearing aids. The patient will need to have a urinalysis, a test of syphilis (RPR), and a pediatric ophthalmology evaluation. If the patient is completely deaf, she or he will also need to have an EKG to rule out a prolonged QT interval (Jervell and Lange-Nielsen syndrome). A genetic screening and CT scan of the temporal bones can also assist with the workup of the case.

Genetic Hearing Loss

Most forms of congenital hearing loss are nonsyndromic and are associated with the autosomal recessive transmission. The most common cause of genetic hearing loss is a defect in the connexin 26 gene, the gene that codes for a gap junction β-2 protein. A table of common syndromes is presented below and should serve as a guide in the astute physician's examination (Table 4–2). For example, Alport's syndrome or Potter syndrome may present with a family history of kidney disease. Heart anomalies should be discovered in the presence of congenital Rubella, DiGeorge syndrome, Hurler syndrome, Patau syndrome (Trisomy 13), Down syndrome (Trisomy 21), and CHARGE syndrome in which coloboma, heart anomalies, choanal atresia, mental retardation, genital anomalies, and external and internal ear anomalies exist.

Table 4–2. Common Syndromes Causing Hearing Loss

Syndrome	Other Characteristics
Alport	Renal dysfunction, ocular abnormalities
Apert	Craniofacial dysotosis, brachycephaly, spina bifida, hypertelorism, syndactyly, cleft palate
Beckwith-Wiedemann	Exophthalmos, macroglossia, gigantism, facial nevus flammeus, midface hypoplasia, hypoglycemia, organomegaly, genitourinary anomalies
Branchio-Oto-Renal	Branchial derived anomalies (cleft palate/lip, cysts, fistulas), renal malformations
CHARGE	Coloboma, heart anomalies, choanal atresia, mental retardation, genital anomalies, ear abnormalities
Crouzon	Premature craniosynostoses, midfacial hypoplasia, ocular deformities, cleft palate
DiGeorge	Hypoplastic thymus, aortic arch anomalies, patent ductus arteriosus (PDA), thyroid agenesis, acrania, microcephaly, micrognathia, cleft palate

Table 4–2. *continued*

Syndrome	Other Characteristics
Fanconi	Aplastic anemia, skin pigmentation, skeletal and renal anomalies, mental retardation
Goldenhar	Unilateral facial hypoplasia, dermoids, vertebral anomalies, micrognathia, cleft lip and palate, laryngeal anomalies
Hurler	Dwarfism, hepatosplenomegaly, mental retardation, hypertelorism, facial deformities, skeletal deformities, short fingers, cardiac anomalies
Klippel-Feil	Fused cervical vertebrae, pectoral girdle deformities, spina bifida, cleft palate
Jervell-Lange-Nielsen	Syncope with prolonged QT interval (cardiac anomalies), family history of death in childhood
Möbius	Absent abductors of the eye, musculoskeletal deformities, cranial nerve palsies, short stature
Osteogenesis Imperfecta	Blue sclera, multiple bone fractures, skeletal deformities, abnormal tooth dentin, cardiovascular and platelet anomalies, macrocephaly
Pendred	Euthyroid goiter, enlarged vestibular aqueduct
Stickler	Pierre Robin sequence (cleft palate, retrognathia, glossoptosis), myopia, retinal detachment, cataracts, marfanoid habitus, arthritis
Treacher Collins	Mandibulofacial dysotosis ("fishmouth"), downward slanting palpebral fissures, coloboma, cleft palate
Usher	Progressive retinitis pigmentosa, mental retardation, vestibular dysfunction
Waardenburg	Pigment abnormalities (white forelock, heterochromic iriditis), craniofacial abnormalities, telecanthus

Nongenetic

Additional causes of congenital hearing loss that are not hereditary include maternal infection, kernicterus, trauma during birth, and medication toxicity. Congenital rubella, syphilis, and cytomegalovirus may be viral causes of hearing loss.

ACQUIRED HEARING LOSS

Acquired hearing loss may be sensorineural or conductive in etiology. The primary cause of acquired hearing loss is noise exposure. Presbycusis is a general term used to describe hearing loss due to aging. Other causes of sensorineural hearing loss include ototoxic medications, autoimmune disorders, sudden sensorineural hearing loss (thought to be viral), head trauma or an acoustic neuroma. Head trauma may also cause a conductive hearing loss. Other causes of acquired conductive hearing loss include otosclerosis, otitis media, obstruction of the ear canal, tympanic membrane perforation, cholesteatoma, or tympanosclerosis.

In noise-induced hearing loss, a temporary loss of hearing may occur which resolves after 24 hours. With repeated loud noise exposure a permanent hearing loss will occur. High-pitched tinnitus frequently accompanies the disorder. Acquiring a history of noise exposure and an audiogram that demonstrates a worsened threshold at 4-kHz frequency typically confirms the diagnosis.

A thorough history of current and past medication use may direct the physician to an ototoxic drug as the cause of the hearing loss. Common medications that may be ototoxic include aminoglycoside antibiotics, platin-based chemotherapeutic agents (cisplatin, carboplatin), and loop diuretics. NSAIDs cause a sensorineural hearing loss (and resultant tinnitus) which reverses after stopping the medication. Close monitoring of a patient's hearing and dose/drug adjustment can reduce the risk of ototoxicity during the use of known deleterious drugs.

Autoimmune disorders, specifically polyarteritis nodosa, systemic lupus erythematosis, and Wegener's granulomatosis may cause hearing loss as an otologic manifestation in middle-aged patients. Laboratory tests, such as immune specific serology, can assist in making the diagnosis, and steroid therapy may be indicated during exacerbations of the condition. Metabolic disorders such as diabetes, hypothyroidism, renal failure, and hyperlipidemia may also cause hearing loss in extreme situations.

PRESBYCUSIS—AGE-RELATED HEARING LOSS

Age-related hearing loss is a high-frequency hearing loss (worst at 8000 Hz) which starts at the age of 40 to 50 years of age. The loss of hearing progresses with time and its progress is dependent on previous exposure to noise and genetic factors.

Symptoms and Signs

The patients are usually brought in by their spouse who complains that the patient cannot hear them or has raised the volume of the television. The patient will have difficulty hearing in noisy environments (eg,

cocktail parties, restaurants, etc) and will have difficulty hearing females and young children with higher
frequency voices. The examination is generally normal.

Diagnosis and What Tests to Order

The diagnosis is by obtaining an audiogram which will
show the hearing loss centered at 8000 Hz. If an asymmetric hearing loss (>10 dB difference in 3 frequencies) is found, an MRI of the internal auditory canals
should be obtained to rule out an acoustic neuroma.

Treatment and When to Refer

The treatment of presbycusis is by using a hearing aid.
The patient should be referred to an otolaryngologist
or audiologist to obtain hearing aids.

SUDDEN SENSORINEURAL HEARING LOSS

Sudden sensorineural hearing loss (SSNHL) is a medical emergency defined as the loss of >30 dB intensity
of hearing in three or more adjacent frequencies. This
loss occurs over a time period of three days or less and
is typically unilateral. Although spontaneous recovery
rates are cited to be between 32 and 70%, and only
10 to 15% of cases are discovered to have a specific
etiology, prompt diagnosis and treatment is imperative.
Reversible causes should aggressively be evaluated
including a perilymphatic fistula (loss of hearing after
pressure [eg, SCUBA diving] or noise trauma), trauma
to the inner ear or ossicular chain, or the presence of

an acoustic neuroma. SSNHL is most commonly identified as being idiopathic and is treated empirically
with systemic and intratympanic steroids. Most cases
may be due to an autoimmune process, or a viral or
vascular etiology.

Symptoms and Signs

The patients will present with a history of sudden loss
of hearing or feeling of a plugged ear and tinnitus
which does not improve after "popping" the ears using
Valsalva. The patient will have a normal ear exam. On
tuning fork testing, the Weber (tuning fork placed in
the midline of the forehead), the sound will lateralize
to the contralateral ear. The Rinne test may show air
conduction louder than bone conduction, but if there
is no hearing present, the sound may not be heard at
all in the affected ear. If a tuning fork is not available,
the patient should be asked to hum. If the patient hears
the humming in the contralateral ear, then a SSNHL
should be suspected.

Diagnosis and What Tests to Order

Every patient suspected of having SSNHL should obtain
an audiogram the same day to make the diagnosis. If
an SSNHL is confirmed, the patient will need an MRI
of the internal auditory canals with gadolinium to rule
out an acoustic neuroma.

Treatment and When to Refer

The patient should be referred for an audiogram and an
otolaryngology visit within 1 to 2 days of presentation.

SSNHL should be treated within 14 days of onset, otherwise the likelihood of hearing recovery is considerably lower. If an audiogram or an otolaryngologist is not immediately available and no contraindications to corticosteroid therapy exist, the patient should be started on prednisone (1 mg/kg/day up to 80 mg daily for 7 days, with an 8-day taper). Although some studies advocate a 14 day course of high dose steroids with a taper over 2 weeks, the senior author's (HRD) experience indicates that a shorter course is equally efficacious.

The patient must obtain an audiogram at the one week time point and if there is no improvement in the hearing, intratympanic steroid therapy should be started under the guidance of an otolaryngologist who performs this treatment or an otologist-neurotologist.

NOISE-INDUCED HEARING LOSS

Patients with acute exposure to very loud sounds (eg, concerts, gun shots, night club, etc) or chronic exposure to loud sounds (eg, factory noise, MP3 players, etc) will develop a sensorineural hearing loss centered around 4000 hertz. As the exposure to the loud sound continues, adjacent frequencies (2000 and 8000 Hz) will also develop a loss.

Symptoms and Signs

The patients will generally present with tinnitus or difficulty hearing in noisy environments (eg, restaurants, cocktail parties, etc). The examination will typically be normal.

Diagnosis and What Tests to Order

The patient should have an audiogram to evaluate the extent of the hearing loss. The diagnosis is by seeing a loss of hearing centered at 4000 Hz.

Treatment and When to Refer

Acute loss of hearing after a very loud noise exposure can be treated with a 5 day course of prednisone (0.5 mg/kg), though its efficacy has not been proven in clinical trials. Prevention of hearing loss with hearing protection and anti-oxidant vitamins is effective. A hearing aid will benefit patients who have difficulty in daily situations.

OTOTOXICITY

Hearing loss can occur as a result of toxicity of certain medications to the cochlea. The most common medications that cause ototoxicity include non-steroidal anti-inflammatory drugs (NSAIDs), aminoglycosides, loop diuretics, and chemotherapeutic agents (most commonly, platin-based drugs). The hearing loss from NSAIDs (most commonly, Aspirin) is reversible after stopping the medication, whereas the hearing loss from the other mentioned drugs is irreversible.

Symptoms and Signs

Patients will most commonly present with tinnitus or hearing loss while on the medication. The examination will be normal. Aminoglycosides are also toxic to the inner ear balance organ (vestibule) and the patients may complain of vertigo or imbalance.

Diagnosis and What Tests to Order

The diagnosis is by performing an audiogram and oto-acoustic emissions testing. The audiogram will typically show a loss of sensorineural hearing in the high frequencies. The otoacoustic emissions (which indicate hair cell function) will show loss of emissions in the high frequencies.

Treatment and When to Refer

The treatment is by stopping the medication and switching the patient to a different drug in a different class of medications. Patients on NSAIDs can be changed to COX-2 inhibitors (eg, celecoxib) if the NSAID is found to be the source of the problem. Patients with a tympanic membrane perforation or a pressure-equalization tube should not be prescribed an aminoglycoside-containing ear drop (eg, Cortisporin®). A fluoroquinolone ear drop (ofloxacin or ciprofloxacin/dexamethasone) should be used instead.

ASYMMETRIC HEARING LOSS

Asymmetric high-frequency hearing loss that is progressive may be indicative of a cerebellar pontine angle (CPA) tumor. The most common CPA tumor is an acoustic neuroma that typically arises from the vestibular portion of the eighth cranial nerve. The presentation may be accompanied by tinnitus, vertigo, and occasionally sudden hearing loss. As discussed previously, a CPA tumor is discovered by distinct audiologic findings and confirmed by an MRI with contrast for this slow-growing tumor. First degree relatives of patients with neurofibromatosis type II should be screened for acoustic neuromas. Other CPA tumors that may present with hearing loss include meningiomas, hemangiomas, arachnoid cysts, epidermoids, or other malignancies. Children with a unilateral hearing loss have a 30% likelihood of failing a grade in school in their 12 years of education; therefore, hearing rehabilitation and preferential seating in class is essential.

POST-TRAUMATIC HEARING LOSS

Trauma to the head that causes a temporal bone fracture may lead to a sensorineural or conductive hearing loss. Fracture through the otic capsule (inner ear hearing or balance organs) will produce sensorineural hearing loss and vertigo. Hemotympanum noted on examination may produce a conductive hearing loss, although patients should also be evaluated for dislocation of the osscular chain after 6 weeks (after the blood resolves). Tuning fork tests, a thorough examination, and an audiogram as described previously will lead to the correct diagnosis. After stabilization of the airway, patients should undergo a complete head and neck examination after experiencing head trauma to rule out cranial nerve or central neurologic injury and to evaluate for facial fractures and cerebrospinal fluid leak. Treatment depends on the type of injury. Tympanic membrane perforations tend to heal and hemotympanum resorbs spontaneously. Surgical reconstruction of the ossicular chain may be necessary if the diagnosis is made.

OTOSCLEROSIS

Otosclerosis is a hereditary condition of progressive conductive hearing loss in which the stapes is fixed onto the oval window. It can be unilateral or bilateral, occurs in females more than in males, and typically presents in patients at the age of 30 to 50 years old. Diagnosis is confirmed via a large air-bone gap noted on audiogram, normal speech discrimination, and a normal physical exam. The audiogram may also demonstrate a Cahart's notch at 2000 Hz at which the bone threshold has a notched dip due to mechanical impedance changes in the middle ear. Treatment is by hearing aid or via surgical ossicular chain reconstruction in which a stapedectomy or stapedotomy is performed and a prosthesis is placed. The patient should be referred to an otologist-neurotologist for evaluation and treatment.

CONDUCTIVE HEARING LOSS

Conductive hearing loss can be caused by any process that impedes the conduction of sound from the auricle to the cochlea. For example, cerumen impaction or a foreign body in the ear canal is a common cause of ear canal obstruction. In addition, congenital malformations of the ear canal, as well as collapse of the ear canal can cause a conductive hearing loss of up to 60 dB. However, the most common cause of conductive hearing loss typically is fluid accumulation in the middle ear. The fluid in the middle ear impedes vibration of the tympanic membrane, reducing the efficiency of sound conduction. Other similar conductive losses may involve tympanic membrane perforation, tympanosclerosis (thickening of the fibrous layer), or atelectasis (loss of the fibrous layer) of the tympanic membrane.

Conductive loss can occur as a result of disruption of sound transmission in other parts of the middle ear or even the inner ear. For example, chronic infections of the middle ear may permanently disrupt the ossicular chain. Or, overgrowth of bone in the stapes region, namely, otosclerosis, reduces mobility of the stapes. Finally, if there is an opening into the inner ear that is uncovered, then some of the sound-induced volume velocity will be shunted away from the cochlea, creating a conductive hearing loss.

Treatment and When to Refer

Generally, conductive loss can be corrected medically, with hearing aids, or surgically, producing nearly normal perceptual performance after correction. The patient should be referred to an otolaryngologist or an otologist-neurotologist if there is persistent conductive hearing loss.

SENSORINEURAL HEARING LOSS

Sensorineural hearing loss (SNHL) usually refers to structural damage in the inner ear, generally due to loss of outer and inner hair cells. The most apparent consequence of outer hair cell damage is loss of sensitivity (an inability to hear soft sounds). This will most commonly occur in the elderly or those with loud noise exposure. Levels of sound and duration of exposure will together act to increase the likelihood of noise-induced hearing loss (Table 4-3).

Table 4–3. Permissible Levels of Sound and Exposure Times to Prevent Noise-Induced Hearing Loss (OSHA Standards)

Number of Hours Per Day	Decibel Level of Sound Exposure
8	90
6	92
4	95
3	97
2	100
1.5	102
1	105
0.5	110
0.25 or less	115

Treatment and When to Refer

Patients with SNHL will generally benefit from hearing aids for rehabilitation. If hearing aids do not help the patients, they may be a candidate for a cochlear implant. A cochlear implant is a device that replaces the function of hearing by directly stimulating the auditory nerve. It is placed via an outpatient procedure and rehabilitation after 6 months will give the patient the ability to understand more than 80% of presented words in a quiet environment.

TREATMENT

Nearly all hearing loss is treatable, either medically, with a hearing aid, or via surgical correction. The treatment plan for specific hearing loss disorders was described previously. However for patients in whom hearing loss is not reversible, methods for bringing the patient back to a functioning level are described below. Hearing aids, both behind the ear, in the ear, and bone-anchored, as well as cochlear implants are discussed.

There are many types of hearing aids, and the best hearing device for a patient should be determined by the nature and degree of their hearing loss. Other factors that are taken into account when fitting a patient with a hearing aid include the shape of the pinna, the size of the external auditory canal, and other ear conditions such as infection or chronic otorrhea. Conventional hearing aids are devices that amplify and filter sound. As technology improves hearing aids gain more ability to specifically amplify deficient frequency groups while producing less feedback and a better signal. These hearing aids can be worn on the body, behind the ear (BTE), in the ear (ITE), in the canal (ITC), and completely in the canal (CIC). As the hearing aid is made less conspicuous, the achievable gain is reduced due to a higher degree of feedback (whistling). The patients who have bilateral hearing loss are best treated with bilateral hearing aids.

For patients with a unilateral profound hearing loss who desires improved sound localization, a contralateral routing of signal (CROS) hearing aid can be considered. The CROS aid consists of a microphone that is located on the side of the head with the poorer hearing ear. The sound is then presented to the better hearing ear to allow the patient to better localize sound. The use of a bone-anchored hearing aid (BAHA) is indicated in patients who do not desire non-implantable hearing aids or the CROS aid. It may be useful in patients with a unilateral deafness, congenital ear malformations, or a chronically draining ear. The sound processor is attached to an implantable titanium post that is located in the bone behind the diseased ear and sends the sound via bone conduction to the hearing ear.

Infants with congenital bilateral sensorineural deafness, children under 18 years of age with severe to profound hearing loss, who have minimal benefit from hearing aids, and adults who do not benefit from hearing aids may qualify for a cochlear implant. Candidacy is also determined by specialized audiologic tests at a cochlear implant center. The implant is a device that digitally converts sound into electrical pulses. The discrete pulses are delivered via a multichannel electrode that is surgically placed into the cochlea. Bilateral cochlear implantation and the hybrid cochlear implant are currently being studied as new methods of electrical sound delivery. Bilateral implantation, although still not accepted as the standard of care for implantation, has demonstrated an improvement in sound localization and the perception of speech in noise. The hybrid implant is a shortened electrode that is partially implanted into the cochlea and is currently under investigation in clinical trials as a device that may be helpful in patients with isolated high-frequency hearing loss. A conventional acoustic hearing aid is worn simultaneously to amplify the preserved low frequency hearing. Other future routes of implantation for hearing loss include implantable piezoelectric middle ear devices, cochlear nerve implantation, and the auditory brainstem implant.

WHEN TO REFER A PATIENT WITH HEARING LOSS

Patients with sudden sensorineural hearing loss (see above) require urgent referral. Patients with asymmetric hearing loss, conductive hearing loss, progressive hearing loss, or any hearing loss in a child will need an evaluation by an otolaryngologist. Patients with acoustic neuromas should be referred to an otologist/ neuro-otologist.

FURTHER READING

Conlin AE, Parnes LS. Treatment of sudden sensorineural hearing loss. *Arch Otolaryngol Head Neck Surg*. 2007; 133:573-581.

Isaacson JE, Vora NM. Differential diagnosis and treatment of hearing loss. *Amer Family Phys*. 2003;68:1125-1132.

Schuller DE, Schleuning AJ. (1994). Hearing loss. In: D. Down, ed. *DeWeese and Saunders' Otolaryngology Head and Neck Surgery* (pp. 453-477). St Louis, Mo: Mosby-Yearbook.

Tabaee A, Roach M, Selesnick SH. (2004). Congenital disorders of the middle ear. In: Lalwani, AK, ed. *Current Diagnosis and Treatment in Otolaryngology—Head and Neck Surgery* (pp. 679-694). New York, NY: McGraw-Hill.

Yueh B, Shapiro N, MacLean CH, Shekelle PG. Screening and management of adult hearing loss in primary care. *JAMA*. 2003;289:1976-1985.

CHAPTER 5

Tinnitus

HAMID R. DJALILIAN
VANESSA S. ROTHHOLTZ
SANAZ HAMIDI

BACKGROUND

Perception of sound in the absence of auditory stimulus is termed as tinnitus. Tinnitus may be the result of hearing loss or sounds produced by adjacent structures or other disease processes. Sounds may be described as ringing, humming, buzzing, roaring, whooshing, chirping, or whistling. Tinnitus affects approximately 37 million Americans and in 10 million it is severe and debilitating. The prevalence of tinnitus in adults worldwide has been estimated to be between 10.1 and 14.5 %, and is more common in people aged between 40 and 70 years old. The most common causes of tinnitus are outlined in Figure 5-1.

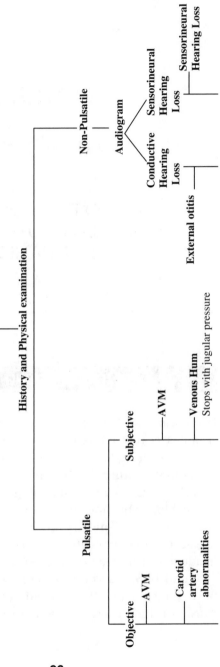

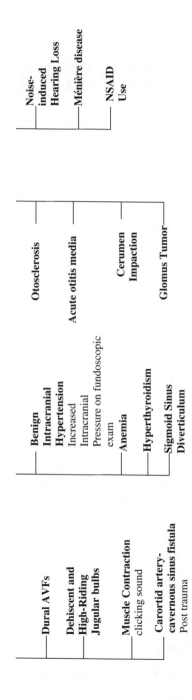

Fig 5–1. Common causes of tinnitus.

Noise-induced Hearing Loss
Ménière disease
NSAID Use

Otosclerosis
Acute otitis media
Cerumen Impaction
Glomus Tumor

Benign Intracranial Hypertension
Increased Intracranial Pressure on fundoscopic exam
Anemia
Hyperthyroidism
Sigmoid Sinus Diverticulum

Dural AVFs
Dehiscent and High-Riding Jugular bulbs
Muscle Contraction clicking sound
Carortid artery-cavernous sinus fistula
Post trauma

TONAL TINNITUS

Most commonly, patients who have tinnitus will complain of a constant or intermittent high frequency (ringing) sound sensation in the ear(s). The patient may complain of a constant hissing, buzzing, or humming sound. The most common etiology for tinnitus is hearing loss. The predominant pathophysiologic mechanism for the development of tinnitus involves the presence of increased auditory cortex activity in the brain as a result of loss of hearing at the periphery. The most common causes include presbycusis, sensorineural hearing loss, cerumen impaction, middle ear infection, tympanic membrane perforation, noise-induced hearing loss, otosclerosis, Ménière's disease, vestibular schwannoma, and ototoxic medications. Tinnitus is more severe in patients with anxiety or depression. An evaluation of these symptoms must be done to evaluate the need for further therapy.

Symptoms and Signs

The patients will generally complain of various tones of sound at different times. The patient will have the symptoms occur more severely at night, because the absence of ambient noise allows the patient to hear the tinnitus more intensely. The examination may reveal abnormalities of the ear canal or the middle ear. However, sensorineural hearing loss and certain types of conductive hearing loss (eg, otosclerosis) can have a normal ear examination.

Diagnosis and What Tests to Order

The diagnosis is by history. An audiogram must be obtained to evaluate the patient's hearing. In the presence of conductive hearing loss or an abnormal tympanic membrane examination, a noncontrast high-resolution CT scan of the temporal bone and an otolaryngology referral is warranted.

Treatment and When to Refer

The treatment of tinnitus includes the treatment of underlying anxiety and depression symptoms. If a hearing loss is present, hearing aids may benefit the patient as well. The patient may benefit from masking therapy (eg, use of a fan or noise generator at bedside). Sound therapy has been found to benefit tinnitus patients and provide the most cost effective therapy. This mode of therapy can be found at www.beyond tinnitus.com.

Acute tinnitus after noise exposure should be treated with prednisone 1 mg/kg/day for 5 days. Patients with unilateral tinnitus or hearing loss should be referred to an otolaryngologist for evaluation for an MRI of the internal auditory canals with gadolinium to rule out an acoustic neuroma. Patients who continue to have difficulty with their tinnitus despite the measures discussed above, should be referred to a tinnitus center.

PULSATILE TINNITUS

The internal carotid artery and the jugular vein both travel within millimeters of the cochlea or the middle ear space. In addition, dural venous sinuses also are very near the structures of the ear. Any change in the flow of blood in these vessels, any anomalous vasculature, or vascular tumor around the temporal bone can cause the sensation of a pulsatile tinnitus. The differential diagnosis of a pulsatile tinnitus is outlined in Table 5–1.

Symptoms and Signs

The patients will generally complain of a pulsatile sensation or the sensation of hearing one's heart beat in

Table 5–1. Differential Diagnosis of Pulsatile Tinnitus

Carotid artery stenosis

Dural arteriovenous fistula

Carotid-cavernous sinus-fistula

Atherosclerotic carotid stenosis

Aneurysm/dissection of the internal carotid artery (ICA)

Fibromuscular dysplasia with ICA stenosis

Cerebral venous sinus thrombosis

ICA aneurysm

Cerebral venous sinus stenosis

Abnormal loop of the anterior inferior cerebellar artery

Glomus tumors

Intracranial hypertension

Meningioma

Sigmoid sinus diverticulum

Anomalous carotid artery or jugular vein

Anemia

Thyrotoxicosis

Venous hum

Pregnancy

Superior canal dehiscence

one or both ears. The patient should be asked for signs of intracranial hypertension including headaches, diplopia, or transient visual loss to rule out benign intracranial hypertension. Finally, the patient should be asked about new life stressors or the possibility of pregnancy. The examination should include evaluation of the ears for a middle ear mass (usually red or purple), auscultation over the carotid arteries in the neck and the mastoids, and gentle compression of the jugular vein for signs of improvement of the symptoms. Finally, fundoscopic examination should be performed to evaluate for signs of intracranial hypertension.

Diagnosis and What Tests to Order

The diagnostic workup of pulsatile tinnitus is aimed at ruling out life-threatening abnormalities. A carotid ultrasound is warranted in any patient with an abnormal neck auscultation, a history of blunt neck trauma or chiropractic manipulation (to rule out a carotid dissection), or in an older patient with atherosclerosis risk factors. An MRI and MRA of the brain and internal auditory canals with gadolinium will help rule out a majority of the abnormalities listed in Table 5-1. In addition, a thyroid panel and hemoglobin test will rule out hyperthyroidism or anemia. A pregnancy test is warranted if the possibility exists in the patient. If benign intracranial hypertension is suspected based on the fundoscopic examination, a lumbar puncture should be performed after imaging of the brain to rule out a mass. A CT scan of the temporal bones to rule out a small glomus tympanicum (paraganglioma of the middle ear cavity) or a sigmoid sinus diverticulum may be warranted if the MRI is normal and the patient has continued complaint. A hearing test will evaluate any possibilities of a conductive hearing loss.

Treatment and When to Refer

The treatment of pulsatile tinnitus depends on the specific etiology. The patient should be referred to an otologist/neuro-otologist for evaluation and management if abnormalities are discovered on the imaging studies. A patient suspected of benign intracranial hypertension should be referred to a neurosurgeon. Dural AV fistulas should be referred to neurointerventional radiology specialists for interventional treatment.

FLUTTERING TINNITUS

Myoclonus in the stapedial muscle, tensor or levetor veli palatine muscles can cause a rhythmic, 60 to 200 per minute, clicking tinnitus. These involuntary jerky movements of these muscles can be seen in the soft palate if caused by the tensor veli palatini.

Symptoms and Signs

The patient most commonly will complain of clicking or fluttering sound that may occur after exposure to certain noises (most commonly occurs in stapedial myoclonus). The patient may also get the tinnitus when not exposed to outside sounds. The physician may be able to see the rhythmic movement of the tympanic membrane or the palate when the myoclonus occurs.

Diagnosis and What Tests to Order

The diagnosis is by the history or examination. A clicking tinnitus that occurs after exposure to sound is classic. A rhythmic movement of the palate or the tympanic membrane also will help. A high resolution MRI of the internal auditory canals with gadolinium to rule out facial nerve pathology (eg, schwannoma) must be obtained.

Treatment and When to Refer

Sudden onset of myoclonus is generally due to increased anxiety or stress, though facial nerve pathology must be ruled out. Stress reduction and alprazolam 0.5 mg po TID will help reduce the patient's symptoms. The patient should be referred to an otologist/neuro-otologist for evaluation and treatment upon diagnosis.

CHAPTER 6

Ear Plugging

ALI SEPEHR
HAMID R. DJALILIAN

BACKGROUND

Ear plugging is a common complaint of patients presenting in a primary care setting. It can be associated with many conditions that will be detailed below. The most common causes of ear plugging and popping are outlined in Figure 6–1.

EUSTACHIAN TUBE DYSFUNCTION

The eustachian tube connects the ear to the nasopharynx and regulates the middle ear pressure and drains the middle ear. Eustachian tube dysfunction (ETD) or blockage occurs due to a combination of anatomic predisposition and mucosal edema secondary to upper airway inflammation (eg, allergic, infectious, or irritative rhinitis). It is most common in children under the age of 5 due to a horizontally oriented tube and

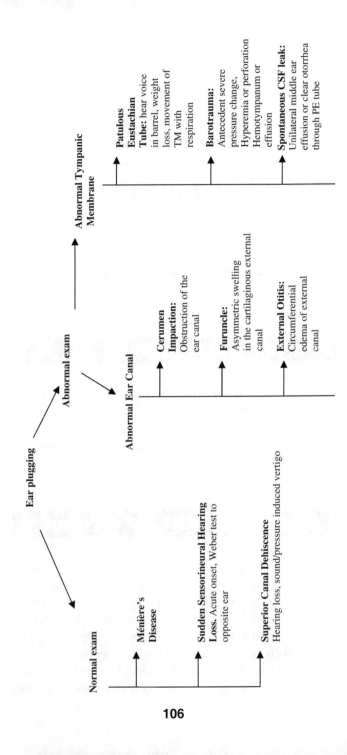

Ear plugging

Normal exam

Ménière's Disease

Sudden Sensorineural Hearing Loss. Acute onset, Weber test to opposite ear

Superior Canal Dehiscence Hearing loss, sound/pressure induced vertigo

Abnormal exam

Abnormal Ear Canal

Cerumen Impaction: Obstruction of the ear canal

Furuncle: Asymmetric swelling in the cartilaginous external canal

External Otitis: Circumferential edema of external canal

Abnormal Tympanic Membrane

Patulous Eustachian Tube: hear voice in barrel, weight loss, movement of TM with respiration

Barotrauma: Antecedent severe pressure change, Hyperemia or perforation Hemotympanum or effusion

Spontaneous CSF leak: Unilateral middle ear effusion or clear otorrhea through PE tube

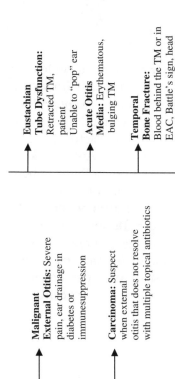

**Eustachian
Tube Dysfunction:**
Retracted TM,
patient
Unable to "pop" ear

**Acute Otitis
Media:** Erythematous,
bulging TM

**Temporal
Bone Fracture:**
Blood behind the TM or in
EAC, Battle's sign, head
trauma

Acute Mastoiditis:
Acute otitis media with
redness, pain, & tender
in post-auricular area

**Malignant
External Otitis:** Severe
pain, ear drainage in
diabetes or
immunesuppression

Carcinoma: Suspect
when external
otitis that does not resolve
with multiple topical antibiotics

Fig 6–1. The most frequent causes of ear plugging.

adenoid hypertrophy. Other risk factors include craniofacial abnormalities (eg, cleft palate and Down syndrome), neuromuscular disease or a nasopharyngeal mass. Immunity is also a factor; therefore, prematurity and bottle feeding are risk factors. Risk factors in adults include allergic rhinitis, chronic sinusitis, smoking, and environmental irritants (eg, dust, pollution, chemicals, etc). Acutely, ETD leads to a negative middle ear pressure and chronically leads to a retraction of the tympanic membrane, middle ear effusion, otitis media, or cholesteatoma. A nasopharyngeal tumor needs to be ruled out in adult patients with unilateral or new onset ETD. Smokers and those of Asian descent are at a higher risk of developing nasopharyngeal cancer.

Symptoms and Signs

The patient will generally present with ear plugging/pressure, a sensation of crackling or popping of the ear, otalgia, hearing loss, tinnitus, and sometimes dizziness (from negative pressure on the round window membrane of the inner ear). The symptoms may be intermittent or constant. A precedent URI or rhinitis (allergic or irritative from smoking or occupational exposure) is generally present. In children, the most common cause of dizziness is ETD. On examination, the tympanic membrane is retracted and there is a hypomobility or immobility of the TM on pneumatic otoscopy. Attention must be given to the pars flaccida (portion of the TM above the malleus) where the only area of retraction may be present. A middle ear effusion may be seen and the patient will be unable (or have difficulty) to "pop" the ear when the patient autoinsufflates with pinched nostrils. Tuning fork testing will generally show a conductive hearing loss: the Weber test lateralizes to the affected side and the Rinne may show that bone conduction is louder than air conduction. If the conductive hearing loss is not great (less than 30 dB), the Rinne may show an air conduction that is louder than bone conduction.

Diagnosis and What Tests to Order

The diagnosis is by the history of ear plugging and the examination findings of retraction of the TM and immobility when the patient attempts to "pop" the ear. Occasionally, the patient will be able to move the TM with Valsalva, albeit with difficulty. A tympanogram and an audiogram will help in the diagnosis. The tympanogram will show a peak in the negative range (less than -100). The audiogram will generally show a conductive hearing loss.

Treatment and When to Refer

The most important aspect of treating ETD is treating the underlying rhinitis. Smoking cessation and nasal saline irrigation (4 puffs QID each nostril) are generally the best treatment in smokers. In nonsmokers, nasal steroid sprays (eg, fluticasone or mometasone 2 puffs each nostril QD) and nasal saline irrigations will help 60 to 70% of the patients. Given the possible role of gastroesophageal reflux disease in this condition, it should be treated if present with a proton pump inhibitor (eg, omeprazole 40 mg QAM before breakfast) for a 2-month duration.

If the patient does not respond to medical therapy after 1 to 2 months, the patient should be referred to an otolaryngologist for nasopharyngoscopy. Myringotomy with tube placement may benefit a subset of these patients. ETD in the presence of recurrent epistaxis or in a patient of Asian descent may indicate a nasopharyngeal tumor. Persistent unilateral effusion in the absence of an antecedent URI or allergic rhinitis may also indicate a nasopharyngeal tumor and requires referral to an otolaryngologist for nasopharyngoscopy. Severe retraction of the tympanic membrane is also another indication for referral to an otolaryngologist.

PATULOUS EUSTACHIAN TUBE

The eustachian tube is normally closed and opens every few minutes in the setting of swallowing, yawning, or an increased upper airway pressure (eg, blowing of nose). Patulous eustachian tube refers to an abnormally open (patent) eustachian tube resulting in an abnormal pathway through which the patient's respiration, phonation, swallowing, and heartbeat directly vibrate the tympanic membrane. Patulous eustachian tube generally occurs in the setting of: (1) weight loss leading to decreased soft tissue around the eustachian tube, (2) neurologic disorders (stroke, multiple sclerosis, motor neuron disease) leading to muscle atrophy, (3) diuretic medications, caffeine, and exercise leading to dehydration and the tissue decongestion, (4) pregnancy hormones or oral contraceptives affecting the mucous/surfactant composition and surface tension which can lead to patency, and (5) adenoidectomy and radiotherapy leading to scar formation in the nasopharynx.

Symptoms and Signs

The patients will generally present with distorted autophony (hearing one's own voice as if speaking in a barrel) or the abnormal detection of self-generated sounds. This heightened sensitivity to self-generated sounds is not muffled as it is in patients with eustachian tube congestion. Despite the abnormally patent eustachian tube, the patient feels that the ears are plugged. On examination one can see movement of the tympanic membrane (TM) with nasal respiration. This movement is accentuated by plugging the opposite nostril and sniffing; and is diminished by laying the patient flat or having the patient bend over (because venous congestion around the eustachian tube will cause closure of the tube).

Diagnosis and What Tests to Order

The diagnosis is by the characteristic symptoms of "sounds like speaking in barrel" and the movement of the TM on nasal respiration as well as the relief of symptoms with lying down or bending over. Continuous tympanometry may be ordered to see the characteristic movement of the TM with respiration, but is generally not necessary.

Treatment and When to Refer

The treatment depends on the etiology. If rapid or extreme weight loss is the etiology some weight gain will cause relief of the symptom. In cases of diuretic use, discontinuation of other diuretics (if possible) and coffee is recommended. Estrogen nasal drops (25 mg of intramuscular premarin in 30 cc of normal saline in a 1-oz dropper bottle, 3 gtt TID in the nose × 4 wks) has been found to help in some patients by causing nasal congestion and congestion at the eustachian tube orifice in the nose. Oral potassium iodide (10 gtt of saturated solution in 1 glass of fruit juice po TID) to induce swelling of eustachian tube opening has been successful in some patients as well. The patient should be referred to an otolaryngologist if the above treatments are not successful or if the diagnosis is unclear for nasopharyngoscopy.

BAROTRAUMA

Barotrauma occurs when there is pressure differentials between the middle and external ears (generally in the setting of eustachian tube dysfunction), such as during flying, sky or SCUBA diving, violent nose blowing or sneezing with the mouth and nose closed, or extreme exertion during breath holding (eg, weightlifting with improper technique). Barotrauma can affect the tympanic membrane and the middle ear causing a conductive hearing loss. It can cause a labyrinthine concussion, intralabyrinthine membrane tears, damage to receptor structures, or at the extreme, a break in the round or oval windows producing a perilymph fistula (PLF) causing progressive sensorineural hearing loss (SNHL) and episodic vertigo. It can rarely cause facial paralysis by inducing hemorrhage in the facial nerve canal.

Symptoms and Signs

The patients will generally present with ear plugging and hearing loss. The patient will relate a history of extreme pressure change such as the inability to clear ears during the descent in SCUBA diving, upon takeoff or landing in an airplane, or other situations described above. The patient generally would have experienced pain and plugging of the ear at the time. The patient may have a constant or fluctuating hearing loss. Tinnitus, episodic vertigo, or disequilibrium may also be present. On examination, blood in the middle ear or a perforation of the tympanic membrane may be present. A hemotympanum or a serous middle ear effusion may be present. Nystagmus or disequilibrium may be seen with pneumatic otoscopy (a seal must be obtained in the ear canal when pneumatic otoscopy is performed).

Diagnosis and What Tests to Order

The diagnosis is by the history of extreme pressure change in the ear and the characteristic findings in the ear exam as described above. An audiogram and tympanogram must be obtained to evaluate the hearing and to check for dizziness on tympanometry.

Treatment and When to Refer

Bed rest, head elevation, and avoidance of any activity that may increase central venous pressures (eg, no Valsalva, sneezing with mouth open, no heavy lifting, or straining). The patient should be referred to an otolaryngologist for possible surgical therapy as soon as possible after the diagnosis.

MÉNIÈRE'S DISEASE

Please see Chapter 9 on vertigo.

SUPERIOR CANAL DEHISCENCE

The inner ear system normally has two areas that are not covered by bone (the round and the oval windows). Absence of bone over the superior semicircular canal

(SSC) possibly from erosion or trauma, acts as a third window, which causes (1) natural pulsations of the CSF to be transmitted to the inner ear; and (2) pressure and noise changes to induce vestibular activity by being dissipated through the vestibular system instead of going through the auditory system.

Symptoms and Signs

The patients generally present with autophony (hearing own voice in head), ear plugging, vertigo with pressure changes, sound-induced vertigo, pulsatile or constant tinnitus, and hearing loss. The patient may also have symptoms such as the ability to hear his or her own eye movement. On examination, the patient may have vertigo or disequilibrium with pneumatic otoscopy or pumping of the tragus.

Diagnosis and What Tests to Order

An audiogram, tympanogram, with acoustic reflexes must be obtained. The diagnosis is best made by using an ultrahigh-resolution (0.5-mm) coronal noncontrast CT scan of the temporal bone which will show the bony defect above the superior canal. The vestibular evoked myogenic potential test will show an abnormally low threshold.

Treatment and When to Refer

The treatment is surgical by plugging of the SSC. Avoidance of precipitating stimuli such as wearing an ear plug for sound-induced vertigo may help. The patient should be referred to an otologist/neuro-otologist for treatment or if the diagnosis is uncertain.

SUDDEN SENSORINEURAL HEARING LOSS (SSNHL)

Patients with SSNHL will most commonly present with a plugging sensation in the ear.

Refer to Chapter 4 on hearing loss for further detail. It is important to consider SSNHL in the differential diagnosis in patients with a sensation of acute plugging of the ear.

SPONTANEOUS CEREBROSPINAL FLUID (CSF) LEAK

A defect in the bony roof of the ear or mastoid (floor of the cranial cavity) can occur spontaneously, after trauma, or from chronic otitis media with cholesteatoma. The defect can be congenital; however, aging and increased intracranial pressure, inflammation, arachnoid granulation, and irradiation are proposed etiologic factors for spontaneous CSF leakage into the temporal bone. Other causes could be a congenital labyrinthine or perilabyrinthine defects. The main problem with a CSF leakage is that it can lead to meningitis. Although a spontaneous CSF leakage will most commonly occur in an older adult (>50 years of age), it can rarely occur in children with anomalous inner ears.

Symptoms and Signs

The patient will present with unilateral ear plugging and unilateral hearing loss. The patient may have occipital headaches, photophobia, nausea, or vomiting. On examination the patient will have a unilateral serous middle ear effusion with no precedent upper respiratory infection or allergy symptoms. The patient may also have a continuous or intermittent clear rhinorrhea or a salty taste in the pharynx. A unilateral clear otorrhea (through a pressure-equalizing tube) may occur that does not respond to antibiotic/anti-inflammatory ear drops. Rarely, the patient may present with recurrent meningitis or spontaneous pneumocephalus.

Diagnosis and What Tests to Order

The best method of diagnosis of a spontaneous CSF leakage is by having a high clinical suspicion in an older adult with a persistently clear middle ear fluid without a precedent URI or allergic rhinitis symptoms. A high resolution, noncontrast CT of the temporal bone in axial and coronal planes will generally show the defect in the floor of the middle fossa (roof of the temporal bone). If there is persistent fluid drainage from a pressure-equalization tube a sample of the fluid can be sent for β_2-transferrin testing. The presence of β_2-transferrin in the fluid is diagnostic of CSF.

Treatment and When to Refer

The patient should be immunized for *Streptococcus pneumoniae* and referred to an otologist/neuro-otologist for repair of the bony defect.

CERUMEN IMPACTION

Cerumen impaction is one of the most common causes of ear plugging. See Chapter 2 on ear pain for more details on diagnosis and management.

MASS OF THE EAR CANAL

A benign or malignant tumor of the ear canal can block the ear canal to cause plugging. If a mass is noted in the ear canal, the patient should be referred to an otolaryngologist.

ABNORMAL TYMPANIC MEMBRANE

Chronic otitis media or a middle ear mass can cause a plugging sensation. If the TM is abnormal, the patient should be referred to an otolaryngologist.

CHAPTER 7

Trauma to the Ear

JAMES M. RIDGWAY
HAMID R. DJALILIAN

INTRODUCTION

Injury of the ear and temporal bone is often initially managed in the primary care and emergency room settings. Clinical findings can include auricular hematoma, tympanic membrane injury, hearing loss, vertigo, facial nerve paralysis, and cerebral spinal fluid leak. An understanding of the differential diagnoses of injuries to the ear and temporal bone, possible symptomatic sequelae, and medical management, are essential for practicing physicians who may encounter such injuries. A complete patient history and examination are essential when approaching the patient with an ear or temporal bone injury.

TRAUMA TO THE OUTER EAR (AURICLE)

Auricular Hematoma

Due to its anatomic location the auricle is uniquely susceptible to blunt, shearing, penetrating, and avulsion injuries. In the circumstance of an auricular hematoma, the injury results from the elevation of the overlying perichondrium from the auricular cartilage with subsequent formation of a hematoma between these two structures. This is commonly observed along the anterior face of the ear where the overlying skin is tightly adherent to the perichondrium. The separation of the perichondrium from the underlying cartilage effectively separates the cartilage from it blood and nutrient supply which can ultimately result in cartilaginous death or infection. Often, the auricular hematoma stimulates scar formation and leads to the classic description of a "cauliflower ear." To prevent this traumatic deformity, evacuation of the hematoma is necessary. Although one may be tempted to simply aspirate the hematoma, this technique is associated with an unacceptably high failure rate.

Treatment and When to Refer

If an otolaryngologist is readily available, consultation should be obtained. If an otolaryngologist is not available, the drainage of an auricular hematoma is performed after complete cleaning of the ear and the injection of local anesthetic (lidocaine 1% with 1:100,000 epinephrine) around the entire ear. Contrary to traditional emergency medicine teachings, injection of lidocaine with epinephrine around the ear is not detrimental. The only time lidocaine with epinephrine is not injected around the ear is when greater than 90%

of the ear is avulsed. The site of incision is preferentially chosen anterior and inferior to the posterior extension of the helix. This affords adequate entry into the hematoma while allowing for a cosmetically concealed incision (Fig 7–1). After complete evacuation of the hematoma, placement of dental rolls on either side of the auricle with through and through nylon suturing is performed so as to secure the bolsters in place and to eliminate the potential space for hematoma reaccumulation. The authors prefer to use Xeroform dressing in this circumstance as it is felt to more readily contour to the natural cartilage framework and is found to harden over 24 to 48 hours for a rigid auricular bolster.

Soft Tissue and Avulsion Injuries

Auricular injuries, in particular crush injuries, often require aggressive wound and antimicrobial therapy. Accurate analysis of the soft tissue injury is essential in the guiding of appropriate management as well as

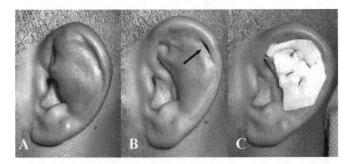

Fig 7–1. The auricular hematoma will show fluctuance and ecchymosis (**A**). The incision is made in the fold between the helix and the antihelix (*arrow*) (**B**). After drainage, the ear should be compressed with through and through sutures (**C**) to prevent reaccumulation of the blood.

meticulous documentation comparing the normal to the injured ear.

Treatment and When to Refer

If an otolaryngologist is readily available, consultation should be obtained. If an otolaryngologist is not available, initial steps in wound treatment include copious irrigation, meticulous debridement of nonviable tissues, and removal of foreign bodies if present. Attention is given to the degree and layer of soft tissue injury, cartilage exposure or involvement, as well as remaining tissue viability. If possible, primary closure of all tissue layers is performed in meticulous fashion. Careful attention in the eversion of skin edges during repair is necessary for optimal cosmetic outcome in this highly visualized area. In the event of segmental defects in which salvageable cartilage is available, a subcutaneous pocket is created in the mastoid region for the banking of de-epithelialized cartilage. Placement of this pocket region adjacent to the site of the auricular defect is critical as the banked cartilage and overlying tissue from the pocket is integrated into the staged repair of the auricle.

In the circumstance of auricular avulsion, microvascular reimplantation is necessary for tissue survival. With the increased success of this technique, it is recommended that the avulsed ear is preserved in a protected ice saline bath until surgical evaluation and potential options have been assessed. Successful reimplantation often requires the use hyperbaric oxygen, anticoagulation, and leech therapies.

Bite Wounds

Soft tissue injury secondary to bite trauma is most commonly associated in canine attack (85–90%), feline

(2-3%), and human assault (2-3%). Of these injuries, auricular trauma and post-traumatic infection can result in extensive morbidity, hearing compromise, and cosmetic deformity. The most common bacteria cultured from the wounds of animal bites are *Staphylococcus aureus*, *Pasturella multocida*, and anaerobic cocci. *Staphylococcus aureus*, anaerobic cocci, *Bacteroides*, and gamma-hemolytic streptococci are isolated from human wounds. Treatment should target the bacteria isolated and the timing of treatment is essential in avoiding further external soft tissue damage.

Treatment and When to Refer

Meticulous wound care is essential as well as broad-range empiric intravenous antimicrobial therapy in the treatment of these contaminated wounds. It is best to not close these wounds tightly to allow a drainage port for the likely infection. Antimicrobial coverage should include *Pasteurella* species as these are most associated with dog and cat bites. Prophylactic antibiotic therapy should be given in all animal or human bites for seven days with amoxicillin-clavulanate (875 mg po BID, in children, 40 mg/kg divide BID). Penicillin-allergic patients can get doxycycline (100 mg po BID, children over 8 years, 2.2 mg/kg po BID). Children under the age of 8 or pregnant women should be treated with erythromycin ethyl succinate 400 mg po Q6hrs (children 40 mg/kg divided QID). Ceftriaxone 1g IM QD (children 75 mg/kg QD) can also be given.

Injuries at high risk for infection include crush, puncture, human and cat bites, delayed presentation, and injury to those with a history of immunosuppression. Such injuries should be treated aggressively and surgical consultation made as soon as possible. Rabies or tetanus prophylaxis should be considered on a case by case basis.

TRAUMA TO THE EAR CANAL

External Auditory Canal Abrasion

See Chapter 3, Ear Drainage.

Trauma of the external auditory canal (EAC) can result from simple attempts in ear cleaning with soft or sharp-tipped devices to temporal bone fractures. Such injuries are often associated with otalgia and hearing loss that can range from mild to severe, depending on the degree of EAC occlusion.

Treatment and When to Refer

The application of otic drops (eg, polymyxin, neomycin, hydrocortisone (Cortisporin Otic Suspension®) or ciprofloxacin/dexamethasone 3 gtt TID to affected ear for 7 days) to prevent otitis externa may be necessary with the signs of infection or frank disruption of canal tissues. If inflammation and occlusion of the ear canal has occurred, placement of a wick may be necessary to aid in the delivery of ototopical antibiotics. In the case of canal stenosis surgical correction may be required. Early stenting of the EAC with multiple otowicks or Xeroform dressing in cases of circumferential injury is essential in the prevention of this complication. For severe injury, an otolaryngology consultation is necessary. All patients should receive a hearing test.

Foreign Bodies

Foreign bodies represent a unique circumstance in trauma of the ear as injury can occur from the object, the patient, or the well-meaning physician. Injury from inanimate objects can occur through initial insertion and resultant infection, expansion (as in hygroscopic seeds), or caustic injury. A practitioner without the benefit of binocular microscope and proper instrumentation is at a significant disadvantage in the attempted removal of a foreign body. Often the ear canal becomes lacerated, the patient traumatized, and the foreign body remains in place. In these circumstances, the patient is best referred to an otolaryngologist for hearing testing and removing the foreign body. This is also true in the case of insect removal. Commonly multiple attempts are made to remove the insect with forceps, suction and irrigation with resultant injury to the canal and tympanic membrane. In these circumstances it is necessary to kill the insect with an organic solvent and then extract it under direct visualization. This is best done with isopropyl alcohol with a few drops into the canal. Lidocaine can also be used to paralyze the live insect, but if the insect is not removed within few hours, it will restart motion in the ear canal.

Alkaline batteries lodged into the external auditory canal constitute a medical emergency as these dangerous objects are capable of extensive liquefactive necrosis. Injuries associated with these devices include extensive tissue destruction, tympanic membrane perforation, hearing loss, and facial paralysis

Treatment and When to Refer

Patients with a deep foreign body of the ear should be referred to an otolaryngologist for hearing testing. Due to the necessity of a microscope and instrumentation for a safe and atraumatic removal, deep, bony canal, or impacted foreign bodies should be referred to an otolaryngologist. Foreign bodies in the cartilaginous canal that are not obstructing the canal may be removed if the primary care/emergency medicine physician can remove the foreign body in one motion in a cooperative child. Manipulation of a foreign body can cause bleeding or edema of the skin and make removal much more difficult and occasionally lead to the need for general anesthesia for its removal. If an alkaline battery is present, at no time should irrigation or otic drops be instilled into the ear canal as this will only facilitate further soft tissue injury. If the question of an alkaline battery in the ear canal exists, but visualization is inadequate, a simple x-ray of the head is more than adequate to confirm the presence of such an object.

TRAUMA TO THE TYMPANIC MEMBRANE

See Chapter 3, Ear Drainage.

Perforation

Injury of the tympanic membrane (TM) can occur from direct or indirect forces with resulting pain and hearing loss. Direct rupture of the membrane commonly occurs during attempts to clean the ear or in children who simply place objects into the ear canal. Cotton-tip applicators, car keys, chop sticks, and hair pins are among the many culprits responsible for direct TM rupture. Indirect injury to the TM occurs from a pressure wave that stretches the membrane beyond its elastic capability and leads to rupture. This form of injury is referred to as barotrauma and is often observed in hand-slap to the ear, explosive injuries (from blast or loud sound), or from barotraumas (eg,

SCUBA diving or flying in a poorly pressurized airplane in the presence of eustachian tube dysfunction).

Examination of the ruptured TM is recommended in a relatively urgent manner with a complete history of events and symptoms recorded. Mechanism of injury, severity of hearing loss, presence of dizziness, otorrhea, blood from the canal, and time line of events are to be elucidated during evaluation. Microscopic evaluation of the tympanic membrane is necessary to determine the degree of injury and the measure of medical intervention. A traumatic perforation will generally have sharp or jagged edges and some blood on the TM. This is in contrast to a perforation from chronic otitis media, which has a rounded appearance and no blood. Gross auditory evaluation with a 512-Hz tuning fork is essential in the primary exam as patients with vertigo, nystagmus, and sensorineural hearing loss of the affected ear classically represent a more severe injury to the ear (a perilymphatic fistula) that requires immediate surgical attention.

Treatment and When to Refer

These patients should be referred for audiometric evaluation including air, bone, and speech discrimination tests soon after the injury. The patient should also see an otolarynologist immediately (same day) if the patient is vertiginous, otherwise same-week consultation is necessary. Most traumatic injuries to the TM are often self-resolving, but require prevention of water entering the ear and the middle ear space due to risk of otitis media.

In the event of a large perforation or a persistent perforation after 3 months of conservative therapy, in-office or intraoperative treatment may be performed. If amenable, the removal of the perforation rim with subsequent application of a paper patch may be performed. In more severe cases a formal tympanoplasty may be necessary for TM reconstruction.

Ossicular Chain Disruption

Disruption of the ossicular chain can occur though penetrating or blunt trauma to the middle ear space. Located behind the tympanic membrane, the malleus, incus, and stapes are bounded by the TM laterally and the oval window medially. These bones are stabilized by various tendons, ligaments, and articulations and allow for vibratory transmissions to the inner ear. Distortion or disruption of the ossicular chain leads to a conductive hearing deficit, which may occur with or without rupture of the tympanic membrane. Discontinuity of the ossicular chain with an associated TM perforation commonly results in minimal conductive hearing loss (CHL) of 35 dB. A maximal CHL of 60 dB is observed with ossicular discontinuity and an intact tympanic membrane. Ossicular disruption most commonly occurs at the incudostapedial joint, but may also occur with dislocation of the incus. More complicated injuries may include fractures of the stapes or even displacement of the stapes footplate through the oval window creating a fistula.

Treatment and When to Refer

Correction of chain discontinuities requires surgical exploration of the middle ear with possible return of dislocated bones to proper positioning, removal of fractured segments and placement of prosthesis, or placement of grafting for repair of oval window injuries. These patients should be referred to an otologist/neuro-otologist.

TRAUMA TO THE TEMPORAL BONE

See Chapter 2, Ear Pain.

General Overview

The temporal bone is subdivided into tympanic, squamous, mastoid, and petrous bones. Traumatic injury to the head can result in fracture of these bones and result in severe injury to the surrounding structures. Temporal bone injuries are separated into otic capsule disrupting and otic capsule sparing. The otic capsule is defined as the cochlea or the vestibule (balance portion of the inner ear). Otic capsule sparing fractures most commonly are the result of a lateral force to the mastoid or ear that produces a fracture line parallel to the long axis of the temporal bone. This fracture passes through the external auditory canal (EAC), the middle ear roof (tegmen tympani), and travels along the anterior surface of the petrous bone. This type of fracture was previously termed longitudinal temporal bone fracture.

Otic capsule disrupting (previously called transverse fractures) are commonly caused by frontal or occipital injuries that create a fracture line perpendicular to long axis of petrous pyramid of the temporal bone. This fracture line violates the otic capsule and results in total sensorineural hearing loss and vestibular compromise of the affected ear. These fractures account for approximately 20% of temporal bone fractures and were previously referred to as transverse fractures.

Complications of Temporal Bone Fractures

There are multiple clinical findings that should alert the physician of temporal bone injury and mandate further evaluation by the clinician. Some clinical findings may be monitored over time whereas others require further, even immediate, medical evaluation. For example, although bruising occurs in most head injuries, specific patterns of distribution are noteworthy. Ecchymosis observed along the mastoid bone, otherwise known as Battle's sign represents violation of the mastoid cortex. Periorbital ecchymosis, commonly referred to as "raccoon eyes," represents a basilar skull fracture in which blood has tracked from the base of the skull, though the soft tissues, and into the periorbital region. Clinical evaluation of patients with such injuries must also include assessment of hearing, presence of dizziness, facial nerve injury, otorrhea, rhinorrhea, and neurologic status.

Hearing Loss and Vestibular Injury

Tuning fork tests and otoscopy are essential in determining conductive, sensorineural, or mixed hearing loss in those with temporal bone injuries. Tuning fork tests are explained in detail in Chapter 1. These findings must be properly documented in all temporal bone injury patients who are able to undergo examination. During otoscopy the clinician should also note the integrity of the TM, the presence of a hemotympanum, or otorrhea. Blood behind the TM is commonly observed in temporal bone fractures that travel through the middle ear space and results in a CHL. If the TM cannot be visualized due to blood, otorrhea, or bone in the canal, the diagnosis of temporal bone fracture, with or without dura injury, must be pursued.

Traumatic injury of the membranous labyrinth (vestibule) may result in nystagmus and the subjective feeling of vertigo. When nystagmus is observed in conjunction with an audiovestibular loss, investigation of an otic capsule disrupting injury is necessary. Other vestibular disruptions may include central injuries to the brain or vestibular nuclei as well as peripheral manifestations such as benign paroxysmal positional vertigo or perilymphatic fistula.

Perilymphatic Fistula (PLF)

Perilymphatic fistulas are characterized by the association of vertigo and fluctuating sensorineural hearing loss. They are the result of shearing forces that disrupt the round or oval window membranes through either sudden increase in transmitted CSF pressures or external forces that impact the TM and ossicles. Such injuries are referred to as explosive or implosive, respectively. Regardless of traumatic mechanism, PLF symptoms commonly manifest within the first 24 to 72 hours postinjury. The patients will have vertigo with coughing, straining, or sneezing. In addition, they will have a fluctuating hearing loss. Many of these patients are mistakenly diagnosed with a postconcussive syndrome and are discharged from medical care with the assumption that their symptoms will spontaneously resolve. Unfortunately, such recovery does not occur and these patients commonly do not return for medical care until years later.

Facial Nerve Injury

Protected by the temporal bone, the facial nerve traverses the longest intraosseous course of any motor nerve in the human. Temporal bone fractures can result in facial nerve palsy. Of extreme importance in these injuries is the time of onset of nerve palsy. Delayed nerve injury represents a gradual nerve weakening that takes hours or even days to develop and requires no intervention other than steroid therapy (prednisone 1 mg/kg for 1 week with an 8-day taper). Immediate nerve injury is the complete loss of nerve function at a specific point in time and will require surgical treatment for restoration of function. Due to the complicated nature of most patients who have sustained temporal bone trauma, the determination of facial nerve injury onset in often difficult as these patients are often unconscious during the primary examination.

CSF Leaks

Traumatic injury of the temporal bone resulting in cerebral spinal fluid (CSF) leaks occurs in approximately 17% of patients. Clinical signs and symptoms of CSF leaks include otorrhea, rhinorrhea, salty taste in mouth, conductive hearing loss, fluid behind the TM, mass behind the TM (encephalocele), and even recurrent meningitis. Each of these clinical findings provides diagnostic clues as to the location of injury along the skull base. CSF otorrhea with associated TM perforation occurs with otic capsule sparing fractures whereas CSF rhinorrhea is associated with an intact TM and otic capsule disrupting fractures. CSF travels through the eustachian tube, as opposed to an injured TM, resulting in rhinorrhea instead of otorrhea. Further evaluation to elicit such findings may include leaning forward or performing Valsalva maneuvers to increase intracranial pressure and thereby increase the CSF leak for clinical detection and fluid collection. Concerns for CSF leaks merit submission of fluid for β-2 transferrin analysis, a CSF specific protein. Otolaryngology and neurosurgical consultation must be obtained for evaluation and treatment.

Encephalocele and Vascular Injury

Injury to the middle cranial fossa can occur creating an open defect and the temporal lobe can herniate as an encephalocele into the middle ear and mastoid. Injury to the great vessels of the head and neck are often associated with penetrating trauma or severe blunt injuries. Any gunshot wounds to the skull base will require angiography for evaluation of the carotid artery.

Treatment and When to Refer

All patients with a temporal bone fracture must have an otolaryngology evaluation.

Fracture and CSF Leak

Temporal fractures resulting in CSF otorrhea or rhinorrhea may be managed with bed rest, head elevation, and stool softeners. The patients are prohibited from straining or sneezing with a closed mouth in attempts to prevent any rise in intracranial pressure. Bed rest may be performed for 7 to 10 days prior to placement of a lumbar drain for additional conservative management. If after 72 hours CSF otorrhea or rhinorrhea persists then surgical management is warranted.

Facial Nerve Injury

The onset of facial nerve paralysis is of paramount importance in the initial management of facial nerve injury. Immediate facial nerve paralysis represents an acute injury which has either severed or severely injured the facial nerve. Such injuries require high-resolution CT imaging of the temporal bone to elucidate the point of injury. In delayed facial nerve paralysis, interventional measures are more conservative with serial diagnostic testing and monitoring of facial nerve degeneration or recovery. In the circumstances in which analysis of the facial nerve is precluded by the treatment of more severe injuries, such injuries are treated in conservative measures analogous to delayed facial nerve palsy.

WHAT TESTS TO ORDER AND WHEN

Pure Tone and Speech Audiometry

All patients who have had head trauma causing rupture of the tympanic membrane, disruption of the ossicles or hemotympanum, or diagnosed temporal bone fractures should have pure tone and speech audiometry tests performed in order to determine if damage to the middle or inner ear has created a hearing loss. The temporal relation from incident to timing of the tests is dependent on the severity of the symptoms. Patients who have symptoms of inner ear dysfunction (vertigo) should have the tests performed in more acute fashion as compared to the relatively asymptomatic patient who presents with a hemotympanum or traumatic tympanic membrane perforation.

Facial Nerve Testing

The complexity in the etiology as well as symptomatology of facial nerve injury requires focused electrodiagnostic studies to elucidate the extent of damage within the facial nerve. The characterization of the injury using electrodiagnostic tests allows for the development of focused surgical treatment plans, prognosis, and possible time course to reinnervation and return to normal function. The tests currently used are limited to patients with complete facial nerve paralysis and for patients in which facial nerve decompression surgery is a possible consideration. The tests are not helpful in patients who have incomplete nerve damage and have maintained some normal function.

Electroneuronography (ENoG aka Evoked EMG)

This test measures the muscle action potential response to facial nerve electrical stimulation. The peak of the amplitude of the action potential of the muscle stimulated is compared between the paralyzed side and the normal side. A reduction in amplitude of more than 90% compared to that of the normal side indicates poor prognosis. If the amplitude remains less than 90% reduced when comparing normal to paralyzed within three weeks, spontaneous recovery is likely. This test is only useful from day 3 to day 21 postinjury.

Electromyography (EMG)

Facial EMG is a test where action potential of the muscle is measured with needle electrodes during active muscle contraction by the patient. The type of electrical activity visualized offers considerable diagnostic information. Electrical silence indicates facial paralysis with the loss of neuromuscular junction. Fibrillation potentials indicate neural degeneration (no regeneration has occurred), whereas polyphasic potentials indicate reinnervation. This test is only useful after 21 days postinjury.

Computed Tomography (CT)

The role of computed tomography (CT) is as temporal bone fractures are commonly discovered during the initial surveillance trauma CT. A high-resolution CT study is indicated in the setting of facial paralysis, cerebral spinal fluid and perilymphatic leaks, suspected vascular injury, disruption of superior external auditory canal, as well as transient or persistent neurologic deficits. For patients with a CSF leak, contrast can be injected intrathecaly to determine the site of the leak.

Angiography

Angiography is reserved for individuals suffering from extensive head trauma in which concerns of hemorrhage, intimal vascular flap, or penetrating injury at the base of the skull is noted during clinical or diagnostics studies. This contrast study allows for the localization of vascular injury as well as interventional therapies necessary for hemostasis.

β-2 Transferrin

This protein study is highly sensitive and specific for a CSF leak as it is only found in CSF, aqueous humor, and perilymphatic fluids. Processing of fluid samples requires 1 cc of fluid and direct transport of the specimen to the laboratory for appropriate processing prior to denaturing of the given protein.

CHAPTER 8

Facial Nerve Paralysis

HAMID R. DJALILIAN
SANAZ HAMIDI
AMIR DEYLAMIPOUR

BACKGROUND

Facial paralysis can be very disconcerting to patients and they often present shortly after the onset of paralysis. Patients most frequently associate facial paralysis with a cerebrovascular accident (CVA); however, a minority of facial paralysis are caused by a CVA. In this chapter, we discuss the most common causes of facial paralysis (Fig 8–1).

BELL'S PALSY

Bell's palsy is a temporary peripheral paralysis of facial nerve that occurs abruptly. Bell's palsy is a term that should be used when other causes of facial nerve paralysis such as malignancy and infections have been excluded. Bell's palsy is thought to be caused by

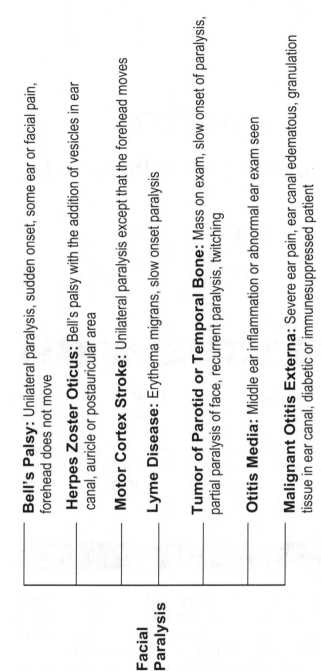

Facial Paralysis

Bell's Palsy: Unilateral paralysis, sudden onset, some ear or facial pain, forehead does not move

Herpes Zoster Oticus: Bell's palsy with the addition of vesicles in ear canal, auricle or postauricular area

Motor Cortex Stroke: Unilateral paralysis except that the forehead moves

Lyme Disease: Erythema migrans, slow onset paralysis

Tumor of Parotid or Temporal Bone: Mass on exam, slow onset of paralysis, partial paralysis of face, recurrent paralysis, twitching

Otitis Media: Middle ear inflammation or abnormal ear exam seen

Malignant Otitis Externa: Severe ear pain, ear canal edematous, granulation tissue in ear canal, diabetic or immunesuppressed patient

Fig 8–1. The most frequent causes of facial paralysis.

herpes simplex virus (HSV) reactivation and edema of the nerve which causes paralysis. With proper treatment, 85% of Bell's palsy patients will have recovery back to normal facial function.

Symptoms and Signs

Patient will generally present with one-sided weakness or complete paralysis of the face which starts suddenly or progress over 2 to 3 days. Paralysis of facial muscles becomes evident as unilateral loss of facial wrinkles in the forehead, inability to close the eyelid, and drooping of the corner of the mouth, taste disturbance, and dry eyes. Also hyperacusis or sensitivity to sound has been reported by 30% of the patients due to the paralysis of the stapedius muscle. On physical examination the unilateral peripheral paralysis of facial nerve leads to the inability of the patient to smile symmetrically, to raise the eyebrows, or to close the eyelids properly.

On history, the onset, rapidity of progress to complete paralysis, previous skin cancers on the face, trauma, and a history of previous facial paralysis should be noted. On physical examination a complete cranial nerve exam and an evaluation of the parotid and the ear should be performed.

Diagnosis and What Tests to Order

Electrical testing using electroneuronography (ENoG) will help in establishing the prognosis of the paralysis. ENoG is only useful after 3 days and before 21 days of the onset of paralysis. This test is only necessary when there is complete paralysis of the face. When incomplete paralysis is present, the likelihood of a normal or near normal recovery is 85%. In this test, a percentage number of degenerated axons on the paralyzed side is given. ENoG results of more than 90% degeneration indicate a poor prognosis. An electromyography (EMG) of the facial nerve is important for understanding the status of the nerve after 21 days postparalysis. Polyphasic potentials indicate regeneration of the nerve. Fibrillation potentials or electrical silence indicate denervation and a very low chance of recovery.

An MRI of the brainstem, temporal bone, and the parotid gland must be obtained when there is a history of recurrent paralysis on the same side, slow onset of paralysis (more than 7 days), a history of facial skin cancers at present or in the past, paralysis duration of greater than 6 months, or an abnormal ear or parotid examination. Brain imaging is necessary when a central cause to the paralysis is suspected. Temporal bone MRI of Bell's palsy patients will generally show some enhancement of the facial nerve without enlargement of the facial canal in the geniculate ganglion area. This enhancement may persist for a few months after resolution of the paralysis.

Lyme disease must be ruled out as a cause of facial paralysis in patients in endemic areas or those who have traveled to the area (New England and midwestern states in the United States) using a Lyme titer. Serum glucose level is ordered if there is a suspicion of diabetes given the higher incidence of Bell's palsy in diabetics.

Treatment and When to Refer

Prednisone (1 mg/kg/d up to 80 mg/d is given for 7 days with a taper over 8 days) in addition to antivirals (acyclovir 800 mg, 5 times a day for 7 days). Valacyclovir (1000 mg BID × 7 days) or famcyclovir (250 mg po TID × 7 days) can be given in place of acyclovir for their more favorable dosing regimen.

Surgical decompression of the facial nerve is recommended in cases where the ENoG shows greater than 95% degeneration within the first 14 days. Surgical decompression must occur before 14 days postparalysis for it to be effective.

Eye care is the most important aspect of caring for facial paralysis. Although it may appear that the patient is tearing, the surface of the eye is generally dry. This occurs because commonly, the lacrimal gland secretion is reduced as a result of the involvement of the greater superficial petrosal branch of the facial nerve. In addition, a patient who can not close his eyes will not be able to moisten the surface of the eye. Tearing is seen because the punctum of the lacrimal duct in the lower eyelid is separated from the globe and the normal muscular contraction that pumps the lacrimal sac is not functional.

Treatment of the Eye: The patients should be advised to keep their eyes moist with artificial tears (one gtt q 1 hour while awake) and to use a lubricant eye ointment (eg, Lacrilube™) to be applied in the eye before sleeping. The patient should be instructed to tape the eye closed when sleeping. Alternatively, the patient can use a moisture chamber which is a clear plastic shield that covers the eye and adheres to the surrounding skin and keeps the eye moist.

Patients with a complete facial paralysis should be referred to an otologist-neurotologist for electrical testing. Recurrent or prolonged (>6 months) facial paralysis, those with an abnormal ear or parotid examination, or those with a history of facial skin cancers should be referred to an otolaryngologist. Patients with an acute onset of central paralysis (forehead sparing paralysis) should be sent to an emergency department with a neurologist consultation for a stroke evaluation.

RAMSAY HUNT SYNDROME (HERPES ZOSTER OTICUS)

Ramsay Hunt syndrome is a combination of facial paralysis similar to Bell's palsy accompanied by development of multiple vesicles on periauricular area, ear canal, tympanic membrane, or the pinna. The etiology of the disease is varicella zoster virus (VZV) infection of the facial nerve. Compared to Bell's palsy, Ramsay Hunt syndrome patients have poorer prognosis in recovery back to normal facial function (55% vs 85% in Bell's palsy), and more severe symptoms (ie, complete paralysis, facial pain).

Symptoms and Signs

Patients usually present with periauricular pain, otalgia, and pain over ear lobes. Vesicles become apparent over the areas described above. Patients with Ramsay Hunt syndrome have a higher incidence of cranial nerve palsies including hearing loss, tinnitus, and vertigo compared to Bell's palsy.

Diagnosis and What Tests to Order

The diagnosis is based on visualization of vesicles and the presence of facial paralysis. See section under Bell's palsy for tests to order.

Treatment and When to Refer

Treatment is similar to Bell's palsy (see above). The patient should be referred to an otologist for electrical testing if complete paralysis is present.

TUMORS INVOLVING THE FACIAL NERVE

Facial nerve neuroma, facial nerve hemangioma, facial and scalp skin cancers, most notably squamous cell carcinoma, can metastasize to the facial nerve. Malignant parotid neoplasms may also involve the facial nerve. Approximately 5% of facial nerve paralysis is due to tumors involving the facial nerve.

Symptoms and Signs

Patients may present with facial twitching which later is followed by progressive facial nerve paralysis. Also, the patient may present with recurrent facial paralysis or a long history (>6 months) of paralysis which was attributed to Bell's palsy in the past. A slow onset of paralysis (over 1 week) is another common finding. Finally, a partial paralysis of the face (eg, single branch) is another warning sign. Tinnitus, hearing loss, and vertigo may be present because some of the patients have associated involvement of the vestibulocochlear nerve. Hearing loss is conductive when the middle ear is involved but sensorineural hearing loss may occur from invasion of the cochlea or extension of the tumor into the internal auditory canal. A complete history and physical examination of the facial movement, parotid gland, and ear must be performed; however, the diagnosis is generally made/confirmed by imaging.

Diagnosis and What Tests to Order

The best imaging modality is an MRI with gadolinium of the temporal bone (internal auditory canal MRI sequence) and the parotid gland. If the patient is unable to have an MRI, a high-resolution CT scan with contrast is recommended. A high-resolution CT of the temporal bones may be obtained for surgical planning. All patients should receive an audiogram to assess for the presence of hearing loss.

Treatment and When to Refer

Treatment is surgical resection of the tumor. The patient should be referred to an otologist/neuro-otologist whenever there is suspicion of a facial nerve tumor.

LYME DISEASE

Lyme disease is a systemic infectious disease caused by *Borrelia burgdoferi*. The disease is transmitted by the *Ixodes* ticks and has been reported in all parts of the US but most notably in the Northeast and the Midwest. Facial palsy is seen in 4.5% of patients with Lyme disease and is bilateral in 25% of patients.

Symptoms and Signs

The patients usually have fever, myalgia, fatigue, and arthralgia. The disease has three stages. The first stage usually presents with a single or multiple annular, erythematous rash that clears in the center and mostly occurs at the site of the tick bite. The rash is called erythema migrans because of its expanding erythematous circle. Carditis and neurologic manifestations of the disease usually manifest weeks to months after the first presentation of the disease. Neurologic symptoms are headache, dizziness, and meningitis besides cranial nerve palsies such as facial palsy. Facial palsy is more common in children. There is generally a history of travel to endemic areas or a tick bite. It would be extremely uncommon in an urban setting with no travel history.

Diagnosis and What Tests to Order

In the presence of a tick bite history and erythema migrans without other symptoms no diagnostic tests are generally required and patients must be treated with antibiotics. Patients with systemic symptoms, for example, facial paralysis, arthralgia, and so forth, should have serologic tests. Serologic tests used for diagnosis are enzyme linked radio immunosorbant essay (ELISA) which should be confirmed with western blot testing.

Treatment and When to Refer

Treatment of Lyme-induced facial paralysis is with cef-triaxone IM/IV 2 g/d (in children, 80 mg/kg IM/IV QD) for 14 days. Localized Lyme disease without neuro-logic or other systemic symptoms can be treated with doxycycline, cefuroxime, or amoxicillin. Moisturizing treatment for the eye as outlined in the Bell's palsy section is recommended in all patients with facial paralysis. Refer the patient to an otolaryngologist if the facial paralysis does not improve. An infectious dis-ease consultation for long-term management given neuroborreliosis is warranted.

TEMPORAL BONE FRACTURE

Refer to Chapter 7 on Ear Trauma

SARCOIDOSIS

Rarely, patients with sarcoidosis can present with facial nerve paralysis and approximately 6% of sarcoidosis patients will develop facial paralysis. The facial paralysis can be unilateral or bilateral. The facial nerve is most commonly involved as a result of parotid gland involvement in sarcoidosis and will be a peripheral paralysis.

Diagnosis and What Tests to Order

An elevated blood acetyl choline esterase (ACE) level, calcium level, and a chest x-ray showing bilateral hilar adenopathy helps with the diagnosis. Tissue biopsy from the affected organ (ie, parotid) showing non-caseating granulomas is diagnostic.

Treatment and When to Refer

Initial treatment with prednisone (1 mg/kg) is recommended. The patient should be referred to an otolaryngologist if facial paralysis does not improve with one week of prednisone.

BILATERAL FACIAL PARALYSIS

Bilateral facial paralysis is defined as the development of the opposite side within 30 days of the onset of the first side. Bilateral facial paralysis is rare (0.3% of all facial paralysis) and is most commonly a manifestation of a systemic disease rather than a localized problem in the facial nerve. The differential diagnosis of bilateral facial nerve paralysis of peripheral origin is in Table 8–1. In a review of the literature, Lyme disease was found to be the etiology in 36% of the cases for facial paralysis, followed by Guillain-Barré syndrome (5%), trauma (4%), sarcoidosis (0.9%), and HIV/AIDS (0.9%).

Diagnosis and What Tests to Order

The initial priority in the evaluation of bilateral facial paralysis is to rule out life-threatening diseases such as leukemia or Guillain-Barré syndrome. Patients suspected of these disorders should be admitted to the hospital. Guillain-Barré patients will generally have a loss of deep tendon reflexes. The workup of the bilateral facial paralysis patient includes a complete blood count, fluorescent treponemal antibody test, anti-HIV

Table 8–1. Differential Diagnosis of Bilateral Peripheral Facial Paralysis

Leukemia	Metabolic diabetes
Trauma skull fractures	Acute porphyria
Infection postinfluenza	Neoplastic acute leukemia
Infectious mononucleosis	Sarcoidosis
HIV infection	Amyloidosis
Lyme disease	Neurologic multiple sclerosis
Guillain-Barré syndrome	Pseudobulbar and bulbar palsy
Syphilis	Parkinson's disease
Brainstem encephalitis	Idiopathic Bell's palsy
HTLV-1 infection	HTLV, human T-cell lymphotrophic virus
Poliomyelitis	

antibody test, serum calcium and glucose as part of a metabolic panel, erythrocyte sedimentation rate, and Lyme titer. Lumbar puncture and an MRI of the brain, temporal bone, and parotid gland with gadolinium are the next steps in the diagnostic workup.

Guillain-Barré syndrome will generally present with progressive ascending weakness or paralysis starting with the legs, trunk, arms, and face. Bilateral or unilateral facial paralysis is seen in 27 to 50% of the cases. Treatment includes plasma exchanges and intravenous immunoglobulins.

Treatment and When to Refer

Given the possible life-threatening causes of bilateral facial paralysis, these patients should be admitted to the hospital for workup and treatment as outlined above. Otolaryngology and neurology consultations will be necessary.

OTITIS MEDIA

The facial nerve courses through the middle ear and occasionally the nerve is not covered by bone. During acute or chronic otitis media, the facial nerve may be involved by infection, which will cause facial paralysis.

Symptoms and Signs

The patient will present with facial paralysis and the signs of chronic or acute otitis media. The tympanic membrane will be erythematous and bulging or perforated. A cholesteatoma may be present.

Diagnosis and What Tests to Order

The diagnosis depends on the exam findings of facial paralysis and acute otitis media on the same side. A CT scan of the temporal bone should be obtained if a cholesteatoma or tympanic membrane perforation is present.

Treatment and When to Refer

The patient should immediately be started on antibiotics (eg, ceftriaxone 2 g IV/IM, children 80 mg/kg IM/IV). A patient with acute otitis media and facial paralysis should be referred to an otolaryngologist immediately for an urgent myringotomy and middle ear culture. A child with facial paralysis and middle ear infection will need general anesthesia for a myringotomy. A patient with cholesteatoma or chronic otitis media and facial paralysis will need urgent referral to an otologist/neuro-otologist for admission and management.

OSTEOMYELITIS OF THE SKULL BASE (MALIGNANT OTITIS EXTERNA)

Skull base osteomyelitis occurs when an infection of the external ear canal (otitis externa) spreads from the skin of the external canal to the temporal bone. It is generally a disease of diabetics or immunosuppressed patients. Facial nerve paralysis occurs as a result of the involvement at the stylomastoid foramen. The most common pathogen is *Pseudomonas aeroginosa*; however, *Staphylococcus aureus*, *Aspergillus*, and *Proteus spp.* have also been reported. The patient will generally present with severe otalgia that is out of proportion to the external otitis. Hearing loss, otorrhea, ear fullness, headache, and facial paralysis may accompany ear pain. On physical examination granulation tissue at the bony cartilaginous junction of the ear canal, edema of soft tissue and lymphadenopathy are occasionally present.

Diagnosis and What Tests to Order

The diagnosis depends on the history, examination, and the technetium-99 bone scan findings. The white blood cell count is often normal but the erythrocyte sedimentation rate (ESR) is elevated. Diagnostic imaging should be performed in an inpatient setting with a technetium-99 bone scan for diagnosis and gallium-67 scan to follow the progression of the disease. The ESR level, gallium scan, improvement of pain and diminishing granulation tissue are markers of resolution. Treatment consists of an initial 6 week course of culture-directed IV antibiotics, placement of an ear wick, the use of otic ear drops, supportive care for cranial nerve palsies, and pain management. A gallium-67 scan is repeated every 3 weeks after the initial 6 weeks of IV antibiotics to monitor for resolution of inflammation. A normal scan marks the end of antibiotic usage. Clinical suspicion must remain high for a malignancy in this scenario and a biopsy of the granulation tissue should be performed if there is no resolution within 1 to 2 weeks.

Treatment and When to Refer

Initial treatment consists of double coverage IV antibiotics against *Pseudomonas spp*. The antibiotics should be changed once culture has been obtained. The patient should be hospitalized immediately if there is suspicion for skullbase osteomyelitis and otolaryngology consultation should be obtained.

CEREBROVASCULAR ACCIDENT (CVA)

Patients with a cerebrovascular accident can present with a facial paralysis. This would occur with a CVA at the level of the motor cortex or at the level of the facial nucleus in the pons. A pontine infarct will have other neurologic deficits, for example, hearing loss, vertigo, among others.

Symptoms and Signs

The patients with a motor cortex CVA will generally present an acute onset of facial paralysis. The patient may have some ipsilateral motor weakness in the upper and lower extremities. The characteristic of motor cortex CVA causing facial paralysis is that the forehead will have normal function whereas the rest of the face will be weak. A pontine infarct will cause a sudden onset of facial paralysis and vertigo. The patient will also have signs of upper and lower extremity weakness. The reason why motor cortex CVA does not cause forehead paralysis is because the cells of the facial nucleus that innervate the forehead receive corticobulbar fibers from both cerebral hemispheres. The cells in the facial nucleus that innervate the lower face receive corticobulbar fibers from the contralateral motor cortex. Also, a motor cortex facial paralysis does not cause decreased lacrimation, taste dysfunction, or decreased salivary flow as in a peripheral paralysis given those are innervated by the parasympathetic system and join the facial nerve outside of the brain-stem. Another sign of a cortical facial nerve paralysis is when the patient moves his or her face with emotion (eg, laughing) but not on volitional motion.

Diagnosis and What Tests to Order

A patient with a central facial paralysis should be sent to the emergency department immediately via ambulance and have a stroke workup and treatment starting with a CT scan of the head.

Treatment and When to Refer

A neurology consultation should be obtained for evaluation for thrombolytic therapy.

FURTHER READINGS

Gevers G, Lemkens P. Bilateral simultaneous facial paralysis—differential diagnosis and treatment options. *Acta Otorhinolaryngol Belg.* 2003;57:139–146.
Gilden DH. Bell's palsy. *N Eng J Med.* 2004;351:1323–1331.

CHAPTER 9

Dizziness and Vertigo

HAMID R. DJALILIAN

BACKGROUND

Dizziness is a common complaint for patients in the primary care or emergency department settings. These patients can be very challenging to diagnose and treat and the average dizzy patient may have seen several physicians before they are diagnosed. Most of this chapter is devoted to the patient with vertigo as it is related to inner ear function. We briefly discuss lightheadedness, imbalance, and multisensory deficit. Figure 9–1 outlines the most frequent causes of vertigo.

OBTAINING A HISTORY IN A PATIENT WITH VERTIGO

Obtaining a proper history is critical in the evaluation of the dizzy patient. The most important part of the history is establishing what exactly patients feel when they state that they are dizzy. The question to ask is,

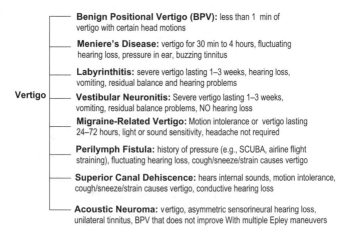

Benign Positional Vertigo (BPV): less than 1 min of vertigo with certain head motions

Meniere's Disease: vertigo for 30 min to 4 hours, fluctuating hearing loss, pressure in ear, buzzing tinnitus

Labyrinthitis: severe vertigo lasting 1–3 weeks, hearing loss, vomiting, residual balance and hearing problems

Vestibular Neuronitis: Severe vertigo lasting 1–3 weeks, vomiting, residual balance problems, NO hearing loss

Migraine-Related Vertigo: Motion intolerance or vertigo lasting 24–72 hours, light or sound sensitivity, headache not required

Perilymph Fistula: history of pressure (e.g., SCUBA, airline flight straining), fluctuating hearing loss, cough/sneeze/strain causes vertigo

Superior Canal Dehiscence: hears internal sounds, motion intolerance, cough/sneeze/strain causes vertigo, conductive hearing loss

Acoustic Neuroma: vertigo, asymmetric sensorineural hearing loss, unilateral tinnitus, BPV that does not improve With multiple Epley maneuvers

Fig 9–1. The most frequent causes of vertigo.

"What exactly does it feel like?" It is best to give the patient a few suggestions. Generally, dizziness falls into one of several categories and the questions to ask are, "Does it feels like there is movement around you (room spins)?" "Does it feel like you are going to pass out?" "Does it feel like you are off balance?" "Does it feel like you are lightheaded?"

The sensation of motion that does not exist is defined as vertigo. For patients to experience vertigo, they must have nystagmus while they are vertiginous. Vertigo cannot occur without nystagmus. Vertigo can be caused by a variety of peripheral, vestibular, or central disorders. Once it is established that the patient is experiencing vertigo, the next most important step in establishing the diagnosis is to ask "How long does the spinning last?" After that, it is important to establish associated symptoms that occur with the vertigo. The questions to ask are, "Is the vertigo associated with hearing loss? Ringing in the ears? Pressure in the ears? Sensitivity to light or sound? Associated with headaches? Is it associated with coughing, sneezing, heavy lifting, or loud noises? Do you have any neck stiff-ness/pain?" Also, it is important to ask, "What makes it start? What makes it stop?" With these questions, the diagnosis of vertigo often can be established without an examination or tests. The examination and tests will only serve to confirm the diagnosis.

EXAMINATION OF THE PATIENT WITH VERTIGO

The examination of the dizzy patient should include orthostatic blood pressure measurements, a complete neurological examination, the Dix-Hallpike (aka Barany) maneuver, as well as an ear, hearing, and extraocular motion exam. The ear examination should focus on abnormalities of the tympanic membrane (eg, drainage, cholesteatoma, tympanic membrane retraction, middle ear mass) and the tuning fork exam should establish if there is asymmetry in the hearing. The extraocular motion exam should be performed to look for conju-gate gaze, double vision, and nystagmus when the eyes are abducted 15°. Physiologic nystagmus can occur when abducting the eyes beyond 20°.

The neurologic exam should include a complete cranial nerve exam and a thorough assessment of the cerebellar/brainstem function. Specific attention must be paid to the Romberg, tandem gait, rapid alternating motion, and finger-nose-finger tests. Patients over the age of 70 generally cannot do the tandem gait, even in the absence of dizziness. Therefore, for those patients, the nontandem gait should be assessed.

The Dix-Hallpike exam is performed by first plac-ing the patient in the sitting position and turning the head 45° in one direction and then lying the patient down quickly while the head is turned. Ideally, the head should hang from the bed by about 30°. However, as most benign positional vertigo (BPV) patients are elderly with cervical osteoarthritis, the head cannot always hang, which is okay. One should then wait for 15 seconds and look at the patient's eyes to look for any signs of nystagmus. The patient is then brought to a sitting position. The head is then turned 45° in the opposite direction and the patient is placed in the supine head-hanging position. The classic nystagmus of posterior canal benign positional vertigo (BPV) (>95% of cases) occurs in a delayed fashion (5–15 seconds), will be rotatory, toward the floor (geotropic), transient (lasting <1 minute), and has a slight up-beat to the pupil as it is turning (in the direction of the posterior semicircular canal). The nystagmus of BPV is generally fatigable but we recommend not retesting the patient multiple times to reduce the discomfort for the patient. It is best to look at a capillary on the conjunctiva to look for the direction of the nystagmus. Potentially, looking at the pupils may miss a rotatory nystagmus. If the patient states that turning to one side brings on the vertigo, the Dix-Hallpike test should begin by turning the head to the opposite direction. This allows for an Epley maneuver to be done after placing the head in the position that leads to the nystagmus without the need to check the opposite ear.

RECURRENT VERTIGO LASTING LESS THAN A MINUTE

Benign Positional Vertigo (BPV)

Short episodes of vertigo (<1 min) are associated most commonly with BPV. BPV is caused by free-floating crystals (otoconia) in the semicircular canals (most commonly the posterior semicircular canal (PSC)). It can occur at any age, but most commonly is found in older adults (>50 yr) or sometimes in younger patients after head trauma or roller-coaster rides. The patient classically complains of vertigo that occurs upon waking or turning in bed. Other presentations include vertigo while turning when driving, or vertigo on getting out of bed or in the middle of the night. To help identify the involved side, the patient should be asked, "Turning to which side brings on your symptoms?" If the patient is unable to remember, one could ask which side of the bed the patient sleeps on and which way they turn to get out of bed. If the patient complains of vertigo when getting out of bed, it is important to know if the vertigo occurs from turning to get up or from going from a lying to a standing position. Dizziness that occurs when going from a lying to a standing position is generally lightheadedness and is associated with orthostatic hypotension, whereas vertigo that occurs when turning is generally associated with BPV. The involved side is the side to which turning brings on the symptoms.

Diagnosis and What Tests to Order

The diagnosis of BPV depends on the history and a positive Dix-Hallpike examination in the absence of other complicating factors (eg, unilateral hearing loss, neurologic deficits, etc). The diagnosis of BPV generally does not require any tests. A videonystagmography (VNG) may be helpful in complicated cases.

Treatment and When to Refer

The treatment of BPV is the performance of the Epley maneuver. This maneuver is simple and takes less than 3 minutes to perform. If the physician is uncomfortable with this maneuver, she or he can refer the patient to

an otologist-neurotologist or to a physical therapist.
The maneuver starts by placing the patient in the Dix-
Hallpike provocative position that brings on the vertigo.

The following is the Epley maneuver for a right-
sided BPV, vertigo when the patient is placed in the
right ear down position (head turned 45° to the right
and then placed in the supine position). The patient
will then experience vertigo in the position (position 1,
Fig 9–2A). The patient's head must be held in place

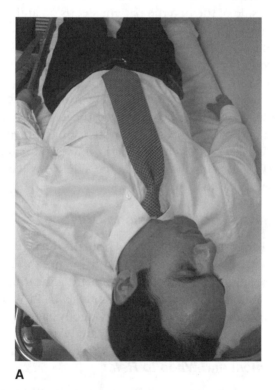

A

Fig 9–2. The Epley maneuver for a right posterior canal
benign positional vertigo. **A.** The patient is placed in the
initial provocative position (position 1), in this case right ear
down. *continues*

while in that position as patients have the tendency to move out of the provocative position. The physician should wait until the vertigo subsides. The head is then turned 90 ° in the opposite (left) direction (position 2, Fig 9–2B). This will place the patient's head in the left ear down position. The patient may or may not experience vertigo in this position. The patient is then asked to turn his or her body so that he or she is lying on the left shoulder and hip. The head is maintained in

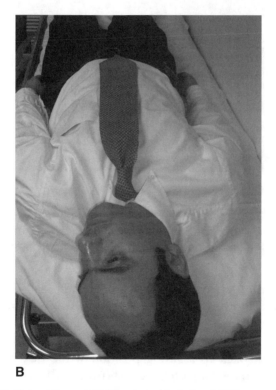

B

Fig 9–2. *continued* **B.** The head is turned 90° away from the initial position into position 2 (in this case turn to the left). *continues*

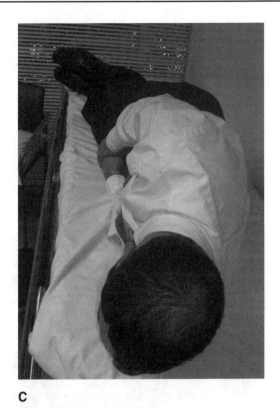

C

Fig 9–2. *continued* **C.** The head is then turned another 90° away from position 2 into position 3, where the nose is pointed somewhat toward the ground. *continues*

the same (left ear down) position. The head is then turned another 90° to the left, which will have the patient's nose pointed toward the ground at a 45° angle (position 3, Fig 9–2C). The patient is then brought back to a sitting position while flexing the neck with the chin on the chest (position 4, Fig 9–2D). After 30 seconds, the head can be taken out of flexion. The maneuver is exactly the opposite for a left-sided BPV (vertigo with the left ear down position on Dix-Hallpike). The patient usually feels vertigo during the

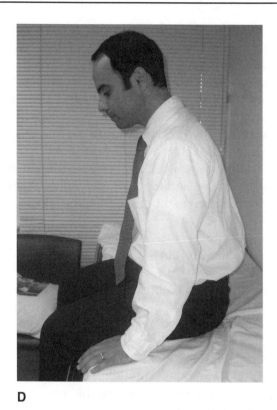

D

Fig 9–2. *continued* **D.** The patient is brought back to the sitting position with the neck flexed.

various positions and the head must be kept in that position until the vertigo subsides (usually ~30 seconds).

A simple way to remember the Epley maneuver is that the head is turned 45 ° in the direction that causes the vertigo and then has to be turned away 90 ° and wait for 30 seconds, and turn away another 90 ° and wait for 30 seconds, and then brought to the sitting position (see Fig 9-2).

After the Epley maneuver, the patient is asked to not lie flat, bend over, or extend the neck for 48 hours.

The patient is asked to wear a soft cervical collar to prevent sudden motion or extension of the neck. After that, the patient may return to normal activities. The patient is asked to follow up in 1 week. The Epley maneuver is successful in 85% of cases on the first attempt. The success rate goes up to 95% when it is necessary to redo the maneuver on the follow-up visit if the patient continues to be symptomatic.

A patient who does not have resolution of the vertigo after two attempts of the Epley maneuver should be referred to an otologist-neurotologist.

Perilymphatic Fistula

The inner ear is composed of two fluid compartments. The endolymphatic compartment is within the membranous inner ear and the perilymphatic fluid surrounds the endolymphatic compartment and fills the rest of the bony inner ear. The inner ear is bone covered and communicates with the middle ear in two areas: the round window and the oval window. If there is a sudden change in atmospheric pressure or in the event of a very strong Valsalva, perilymphatic fluid may leak into the middle ear through those windows, called a perilymphatic fistula (PLF).

Symptoms and Signs

The leakage of this perilymphatic fluid causes short bouts of vertigo (generally <1 min) and a fluctuating hearing loss and will most commonly occur with a change in pressure (eg, blowing of nose, sneezing, coughing, lifting something heavy, straining for stool, going up or down in an elevator or plane, or SCUBA diving). These actions also are the ones that generally cause the PLF to start. One more characteristic of patients with PLF is sound-induced vertigo. The patients will complain of loud sounds causing vertigo, especially when the sound is presented in the affected ear. PLF may also occur as a result of temporal bone fractures or cholesteatomas that have eroded into the structures of the inner ear.

A patient suspected of having a PLF should have a complete exam as described earlier. A pneumatic otoscope should be placed in the ear canal and, using a large speculum, a seal should be obtained. The pressure in the ear canal should then be fluctuated using the pneumatic otoscope to see if that will cause vertigo. Alternatively, pumping the tragus can also cause vertigo in these patients.

What Tests to Order and When

If PLF is suspected, an audiogram and a videonystagmography (VNG), including a fistula test, should be obtained. The audiogram may show an asymmetric hearing loss and the VNG may show a positive fistula test (vertigo when placing negative pressure in the ear canal). Because patients with PLF have very similar symptoms to those with superior canal dehiscence (SCD), an ultrahigh-resolution CT scan of the temporal bone (0.5-mm slice thickness) with sagittal reconstruction images should be obtained to rule out SCD. If an asymmetry in the vestibular function on VNG or in hearing is found, an MRI of the internal auditory canal should be obtained to rule out an acoustic neuroma.

Treatment and When to Refer

A patient suspected of having PLF or upon diagnosis should be referred to an otologist-neurotologist for evaluation and treatment. The treatment of this disease is surgical sealing of the round and oval windows. Until the patient gets definitive treatment, she or he should refrain from activities that cause the vertigo (eg, blowing of nose, sneezing, coughing, lifting something heavy, straining for stool, going up or down in an elevator or plane, or SCUBA diving). The patient should be prescribed a stool softener to prevent straining. This will prevent further loss of perilymphatic fluid, which would cause further hearing loss and loss of vestibular function.

Superior Canal Dehiscence

Chronic pulsations of the dura or aggressive arachnoid granulations may cause erosion of the bone overlying the superior canal causing superior canal dehiscence. Superior canal dehiscence (SCD) is a recently recognized disorder that is characterized by bouts of vertigo (generally <1 min) or sensations of movement of space around them (generally <5 sec), hearing loss, autophony (sensation of hearing themselves in that ear), pulsatile tinnitus, and sensation of plugging in the ear. One other symptom related to SCD is the sensation that patients can hear their own eye movement. The vertigo or sensation of movement is generally pressure-related or loud-sound related. The symptoms of SCD are very similar to those of PLF.

Diagnosis and What Tests to Order

The diagnosis is by ultrahigh-resolution CT scan of the temporal bone (0.5-mm slice thickness) with sagittal reconstruction images. A vestibular-evoked myogenic potential (VEMP) test or a fistula test is often positive in these patients. The audiogram may show a conductive or a sensorineural hearing loss. It is not uncommon to have a patient with SCD who has had a surgery performed for a PLF without improvement due to a lack of proper diagnosis and the similarities of the two disorders.

Treatment and When to Refer

A patient suspected of having SCD should be referred to an otologist-neurotologist for evaluation. Treatment is surgical plugging of the involved superior canal.

Acoustic Neuroma

Schwannomas of the vestibular nerves are most commonly called acoustic neuromas (AN). These tumors generally are very slow growing and most commonly present in the 5th to 7th decades. These tumors can occur in younger patients though and can occur bilaterally as part of neurofibromatosis type II in teenagers.

Symptoms and Signs

The most common symptoms are unilateral tinnitus, asymmetric hearing loss, sudden hearing loss, distortion of sounds in the ear, and vertigo. The vertigo in AN patients can vary between episodes lasting less than a minute to constant vertigo/imbalance. Large tumors will cause facial paresthesias or paralysis of cranial nerve IX or X. An AN will almost never cause facial paralysis.

Diagnosis and What Tests to Order

An audiogram should be obtained in all patients who present with vertigo or any hearing related complaints. A VNG may be necessary if the diagnosis is not clear from the history. An MRI of the internal auditory canals with gadolinium should be obtained in patients with asymmetric hearing loss, atypical vertigo, sudden hearing loss, or patients with unilateral tinnitus lasting more than 6 months. Because AN can present in a very similar manner as BPV, an atypical BPV patient who does not respond to three Epley maneuvers should have an MRI to rule out an AN. The gold standard for diagnosis is an MRI of the internal auditory canals (IAC). A brain MRI may miss a small AN in the internal auditory canal; therefore, a dedicated IAC MRI needs to be obtained for evaluation. Auditory brainstem response testing is useful for diagnosing large tumors, but may miss small tumors

Treatment and When to Refer

There are three options in the treatment of acoustic neuromas: watchful waiting with yearly MRIs, surgical resection, and stereotactic radiation therapy. Upon diagnosis of an AN, the patient should be referred to an otologist-neurotologist.

Migraine-Associated Vertigo (MAV)

Thirty percent of patients with migraine will experience vertigo. The vertigo may occur at the time of the headache or at other times. The criteria for diagnosis of migraine-associated vertigo include the diagnosis of migraine by the International Headache Society criteria, recurrent vestibular symptoms (vertigo, head motion intolerance), episode, and at least one of the following during at least two vertiginous attacks: migrainous headache, photophobia, phonophobia, or visual or other auras.

Symptoms and Signs

Patients may complain of vertigo lasting less than a minute, a few minutes, or a few hours, sometimes lasting up to 24 to 48 hours. Sometimes the patient may present with several weeks of motion intolerance and a sensation that their visual fields move with head motion. The patient generally will have sensitivity to light or sound during the episodes and will have relief with sleep. Headache must not be present for a diagnosis of MAV. The history of migraine headaches or auras/scotomas in the past or a strong family history of migraine (eg, first degree relative) often will be found.

Diagnosis and What Tests to Order

An MRI of the brain is indicated when there are neurologic deficits or signs of severe headaches. A VNG may be necessary to rule out peripheral causes of vertigo.

Treatment and When to Refer

Although MAV generally may respond to abortive medications such as triptans (eg, sumatriptan 25–100 mg po × 1), the need for frequent treatment (up to daily) has led to the recommendation of prophylactic therapy for these patients. Prophylactic treatment regimens are outlined in Table 9-1. Referral to a neurologist or an otologist/neuro-otologist for patients who do not respond to standard therapy or for long-term management is indicated.

Table 9–1. Prophylactic Regimens for Migraine-Related Vertigo

Drug	Dosing Regimen	Side Effects
Nortriptyline	25 mg po QHS for 3 weeks, then increase by 25 mg every 3 weeks up to 75 mg QHS	Dry mouth, weight gain
Topiramate	25 mg po QD, increase by 25 mg every week up to 150 mg po QD	Weight loss, tingling in fingers, word-finding difficulties
Atenolol	50 mg po QD, increase to 100 mg po QD after 2 weeks	Fatigue, impotence
Verapamil SR	120 mg po QD, increase up to 240 mg po QD after 2 weeks	Constipation
Venlafaxine	12.5 mg po QD, increase every week by 12.5 mg up to 75 mg po QD	Nausea, somnolence, QT prolongation

RECURRENT VERTIGO LASTING 30 MINUTES OR MORE

Ménière's Disease

Symptoms and Signs

Ménière's disease is characterized by episodic vertigo lasting 30 minutes to several hours (typically 2–3 hrs), fluctuating progressive hearing loss, pressure sensation in the ear (not relieved by Valsalva), and a roaring tinnitus. The disorder is caused by an increase in the endolymphatic fluid pressure. The episodes of vertigo typically are triggered by stress, increased salt, caffeine, or alcohol intake.

Diagnosis and What Tests to Order

The diagnosis is generally clinical. A low-frequency sensorineural hearing loss on audiogram or a loss of vestibular (caloric) function on a VNG will confirm the diagnosis. An MRI of the IAC with gadolinium must be obtained to rule out an acoustic neuroma in cases of asymmetric hearing loss or asymmetric vestibular function (>25% weakness on caloric testing).

Treatment and When to Refer

The treatment includes stress reduction (daily exercise and meditation), low salt diet (<2000 mg sodium/day), and elimination of caffeine and alcohol. A diuretic (hydrocholorothiazide 37.5 mg/triamterene 25 mg q.a.m.) will help in cases of at least weekly vertigo or those who do not respond to conservative therapy. Referral to an otologist-neuro-otologist is necessary after diagnosis for long-term medical or surgical management.

Labyrinthitis

Labyrinthitis is a rare disorder characterized by severe sustained (>7 d) associated with hearing loss and almost always accompanied by vomiting (due to the severity of the vertigo). The vertigo generally lasts 2 to 3 weeks. It is thought to be viral but can occur as a result of bacterial invasion through the round window after an acute otitis media. These patients will always have a residual loss of hearing and balance function after labyrinthitis. Therefore, a patient who presents with a history of labyrinthitis in the past must have some residual hearing loss in the affected ear. The patient will have nystagmus with the fast component towards the affected ear present.

Diagnosis and What Tests to Order

The diagnosis of labyrinthitis requires severe sustained vertigo that lasts more than 7 days that is accompanied by sensorineural hearing loss. The ear examination will be otherwise normal. Generally, though, patients will present during the first 24 hours and the diagnosis has to be made based on the severity of the vertigo, vomiting, and hearing loss. A tuning fork examination will help determine whether hearing loss is present. An MRI of the internal auditory canals must be obtained to rule out an acoustic neuroma.

Treatment and When to Refer

The patient may require admission for IV fluids as the nausea and vomiting may be excessive. On an outpatient basis, an intramuscular injection of a benzodiazepine (eg, diazepam 5 mg) and corticosteroids (eg, dexamethasone 0.1 mg/kg) will help acutely in the relief of nausea. Oral corticosteroids (eg, prednisone 0.5 mg/kg) for 5 days will help reduce the nausea associated with the severe vertigo. Oral benzodiazepines (eg, diazepam 5 mg po tid) will also help reduce the vertigo. The patient should be referred to an otologist-neurotologist after diagnosis.

Vestibular Neuronitis

Vestibular neuronitis results from a viral infection of the vestibular nerve. The virus involved is not known.

The patients present in exactly the same manner as those with labyrinthitis with the exception that patients with vestibular neuronitis do not have hearing loss.

Diagnosis and What Tests to Order

The patients have severe sustained vertigo lasting longer than 1 week (typically 2–3 weeks). An MRI of the internal auditory canals with gadolinium to rule out an acoustic neuroma must be obtained. The MRI may show enhancement of the vestibular nerves.

Multiple Sclerosis (MS)

Ten percent of MS patients present with vertigo and 30% of them will experience vertigo at some time during their disease. The vertigo can be short (<1 min) or can be sustained and longer than 24 hours. MRI of the brain and an appropriate history with loss of neurologic function and subsequent recovery help with the diagnosis. Further testing including lumbar puncture will confirm the diagnosis. A patient suspected of having MS should be referred to a neurologist for confirmation of diagnosis and treatment.

Pontine Infarction

Patients with lacunar infarcts of the pons can present with vertigo, which may or may not be associated with other neurologic dysfunctions. Most commonly, these patients will present with sudden onset of severe imbalance. Patients often will have a history of hypertension, cardiac valve replacement, arrhythmia, or atherosclerosis.

An MRI of the brain is indicated to rule out an intracranial mass. Small lacunar pontine infarcts usually do not appear on an MRI of the brain. Larger infarcts will appear on an MRI but will have other neurologic deficits. The diagnosis is clinical. Management of the cardiovascular risk factors is needed. Physical therapy and use of assistive devices will help in long-term management.

LIGHTHEADEDNESS

Lightheadedness generally occurs due to a drop in cerebral blood flow during positional changes. It can be caused by hypovolemia, long-standing hypertension (loss of elasticity of cerebral arteries/arterioles), long-standing diabetes (neuropathy at carotid bulb), atherosclerotic coronary artery disease, beta-blockers, or other antihypertensives. When the patient goes from a lying to a sitting or a sitting to a standing position, venous blood pools in the legs. This leads to a drop in arterial blood pressure in the carotid bulb which leads to a sympathetic stimulation of the heart. This requires the heart to beat faster and more efficiently to pump blood from the dependent lower extremities against gravity to maintain cerebral blood flow within a second. Any condition that adversely affects this system will cause a delay in the maintenance of cerebral blood flow and lead to a sensation of lightheadedness.

Symptoms and Signs

The patient most commonly will complain of "dizziness" when she or he stands or sits up quickly. The patient will have a sensation of near-fainting and a dark visual field for a few seconds. The patients will not have any true vertigo (motion of room about them). The patient should be questioned about physical activity (perspiration) and fluid and caffeine intake. A dark yellow color to the urine or constipation may indicate chronic hypovolemia. On examination, orthostatic systolic blood pressure may show a drop of 20 mm Hg and an increase of heart rate of 20 beats per minute. However, it must be noted that orthostatic blood pressure checks measures radial artery blood pressure changes, not cerebral blood pressure changes. Therefore, a normal orthostatic blood pressure check does not rule out the diagnosis of orthostasis as the cause of lightheadedness.

Diagnosis and What Tests to Order

The diagnosis is by history and a review of the patient's medications. Diuretics, beta-blockers, a long-standing hypertension or diabetes mellitus history, or evidence of coronary artery (or peripheral vascular) disease is strongly suggestive. If the patient denies these symptoms, a cardiovascular (eg, echocardiography) and diabetes (eg, fasting blood glucose or hemoglobin A1c) workup is warranted. Ankle-brachial blood pressures may indicate evidence of peripheral vascular disease.

Treatment and When to Refer

Treatment of lightheadedness consists of behavioral and medication modification. If the patient's problem primarily stems from perspiration, exercise, fever, vomiting, diarrhea, and poor hydration, drinking liquids containing electrolytes (eg, sports drinks, Gatorade®, etc.) will generally suffice. Patients who consume significant caffeine (greater than 3 caffeinated beverages) per day should gradually decrease their caffeine intake and switch to decaffeinated beverages slowly. The caffeine content of newer caffeinated drinks (eg, espresso, cappuccino, etc) can sometimes be equivalent to 6 to 8 caffeinated carbonated beverages (eg, Pepsi or Coca-Cola). This high caffeine intake can cause significant diuresis and chronic hypovolemia. The patients should be asked to drink enough water per day until their urine becomes clear.

Patients with hypertension should have their medications reviewed. Diuretics and beta-blockers should be changed to other anti-hypertensives if possible. Support stockings used for venous insufficiency (eg, Jobst stocking) should be used in these patients to help decrease venous pooling in the lower extremities upon sitting or standing. The patient should be instructed to get up slowly out of bed or from a chair and to contract his or her muscles in all four extremities to increase venous return to the heart. Patients at risk for falls should be provided a physical therapy consultation for a possible use of a cane or walker. Muscle strengthening and balance training tends to help these patients.

IMBALANCE

The body's balance is controlled using 3 systems: (1) visual; (2) vestibular; and (3) proprioception. The input from these 3 systems comes into the cerebellum and the brainstem which will direct muscular movement in the eyes, trunk, and lower extremities to keep the body upright and the visual field fixed. Any disturbance of this system can lead to a sensation of motion. With the exception of acute loss of vestibular function (labyrinthitis, vestibular neuritis, or acoustic neuroma) significant imbalance and falls are almost always caused by disturbance at the level of sensory integration (pons and cerebellum). Most commonly, this disturbance is due to a mass effect or a lacunar infarction at the brainstem level.

Symptoms and Signs

The patients will complain of loss of balance when walking. These patients will generally have a long-standing hypertension history, which predisposes them to lacunar infarctions at the pontine level. A history of diabetes mellitus may be present. The patient may have had an acute loss of balance or may have a chronically progressive loss of balance. A full neurologic examination should be performed including Romberg, tandem gait, rapid alternating motion, heel-knee-shin, and finger-nose-finger. Proprioception should also be checked. Any history of joint replacements should be obtained as it will cause a loss of proprioception in that joint and worsened balance.

Diagnosis and What Tests to Order

The diagnosis is clinical and will be clear on tandem or normal gait. All patients with a loss of balance should undergo an MRI of the internal auditory canals with gadolinium should be obtained to rule out mass lesions or an Arnold-Chiari malformation (herniation of cerebellum below foramen magnum). If multiple sclerosis is suspected, a brain MRI should also be obtained. If acute cranial neuropathies are present or a cerebral vascular accident (CVA) is suspected, the patient should be sent to the nearest emergency department via ambulance for a CVA workup.

Physical therapy for muscle strengthening, balance therapy, and gait training will help reduce the chance of falls which can lead to fractures. The patients commonly will need an assistive device (eg, cane or walker) to help maintain their balance when walking.

PART II

Diseases of the Nose and Sinuses

CHAPTER 10

History and Examination of the Nose

EDWARD C. WU
VANESSA S. ROTHHOLTZ
HAMID R. DJALILIAN

The primary care physicians encounter patients with sinonasal-related chief complaints on a daily basis. The history of the condition can be long and complicated. It is imperative to acquire a detailed history along with a comprehensive exam of the nose and sinuses to arrive at an accurate diagnosis and solid treatment plan.

HISTORY

There are a number of common patient complaints that warrant a detailed history of the nose and sinuses (Table 10–1). For each symptom, it is helpful to ask about the onset, duration, recurrence, variability, location and quality of pain if present and the impact of the condition on the patient's life. For a patient presenting with nasal discharge, it is important to ask

Table 10–1. Indications for Obtaining a More Detailed Sinonasal History

- Rhinorrhea/discharge (ie, allergies, sinusitis, coryza)
- Congestion/airway obstruction (ie, anatomic, mass)
- Sneezing, itchiness, dryness (ie, allergies)
- Pain and tenderness in nose or surrounding areas (ie, sinusitis, mass)
- Masses and polyps
- Nose bleeding (epistaxis)
- Loss of sense of smell (anosmia)
- Trauma to nose
- Halitosis—suggests possible nasal mass
- Questionable foreign body

about the color, texture, and presence of a foul odor. Specific questions in the sinonasal history are listed in Table 10–2.

As with any history acquired, it is important to ask the patient about current and past health conditions, surgical history, history of trauma, and family history. One should also inquire about allergies to medications, current and past medications, tobacco use, alcohol ingestion, illicit drug use, social history, and occupational history, including exposure to chemicals. Intranasal over the counter vasoactive medications, such as Afrin, may cause rhinitis medicamentosa, which is the occurrence of nasal congestion from the overuse of these agents. The information garnered from these questions will serve to place a proper context to the current complaint. As always, make sure to review the systemic patient history carefully to note any potentially missed points of interest (Table 10–3).

Table 10–2. Questions To Be Addressed When Obtaining a History for a Sinonasal Complaint

General Questions

- When did the problem start?

- How long has the problem lasted?

- Is this a new, recurring, or chronic problem?
  - Any prior physician visits?
  - Previous treatments attempted?
  - Duration of prior treatments?

- Do the symptoms vary?
  - How often do the symptoms change? Seasonally? Time of day? In different environments? Improve? Worsen? Under what conditions?

- Is the problem unilateral or bilateral?
  - On which side did the problem originate?

- Have any home remedies or alternative medicine treatments been attempted?
  - If so, how successful were they?

- How bothersome is the problem?

- Is the problem seriously affecting daily life?

- If there is discharge, what is the color, texture, and is there odor?

- If there is pain, how painful is it on a scale of 1 to 10?

EXAMINATION

After the completion of a thorough history, the examination of the nose should be performed starting with the most comfortable maneuver and ending with the least comfortable maneuver. It can be challenging to examine such a cavernous area, but the task is made easier with the correct instruments and a dependable light source.

Table 10–3. Specific Questions to Be Asked of Patients in Other Components of the History

- Allergies (specific allergens or environments)
  - Is the patient allergic to animals and pets? Dust? Pollen?
- Medication and drug use
  - Does the patient take medications for the relief of symptoms?
  - Does the patient take medications that may be causing the symptoms?
- Smoking
  - Does the patient smoke?
  - Is the patient frequently exposed to secondhand smoke?
- Occupation
  - Is there anything in the workplace that could be causing the problem(s) such as allergens or chemical exposure?
- History of previous illness
  - Is there anything that may be related to the nasal symptoms such as cough, headache, or fever?
- Chronic health problems
  - Inquire about snoring, sleep apnea, prior stroke, diabetes, hypertension
- History of previous surgery
  - Has the patient ever undergone procedures to alleviate nasal problems?
  - Has the patient undergone reconstructive surgery of the nose?
  - Has the patient undergone cosmetic surgery of the nose?
  - Has the patient experienced any abnormal bleeding after routine surgery?
- History of trauma to nose and surrounding areas
- Family history
  - Bleeding disorders
  - Wegener's granulomatosis
  - Osler-Weber-Rendu syndrome
  - Telangiectasias elsewhere
  - Nasal carcinoma
  - Ethnicity
- Environment/Recent Travel

It is wise to take a step back and examine the patient's general appearance as a whole. Note the physical structure and surface anatomy of the nose. Determine the presence of deformities, asymmetries, unusual texture and color, or other abnormal physical features. Observe the external appearance of the patient's nasal septum.

After informing the patient of your intent, tap the frontal sinus (over the glabella) and maxillary sinus areas (lateral to the nose) with the tip of your finger or finger joints. Note any tenderness or fullness that may indicate acute sinusitis. Patients who suffer from chronic sinusitis will not have any tenderness on this procedure.

Moving onto the intranasal examination, place the thumb of your nondominant hand gently on the tip of the patient's nose and the fingertips of the same hand on the patient's forehead for stability and control of the movement of the head. Lift the nose upward so that the anterior and inferior surfaces are visible through the widened nostrils. From this view, using an otoscope as a light source, you should clearly see the anterior aspect of the patient's inferior turbinate, the anterior aspect of the septum, and the degree of patency of the anterior aspect of the patient's nasal cavity (Fig 10-1). For children and adults, first look into the anterior nose using the light of the otoscope. For adults, it may be more appropriate to use a nasal speculum. For more posterior exposure, prolonged, or endoscopic examination of the nose, it may be useful to apply a vasodilator and local anesthesia (eg, 4% lidocaine with oxymetazoline) in droplet or spray form prior to examination. This improves patient comfort and may have the added effect of decongesting the nose thereby facilitating an improved exam.

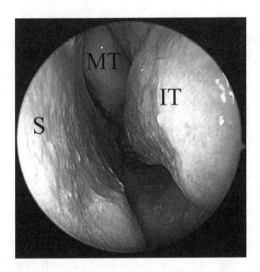

Fig 10–1. Anterior rhinoscopy view of the left nostril. The nasal septum (*S*) occupies the medial nasal cavity. The inferior turbinate (*IT*) and the middle turbinate (*MT*) are seen in the lateral nasal cavity. The IT has a thicker and boggier mucosa than the thinner and smoother mucosa of the MT. Picture courtesy of Quoc A. Nguyen, MD.

Prepare for inspecting the posterior aspect of the nasal cavity by placing the widest available speculum onto the otoscope. Have the patient tilt the head back. Carefully insert the otoscope into the patient's nose without contacting the nasal septum. Look deeper until the inferior and middle turbinates (lateral), nasal septum (medial), and nasal passage are more visible. Keep in mind that it is rather rare to find a noticeably straight nasal septum, as the nasal septum is a common site of continuous minor trauma that would result in deviations. In those patients with recurrent epistaxis, particular attention should be paid to the antero-inferior area of the patient's septum, also known as Little's area where Kiesslebach's plexus is located. In this location, epistaxis most frequently originates, and the presence of telangiectasias and dried blood should be noted. The nasal septum should be examined along its length, looking for perforations, any deviations anteriorly or posteriorly, nasal septal spurs and evidence of past or current bleeding.

At the same time, observe the red nasal mucosa. Note the color and whether there are any abnormalities, including damage, dryness, swelling, bleeding, and exudate (mucus, pus, or both) emanating from the posterior nasal cavity, the frontal sinus duct or the middle meatus located directly underneath the middle meatus on the lateral nasal wall.

At this point, it is also possible to see abnormalities such as benign nasal polyps (pale and semitranslucent grapelike masses) (Fig 11–2 in Chapter 11), dense masses, and ulcers. It is sometimes difficult to distinguish between a boggy turbinate, a diseased turbinate and a chronic polyp. Determining a diagnosis may be achieved by palpating the structure lightly with a cotton tipped-applicator. A turbinate should be sensitive to the touch and hard on palpation given it is bone covered by mucosa. A polyp, however, will be spongy in character with few if any nerve endings and painless.

If inspection and removal of a questionable foreign body is necessary, do so carefully. It may be dangerous to carelessly apply additional force against it, thereby displacing it further into the nose, or worse, past the nose and into the airway. This is particularly dangerous in uncooperative children, and any questionable foreign body should be referred to a specialist right away. If the presence of an intranasal button battery is suspected, this must be removed immediately because its caustic qualities can quickly turn irreparably destructive.

It may be worthwhile to note a simple test for the sense of smell. Take coffee grounds or any strongly odorous but safe and readily available material and hold it right beneath the patient's nostrils. Be mindful not to place a noxious substance (eg, ammonia or alcohol) beneath the patient's nose because it will stimulate the trigeminal nerve and not the olfactory nerve. In the absence of decongestion, the smell should be clear in a normal individual.

One of the main methods by which direct imaging of the nose is attained is through nasal endoscopy (flexible or rigid rhinoscopy), where an endoscope is inserted through each of the nares to view the posterior portion of the interior nose. The major advantage of using nasal endoscopy in addition to simple physical examination is to elucidate the progression and location of localized disease within the nose, which leads to better diagnosis, pathologic analysis, assessment, and treatment of the disorder. Nasal endoscopy is generally performed by otolaryngologists.

IMAGING

In the past, x-rays have been the primary imaging test for visualizing the paranasal sinuses. Sinus x-rays have high false positive and false negative rates and are not used much anymore. For the otolaryngologist, computer tomography (CT) imaging of the sinuses are routinely ordered to assist in the evaluation of the paranasal sinus anatomy. It provides additional information about the extent and location of disease as well as proximity to key peripheral structures such as the orbit and cranial base. Coronal views without contrast are typically ordered as the drainage ports (ostiomeatal complex) of the sinuses are visualized better on coronal images. They assist in treatment and surgical planning, if necessary. Magnetic resonance imaging (MRI) is reserved to clarify the extent of a sinonasal mass suspicious for a neoplasm.

WHEN TO REFER

Recognizing sinonasal disorders that need to be evaluated and treated by a specialist is very important. Any nasal mass, chronic sinusitis and nasal polyposis should be referred for further workup. A CT of the sinus in axial and coronal views without contrast prior to referral is often helpful to determine the extent of the disease. A foreign body in the nasal cavity that cannot be removed under direct visualization in an office setting due to lack of proper instrumentation should be referred to an otolaryngologist for evaluation and removal. CSF rhinorrhea is another dangerous condition that should be viewed with a high index of suspicion. Cerebrospinal fluid is frequently suspected when persistent, unilateral, clear fluid that occurs post-traumatically or spontaneously, especially in obese patients. Chronic epistaxis can be referred on an outpatient basis for thorough workup provided a patient's hematocrit and vital signs are stable, and the treatment of any underlying medical cause is exhausted. Finally, any sinonasal disorder that involves vision changes or mental status changes should be sent to the emergency room for a complete evaluation and an urgent otolaryngology consultation.

CHAPTER 11

Nasal Obstruction

PAUL SCHALCH
HAMID R. DJALILIAN

BACKGROUND

Nasal obstruction is a very common complaint in both adult and pediatric patients. It is often self-treated with home remedies and over-the-counter medications. Patients usually seek help from their primary care physicians when these first-line interventions have failed. The most frequent causes of nasal obstruction are outlined in Figure 11–1.

EVALUATION

In general, the causes of nasal obstruction can be divided into reversible (or functional) and fixed (anatomical, structural). The main distinction is made based on the information obtained from a careful history and the findings on physical exam, as well as therapeutic trials with topical decongestants.

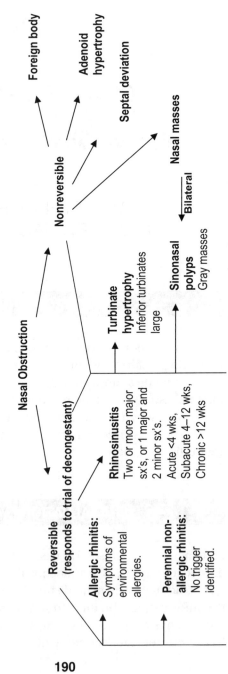

Nasal Obstruction

Reversible
(responds to trial of decongestant)

Nonreversible

Foreign body

Adenoid hypertrophy

Septal deviation

Nasal masses

Turbinate hypertrophy
Inferior turbinates large

Rhinosinusitis
Two or more major sx's, or 1 major and 2 minor sx's.
Acute <4 wks, Subacute 4–12 wks, Chronic >12 wks

Allergic rhinitis:
Symptoms of environmental allergies.

Perennial non-allergic rhinitis:
No trigger identified.

Bilateral

Sinonasal polyps
Gray masses

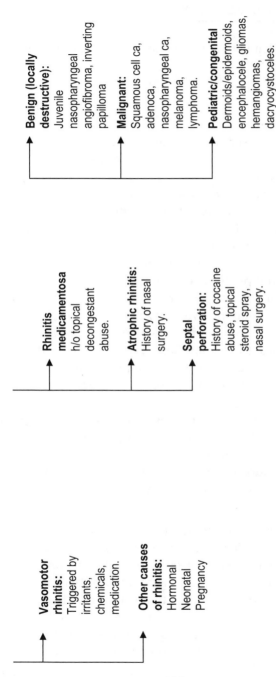

Vasomotor rhinitis:
Triggered by irritants, chemicals, medication.

Other causes of rhinitis:
Hormonal
Neonatal
Pregnancy

Rhinitis medicamentosa
h/o topical decongestant abuse.

Atrophic rhinitis:
History of nasal surgery.

Septal perforation:
History of cocaine abuse, topical steroid spray, nasal surgery.

Benign (locally destructive):
Juvenile nasopharyngeal angiofibroma, inverting papilloma

Malignant:
Squamous cell ca, adenoca, nasopharyngeal ca, melanoma, lymphoma.

Pediatric/congenital
Dermoids/epidermoids, encephalocele, gliomas, hemangiomas, dacryocystoceles. Choanal atresia, other craniofacial abnormalities.

Fig 11–1. The most frequent causes of nasal obstruction.

191

The elements of the history for nasal obstruction are:

1. Onset
2. Duration
3. Constant versus intermittent, day versus night-time (including impact on quality of sleep)
4. Laterality
5. Ameliorating (eg, use of breathing strips) and worsening factors (supine position)
6. Use of medications (topical and systemic), drugs (cocaine) and tobacco
7. Previous surgery, trauma, foreign bodies (in children and psychiatric patients)
8. Concurrent allergies or allergy-related conditions (asthma, conjunctivitis, eczema)
9. Presence and nature of discharge and/or bleeding
10. Associated symptoms (loss of smell, postnasal drainage, otalgia, clogged or "popping" ears, chronic cough, headaches, vision problems, epiphora, fever, etc)
11. Associated conditions (pregnancy, rheumatologic disease, diabetes, gastroesophageal reflux, cystic fibrosis, syndromes and congenital malformations)
12. Occupational exposure to sawdust, toxic fumes, heavy metals, and radiation.

The physical exam should include careful observation for nasal deformities (eg, crooked nose), elongated midface (indicating adenoid hypertrophy), mouth-breathing, overbite, and gross cranial nerve deficits (which may indicate the presence of a tumor or any other invasive/destructive lesion). A thorough head and neck exam with proper documentation is essential in establishing the etiology of nasal obstruction.

Anterior Rhinoscopy

Anterior rhinoscopy requires good technique and a good understanding of the nasal anatomy. Common causes of nasal obstruction that can be diagnosed with anterior rhinoscopy include septal deviation, septal perforation, turbinate hypertrophy, mucosal discoloration, inflammation, ulceration, crusting, presence of discharge, and polyps or masses/tumors in the nasal cavities (Fig 11–2).

Alternatively, a flexible or rigid fiberoptic scope, which may or not be available in the primary care setting, can be used to visualize the nasal passages, the patency of the choanae, and the adenoid pad directly. This enables the examiner to have a better view of the nasal anatomy and rule out the presence of any masses not visible on anterior rhinoscopy.

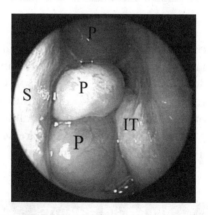

Fig 11–2. Nasal polyps on anterior rhinoscopy will appear as gray glistening masses that are compressible and have few sensory receptors. The "P" indicates the polyps which are positioned between the inferior turbinate (*IT*) and the nasal septum (*S*). Picture courtesy of Quoc A. Nguyen, MD.

Therapeutic Trial with Topical Decongestant

A therapeutic trial of topical decongestants (eg, oxymetazoline, phenylephrine, or neosynephrine) may help in discerning if the cause for nasal obstruction is reversible vs. fixed. Reversible nasal obstruction that responds to decongestants can be secondary to allergic, inflammatory or infectious etiologies, with or without an underlying anatomic defect. Reversible nasal obstruction indicates mucosal disease, which can generally be treated medically. Fixed nasal obstruction, in turn, indicates the presence of defects or masses that should be evaluated by an otolaryngologist for possible surgical correction.

REVERSIBLE CAUSES OF NASAL OBSTRUCTION

Reversible nasal obstruction is usually bilateral and may be accompanied by mucosal manifestations such as inflammation, purple or pale discoloration, and may also include enlargement of the inferior turbinates. When the response to topical decongestants is positive and anterior rhinoscopy reveals no septal deviation or any masses in the nasal cavities, there are several possible diagnoses that should be considered.

ALLERGIC RHINITIS

Patients with allergic rhinitis generally present with nasal obstruction, clear rhinorrhea, postnasal drip, sneezing, and itching of the nose, nasopharynx, pharynx, or eyes. The symptoms may or not be seasonal in nature.

Symptoms and Signs

The cardinal symptoms are nasal obstruction, rhinor-rhea, itching, and sneezing. Physical findings include edematous, bluish-discolored turbinates, polypoid mucosa or polyps (gray, glistening masses in the nasal cavity) obstructing the nasal cavity, crease above the nasal tip (caused by the constant rubbing of the nose in an upward fashion, also known as the "allergic salute"), allergic shiners, Morgan-Dennie lines (lines under the lower eyelid), watery rhinorrhea, and more systemic manifestations such as eczema, ocular, or generalized pruritus, dermatographism (edema/ery-thema of the skin upon scratching), and asthma.

Diagnosis and What Tests to Order

A detailed history that establishes the temporal rela-tionship between environmental factors and the oc-currence of symptoms is helpful for the diagnosis. More specialized allergic testing and immunoglobulin E measurements are usually reserved for moderate to severe cases that are unresponsive to empiric therapy.

Treatment and When to Refer

Treatment of allergic rhinitis is best done using topical nasal steroid sprays, topical antihistamines, or oral antihistamines. Topical nasal sprays (eg, fluticasone or mometasone) should be used 2 puffs each nostril qd [children 2–11 yo, 1 puff each nostril qd]. Fluticasone furoate is approved for ages 2 years and above, whereas fluticasone propionate is approved for ages 4 and above. Topical antihistamines (olopatadine [Patanase®] or azelastine) should be used as 2 puffs each nostril

BID (patients 12 years of age and above). The patient should be instructed to spray the lateral wall of the nose and not the nasal septum. Spraying the septum is less effective. In the case of nasal steroids, spraying the septum will lead to a higher chance of epistaxis and rarely, septal perforation. Topical anti-histamine, and oral antihistamines are useful when patients also suffer from other symptoms such as pruritus in the eyes or skin. The less-sedating or nonsedating oral antihistamines in order of efficacy are levocetirizine (Xyzal®) 5 mg po qd [children 6 to 11, 2.5 mg po qd], cetirizine 5–10 mg qd [children 1 to 5 yo, 2.5 mg po qd]; fexofenadine 180 mg po qd [children 2–11 yo, 30 mg po qd; children 1–2 yo; 15 mg po bid]; loratadine 10 mg po qd [children 2–5 yo, 5 mg po qd]. Cetirizine is not classified as a nonsedating oral antihistamine. Sedating oral antihistamines (eg, diphenhydramine, dimenhydrinate) are generally more effective than their nonsedating counterparts, but their duration of efficacy is shorter and due to their sedating side effects they are not used commonly. Montelukast (10 mg po qd; for children less than 15 years old, 5 mg po qd) can also be used in patients with as an adjunctive therapy or as monotherapy especially in patients with asthma and allergic rhinitis. Ocular symptoms can be treated with olopatadine one gtt BID each eye (patients aged 3 years or older).

Environmental control and avoidance of exposure to allergens is always useful in controlling symptoms and decreasing the requirements of both topical and oral medications. Simple measures such as not allowing pets (especially cats) in the bedroom, closing the bedroom windows, HEPA filters, and using mattress covers and hypoallergenic linen may in fact be quite effective.

The patient should be referred to an otolaryngologist if an adequate trial of nasal steroid spray and antihistamines fails to control the patient's symptoms. More specialized immunotherapy should be reserved for severe cases that do not respond to environmental control and topical and oral medications. Patients with asthma and allergic rhinitis will require a referral to an allergist.

PERENNIAL NONALLERGIC RHINITIS

Perennial nonallergic rhinitis will present with persistent nasal obstruction, with or without sneezing. It can be caused by a variety of factors including irritative, hormonal, and vascular factors. The main distinguishing feature is the lack of a clear relationship with any potential environmental triggers. In many cases, there are no identifiable triggers for the symptoms. An IgE-mediated mechanism cannot be demonstrated.

Symptoms and Signs

The patients will most commonly present with nasal obstruction. The patients will commonly have post nasal drainage without other systemic manifestations of allergic disease. The symptoms are present throughout the year, independent of any seasonal patterns.

Diagnosis and What Tests to Order

The diagnosis is made by a detailed history that fails to reveal a causal relationship with traditional environmental triggers, as well as any seasonal patterns. Occasionally, a pattern of exposure to non-traditional environmental triggers can be established, such as solvents, detergents, fuels, bleach, etc).

Treatment and When to Refer

Topical nasal steroids have been showed to be beneficial in the treatment of perennial nonallergic rhinitis. A similar regimen of fluticasone, mometasone, budesonide, flunisolide, or triamcinolone, consisting of 2 puffs per nostril once to twice a day should be prescribed. Avoidance of any environmental factors, including second-hand smoking, if any are identified is also important. Isolated rhinitis, without other symptoms such as itchy eyes or nose or sneezing can be treated with anticholinergic nasal sprays, such as ipratropium bromide 0.03%, 2 puffs per nostril TID.

VASOMOTOR RHINITIS

See Chapter 13, Nasal Discharge.

RHINITIS OF PREGNANCY

Rhinitis of pregnancy and other hormonally mediated types of rhinitis present in the setting of hormonal changes and usually subside upon delivery or cessation of hormone therapy. It affects 5 to 32% of pregnant women.

Symptoms and Signs

The patients will present with bilateral nasal obstruction which generally starts toward the end of the first trimester. The examination will reveal enlarged inferior turbinates and clear drainage in the nose.

Diagnosis and What Tests to Order

Diagnosis is based on the presence of rhinitis in a pregnant patient without previous symptoms of rhinitis.

Treatment and When to Refer

Topical nasal steroids have been used for treatment. Budesonide is the only nasal steroid that can be used in pregnancy. The bioavailability of budesonide is 13 to 29%, which is one of the highest in the nasal steroid class. Therefore, the authors generally do not recommend nasal steroids in pregnant patients. Referral is warranted for nasal endoscopy if unilateral nasal obstruction or drainage exists or if other symptoms (eg, unusual symptoms, purulence not responsive to antibiotics, etc.).

NEONATAL NASAL OBSTRUCTION

Neonatal nasal obstruction can be caused by choanal atresia, stenosis of the piriform aperture, rhinitis medicamentosa, or allergic rhinitis (secondary to milk, wheat, etc).

RHINOSINUSITIS

See Chapter 13, Nasal Discharge.

RHINITIS MEDICAMENTOSA

Rhinitis medicamentosa occurs as a result of prolonged use (more than 5–7 days) of nasal sympathomimetic decongestant spray (eg, oxymethazoline, neosynephrine or phenylephrine) abuse. Longer term use of these sprays causes a rebound effect with increased nasal congestion and the duration of efficacy of the spray becomes shorter. The patient will then use the spray more frequently throughout the day to stop the nasal obstruction. A careful history of use, frequency, and duration of any over-the-counter decongestant sprays is essential. The nose appears congested, the mucosa and turbinates may be hyperemic or pale and boggy. There is scant clear mucous present. Management is with a gradual discontinuation of topical decongestants over one month, and topical steroid sprays (fluticasone or mometasone 2 puffs per nostril BID for one month, then decreased to two puffs daily in each nostril and eventually stop after 3 months of therapy). It is important to note that these patients generally have an underlying cause for nasal obstruction (most often allergic rhinitis) for which they originally began self-medication with the topical decongestant medication. Treatment of the underlying condition (eg, with nasal steroids) is critical, while gradually tapering off the nasal decongestant. Referral is necessary if there is no improvement of the symptoms after one month of treatment.

ATROPHIC RHINITIS

Atrophic rhinitis, also known as empty nose syndrome, occurs as a result of overzealous resection of the inferior and middle turbinates in patients who undergo nasal surgery. Septal perforation can also occur after nasal surgery (septoplasty). Empty nose syndrome and septal perforation can also be found in patients with a history of cocaine abuse, which causes ischemia of the mucosa and subsequent destruction, as well as autoimmune disorders such as systemic lupus erythematosus and malignancies such as lymphoma. The destruction of the mucosa leads to the loss of the normal physiology of the nose (moistening and warming of the inspired air, as well as mucocilliary clearance). The abnormal mucosa causes excessive crusting of the nasal cavity, turbulent airflow, and ensuing nasal obstruction. Detailed surgical and social history data is the cornerstone of diagnosis. Management consists of scheduled debridements under endoscopic guidance and daily buffered saline irrigations (3–4 puffs, 4 times a day) to minimize crusting.

FIXED NASAL OBSTRUCTION

Fixed nasal obstruction is oftentimes caused by anatomical defects or masses, which may be uni- or bilateral. In most cases, surgical treatment is indicated. There are, however, exceptions to the rule. A trial of topical decongestant sprays notably fails to produce any transient improvement. The presence of masses may or not be evident on anterior rhinoscopy and, frequently, imaging is required to rule out their presence.

NASAL SEPTAL DEVIATION

Septal deviation is one of the most common causes of nasal obstruction. A perfectly straight septum is rather uncommon, and anterior and/or posterior deviations,

S-shaped septa, and septal spurs can be diagnosed on anterior rhinoscopy in patients without any history of surgery or trauma, and also in patients without any complaints of nasal obstruction. Septal deviation, in fact, might only cause nasal obstruction in conjunction with other anatomic and functional factors or abnormalities, such as inferior turbinate hypertrophy, allergy or inflammation, and even the normal nasal cycle (alternating hypertrophy of the inferior turbinates every 3-4 hours, regulated by the autonomic nervous system). Detailed history of trauma to the nose, including potential nasal fractures, should be obtained, as the septum may be concurrently fractured and dislocated toward one side of the nose.

Consider also patients who have undergone cosmetic surgery of the nose (rhinoplasty), who may have collapse of the lateral nasal wall, causing either fixed (constant) or dynamic (collapses when taking a deep breath through the nose) obstruction of the nose. Up to 10 to 15% of patients that undergo rhinoplasty have some degree of nasal obstruction, which occasionally requires revision surgery.

Symptoms and Signs

Nasal obstruction is usually unilateral, although it may be bilateral in the case of bilateral septal spurs or S-shaped septa. Examination will commonly reveal the deflection of the nasal septum to one or both directions. Though uncommon, the septal deviation may be located only posteriorly in the bony portion of the septum.

Diagnosis and What Tests to Order

Septal deviations can usually be diagnosed on anterior rhinoscopy, although more posterior spurs may only be evident during nasal endoscopy. Imaging (CT scan) is usually not necessary for diagnosing septal deviation, but is probably the best imaging modality if an imaging is to be obtained to evaluate fixed nasal obstruction. Plain films have no role in diagnosing septal deviation.

Treatment and When to Refer

The treatment of septal deviation is generally surgical, in the form of a septoplasty, which may be performed in conjunction with reduction of the inferior turbinates, if these are found to contribute to the nasal obstruction.

Inferior Turbinate Hypertrophy

Bilateral inferior turbinate hypertrophy is a common finding in patients with underlying allergic disorders. It is caused by the hypertrophy of the submucosal tissues and enlargement of the venous sinuses of the turbinates. Unilateral hypertrophy can also be a compensatory mechanism in cases of significant septal deviation, contralateral to the narrowed side. Care must be taken not to confuse this unilateral hypertrophy with the previously mentioned nasal cycle. Hypertrophic turbinates in the context of allergies usually have a purplish discoloration, and on occasion so-called "mulberry" changes. Hypertrophy of the inferior turbinates, however, might be an isolated anatomic abnormality without an underlying cause, and may not always respond to a trial of decongestants.

Symptoms and Signs

Uni- or bilateral nasal obstruction, may be fluctuating, and is generally worse when lying down because of pooling of blood in the venous sinuses of the turbinates. Examination will reveal the changes described above.

Diagnosis and What Tests to Order

Inferior turbinate hypertrophy can be diagnosed on anterior rhinoscopy. The inferior turbinates appear inflamed, swollen, and sometimes have a blue or pale appearance. A careful history of allergies, use of topical decongestants and other drugs, and recent hormonal changes should be elicited from all patients because it constitutes a common manifestation of various types of rhinitis.

Treatment and When to Refer

Inferior turbinate hypertrophy again constitutes a special case. Although it is an anatomic problem, oftentimes it improves with medical management in the form of topical nasal steroids and treatment of underlying conditions. The patient should be referred to an otolaryngologist when there is persistent obstruction not responsive to topical steroid sprays, for evaluation for possible surgical treatment.

NASAL MASSES

Nasal masses presenting as obstruction may be uni- or bilateral, benign or malignant, congenital or acquired. The importance of accurate diagnosis and appropriate workup and referral cannot be overemphasized in the case of neoplasia, regardless of its benign or malignant nature. In some cases, masses are localized in the posterior aspect of the nasal cavity or nasopharynx, anterior rhinoscopy will be unremarkable and nasal endoscopy as well as imaging studies are required to establish a diagnosis. Congenital and pediatric nonreversible nasal obstruction constitutes a special group of diagnoses which are described in a separate section (see below).

BILATERAL NASAL MASSES

Bilaterally enlarged inferior or middle turbinates can sometimes be confused with nasal masses. Inferior turbinates are distinguished by the fact that they have smooth nasal mucosa covering them and they are attached to the lateral aspect of the nasal cavity. Even though they are bilateral structures, the turbinates fluctuate in size throughout the day, exhibiting alternating enlargement over periods of 30 minutes to 3 hours. This changing appearance should be kept in mind whenever there is uncertainty about the findings on anterior rhinoscopy. Sinonasal polyps constitute changes of diseased mucosa, be it due to inflammatory or allergic causes. Polyps have a gray appearance (see Fig 11-2).

Symptoms and Signs

Patients usually have symptoms consistent with allergic rhinitis or rhinosinusitis (see previous sections). Polyps have a pale, grayish appearance, and are usually readily visible on anterior rhinoscopy. On occasion, they even protrude from the nasal cavities, or are visible on examination of the oropharynx, protruding beyond the soft palate (also known as antrochoanal polyps). Careful history documenting symptoms of asthma, aspirin intolerance, chronic sinusitis, allergic rhinitis, cystic fibrosis, and Churg-Strauss syndrome should be obtained in order to determine the presence of these and other underlying conditions and institute treatment, as indicated.

Diagnosis and What Tests to Order

Diagnosis is usually made based on the characteristic appearance of polyps, and their bilateral nature. Any child under 18 years of age, with a history of nasal polyps should be evaluated with a sweat chloride test, given the common occurrence of nasal polyps in cystic fibrosis.

Treatment and When to Refer

Treatment of nasal polyps is generally geared toward treating the underlying inflammatory/allergic conditions. Nasal steroid sprays (fluticasone or mometasone: one [for children] to two puffs [for adults] per nostril, once a day), or a short course of prednisone (0.5 mg/kg/d for 5 days) will help in reducing the size of the polyps. Polyps may shrink once appropriate pharmacotherapy for either allergic or inflammatory conditions is instituted. Chronic sinusitis, however, might require endoscopic sinus surgery with removal of extensive polypoid disease. Treatment of underlying conditions is essential, as nasal polyps tend to recur. The patient should be referred to an otolaryngologist if there is no response to conservative medical treatment. A coronal (noncontrast) CT of the sinuses prior to referral will expedite the patient's care.

UNILATERAL NASAL MASS

Unilateral nasal masses can represent benign or malignant tumors. Benign tumors tend to be locally destructive, so prompt diagnosis is imperative.

Symptoms and Signs

Unilateral nasal obstruction that does not resolve with topical medications in the absence of septal deformities is the cardinal symptom. Additionally, patients may report unilateral rhinorrhea, which may be clear or purulent, or recurrent epistaxis. Symptoms specific of cranial nerve deficits (eg, facial paresthesia), epiphora, proptosis, diplopia, cheek mass or deformity, loose maxillary teeth or dentures that fit poorly are suggestive of a locally destructive or malignant process. Middle ear effusion (generally serous, yellow-tinged) and tympanic membrane retraction could indicate eustachian tube dysfunction as a result of inflammatory nasal disease or, if unilateral, the presence of a mass in the nasopharynx. The presence of posterior nasal discharge and any masses that cause asymmetry of the palate or that protrude from the nasopharynx should also be ruled out with a careful oropharyngeal examination.

Multiple and often bilateral lymphadenopathy (<1 cm) could be suggestive of an infectious/inflammatory cause of nasal obstruction, whereas a single, enlarged neck mass(es) (>1 cm) could be suggestive of a malignant tumor in the upper aerodigestive tract.

Diagnosis and What Tests to Order

Anterior rhinoscopy may confirm the presence of a tumor; however, in many cases anterior rhinoscopy might be non-diagnostic. If available, nasal endoscopy should be performed in all cases in order to visualize the middle meatus area (under the middle turbinate) and the nasopharynx posteriorly. Imaging should only be obtained after nasal endoscopy has been performed. CT scan of the sinuses with contrast and gadolinium-enhanced MRI are two diagnostic modalities that are essential in confirming the diagnosis of tumor, evaluating the extent of disease, and its possible malignant nature (bone destruction, intracranial spread). Biopsies of nasal masses are, in general, discouraged as a first step in diagnosis without any imaging data, for some masses might be highly vascularized, and, particularly in the case of pediatric nasal masses, some might have a connection with the subarachnoid space (see section on pediatric nasal masses, below).

Benign, locally destructive neoplasms include inverting papilloma (HPV-caused papilloma with 10% malignant transformation rate) and juvenile nasopharyngeal angiofibroma (almost exclusively in adolescent males, who present with nasal obstruction or recurrent epistaxis). Malignant tumors include, among others, squamous cell carcinoma, nasopharyngeal carcinoma, adenocarcinoma, melanoma, and lymphoma.

Treatment and When to Refer

Patients with unilateral nasal masses should be referred to an otolaryngologist for evaluation as soon as possible. A CT scan of the sinuses with contrast will assist in expediting the patient's care.

NONREVERSIBLE CONGENITAL AND PEDIATRIC NASAL OBSTRUCTION

ADENOID HYPERTROPHY

Adenoid hypertrophy is one of the most common causes of nasal obstruction in the pediatric population. The adenoid pad, located high in the nasopharynx, grows significantly between the ages of 2 and 5 years, and involutes thereafter.

Symptoms and Signs

Patients with long-standing adenoid hypertrophy develop so-called "adenoid facies," with elongated, flattened midface, infraorbital shiners, overjet of maxilla and open mouth due to chronic mouth breathing (Fig 11–3). Patients (or their caregivers) usually report nasal obstruction and congestion with or without clear rhinorrhea. The patient may also have snoring or sleep apnea. Sleep apnea can be manifested by restless sleep, enuresis, breathing pauses, choking episodes at night, constant need for napping, and even behavioral problems. Older children with adenoid hypertrophy may have concomitant otitis media with effusion and tonsillar hypertrophy, with their associated symptoms. Symptoms of allergic disorders such as sneezing, clear rhinorrhea, watery eyes should be investigated.

Diagnosis and What Tests to Order

In many instances the diagnosis is clinical. Lateral neck x-rays are useful in identifying adenoid hypertrophy,

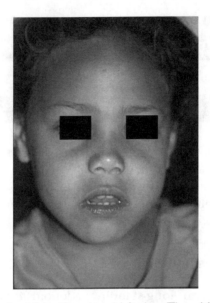

Fig 11–3. A child with adenoid facies. The child has the sunken midface, open mouth (due to nasal obstruction), dry lower lip, and green drainage from the nostril (due to chronic sinusitis). Picture courtesy of Carol MacArthur, MD and Gurpreet S. Ahuja, MD.

which is graded according to the degree of obstruction of the nasopharynx (grade I: <25%, II: 25–50%, III: 50–75%, and IV: >75%). It is recommended to perform x-rays when referring a patient for further treatment to an otolaryngologist and to send the studies with the patient, in order to avoid the need for repeat studies.

Treatment and When to Refer

Treatment of nonreversible causes of nasal obstruction in the pediatric population is usually surgical. Exceptions, however, include observation and medical management in the case of turbinate hypertrophy, adenoid hypertrophy and septal deviation in children. The adenoid pad usually involutes after the fifth year of life. The nasal obstruction may actually resolve as a result of this, together with the widening of the nasopharyngeal space as a result of growth. The impact of nasal obstruction in the craniofacial development and the quality of sleep should be carefully assessed before opting for the more conservative approach.

NASAL FOREIGN BODIES

Foreign bodies should always be in the differential diagnosis, particularly in cases of unilateral nasal obstruction and foul nasal discharge in children as well as patients with psychiatric or developmental conditions.

Symptoms and Signs

Foreign bodies in the nose can present as unilateral nasal obstruction and unilateral discharge. At this point it is imperative to establish the nature of the foreign body.

Diagnosis and What Tests to Order

The diagnosis is clinical. History by the parents or caregivers is the most important element of diagnosis. Anterior rhinoscopy may or may not reveal the presence of a foreign body. If the nasal mucosa is significantly swollen, a topical nasal decongestant should be administered (oxymetazoline, neosynephrine, phenylephrine, 2–3 puffs per nostril) to facilitate visualization. This will also help in terms of reducing the amount of epistaxis in case attempts to retrieve the foreign body are made, which may result in trauma to the nasal mucosa. Long-standing foreign bodies (more than a few days) will have significant amount of dry drainage around the foreign body.

Treatment and When to Refer

When a foreign body is not visualized on anterior rhinoscopy but there is strong suspicion for the presence of one in the nose, nasal endoscopy should be performed by an otolaryngologist. Retrieval of a nasal foreign body can be attempted in the office if the right instruments are present, the foreign body is readily visible, and the patient is reasonably cooperative or easily restrainable. Multiple unsuccessful attempts can cause significant inflammation, which might make further attempts for removal even harder, and cause significant epistaxis or injury to the patient. In this case, nasal foreign body removal should be performed by an otolaryngologist under endoscopic visualization in the operating room or under sedation. Round alkaline batteries (watches, calculators) need to be removed immediately because they cause significant caustic burns of the nasal mucosa, with ensuing scarring.

CONGENITAL NASAL OBSTRUCTION

Congenital causes of nasal obstruction (present at birth) include choanal stenosis and atresia, piriform aperture stenosis, midline masses such as encephalocele, dermoids and epidermoids, gliomas, hemangiomas, and dacryocystoceles with intranasal cysts. A rather uncommon cause nowadays is the presence of congenital syphilis, which causes nasal obstruction with mucopurlulent rhinorrhea and flattening of the nasal dorsum ("snuffles"). Any evident facial malformations, asymmetry, sinuses, or masses over the dorsum of the nose should also be documented.

Symptoms and Signs

The presence of a mass may be evident. Difficulty breathing, even respiratory distress, more pronounced during feeding, is common in neonates because they are obligate nasal breathers until about 5 months of age. Respiratory distress and cyanosis are usually relieved when crying. Attention should be paid to the presence of uni- versus bilateral obstruction, as well as epiphora and dacryocystitis. Tumors that are connected to the subarachnoid space characteristically grow in size when the child is crying, which often happens during physical exams (Furstenberg's sign).

Diagnosis and What Tests to Order

Imaging study modalities for the workup of nasal obstruction include computed tomography (CT) and magnetic resonance imaging (MRI). CT is the best modality for studying osseous anatomy, that is, facial bones, sinuses, and septum (including the choanae), evaluating the presence of mucosal thickening, and inspissated secretions in the sinuses. MRI is the best study modality whenever greater detail of the soft tissue structures is needed. MRI is also the modality of choice when diagnosing congenital midline masses, vascular malformations/hemangiomas, and sinonasal as well as anterior skull base tumors.

Treatment and When to Refer

Biopsy of any nasal mass should not be performed until evaluation by an otolaryngologist is completed, due to the potential disastrous consequences of biopsying a vascular mass such as a hemangioma or any mass with a subarachnoid connection which may contain cerebrospinal fluid and potentially brain tissue (eg, encephalocele). A more extensive review of pediatric craniofacial syndromes is beyond the scope of this text. Any pediatric nasal mass should be referred to an otolaryngologist for evaluation and treatment.

FURTHER READING

Anon J, Jacobs M, Poole M, et al. Antimicrobial treatment guidelines for acute bacterial rhinosinusitis. *Otolaryngol Head Neck Surg.* 2004;130:1–45.

Corey JP, Houser SM, Ng BA. Nasal congestion: a review of its etiology, evaluation, and treatment. *Ear Nose Throat J.* 2000;79:690–693,696,698.

Máspero J, Rosenblut A, Finn AJ, Lim J, Wu W, Philpot E. Safety and efficacy of fluticasone furoate in pediatric patients with perennial allergic rhinitis. *Otolaryngol Head Neck Surg.* 2008;138:30–37.

CHAPTER 12

Epistaxis

ROHIT GARG
HAMID R. DJALILIAN

Reported to affect 60% of the population at one time or another in their lifetime, epistaxis, or nasal bleeding, is a commonly occurring phenomenon. Epistaxis severity ranges from minor self-limited bleeding to life threatening massive brisk bleeding. Only approximately 5% of patients with epistaxis seek medical attention with their primary care physician or local emergency department to control or stop the hemorrhage.

Nose bleeding usually occurs due to mucosal disruption, with consequent exposure and breaking of underlying vessels. There are two categories of epistaxis: anterior and posterior. Anterior epistaxis constitutes 90 to 95% of cases and primarily involves the Kiesselbach plexus located in the anterior aspect of the nasal septum. Bleeding from this area tends to be of a venous or capillary origin and thus presents as a constant ooze. It is most commonly caused by excessive drying of the septum (due to air dryness, aging, or septal deviation) or digital manipulation (nose picking in children). Posterior nasal bleeds are less common and tend to be more profuse and brisk, often times with an arterial origin (sphenopalatine artery or one of its tributaries). Posterior nasal bleeding will generally only occur in the setting of hypertension or coagulopathies. The most common causes of epistaxis are listed in Table 12–1.

Table 12–1. Differential Diagnosis of Epistaxis

Local dryness (summer or winter season, elderly)

Epistaxis digitorum (nose picking) [child, dryness, anterior]

Foreign bodies (peds, unilateral nasal drainage before bleeding)

Sinunasal neoplasms ([anterior or posterior] smoker, woodworker, decreased V2 sensation, mass seen, bleeding always on the same side)

Irritants (smoker, job exposure)

Medications (nasal steroids, anterior)

Juvenile nasopharyngeal angiofibroma (anterior or posterior, peripubertal male, recurrent)

Septal deviation (deviation seen)

Septal perforation (perforation seen)

Trauma (acute trauma)

Vascular malformation or telangiectasia (HHT)

Hemophilia

Hypertension

Leukemia

Liver disease (eg, cirrhosis)

Medications (eg, aspirin, anticoagulants, nonsteroidal anti-inflammatory drugs)

Platelet dysfunction

Symptoms and Signs

Although diagnosis of nasal bleeding is often clearly evident, a complete history and physical examination is crucial. Anterior bleeding is usually clinically obvious, however, posterior epistaxis may be asymptomatic or present insidiously. Important aspects to address in the history include the following: (1) Source of bleeding—unilateral or bilateral, anterior or posterior (it is important to ask the patient if the bleeding is anterior or posterior when the patient is sitting or standing straight and not pinching the nose); (2) Amount of bleeding (eg, tablespoon(s), cup, or pitcher of blood [number of tissues used for cleaning the blood is not a good indicator of amount]); (3) Duration of bleeding; (4) First episode or recurrence; (5) Trauma to the nose; (6) Possible foreign body insertion; (7) Airway issues: dyspnea; (8) Hematemesis, hemoptysis, melena (posterior nasal bleeds may present silently with symptoms related to swallowed blood); (9) Past medical history: hypertension, easy bruising, bleeding disorders, or drug or alcohol abuse; (10) Medications that promote bleeding (ie, anticoagulants, NSAIDs); and (11) Family history of bleeding disorders. Often, the patient will state that the bleeding started on one side and subsequently involved the other side, which indicates that the blood is going through the nasopharynx to the other side. The patient may also state that the bleeding was first anterior and then became posterior. This occurs because the patients will often tilt their head back during the bleeding and the blood streams to the back of the nose.

Physical examination should also be performed in a methodical and meticulous manner to ascertain the bleeding source. Prior to examination of the nose, the blood pressure and heart rate must be checked. In examining the nose, best visualization is accomplished with a nasal speculum and headlight or mirror. In a primary care setting, an otoscope may be used as a light source. The anterior septum and anterior nasal cavity should be inspected for any obvious bleeding sites that may be amenable to direct pressure or cautery. Gentle suctioning using a 10 or 12 French Frasier suction tip may be used to remove large clots that obstruct complete examination. The oral cavity and posterior oropharynx should also be thoroughly inspected. Any blood in the posterior pharynx should be suctioned with a Yankauer suction or irrigated with gargling. A constant and steady drip or ooze in the posterior pharynx after clearing usually signifies a posterior origin of the bleed.

What Tests to Order

First time or infrequent self-limited epistaxis does not require any further workup or laboratory analysis. However, in cases of recurrence, significant blood loss, or suspicion of malignancy, a complete blood cell count should be obtained. In cases where a coagulopathy is suspected, additional blood work should include prothrombin time (PT/INR), partial thromboplastin time (PTT), and bleeding time. In cases of brisk bleeding or significant blood loss, blood typing and cross-matching may also be necessary.

CT scan with contrast can be ordered when there is a suspicion for nasal mass or malignancy as a cause of the bleeding. These would include recurrent epistaxis in a peripubertal male (to rule out a juvenile nasoparyngeal angiofibroma), smoker, patient with a history of woodworking (increased risk of sinunasal malignancies), Asian patient (high risk of nasopharyngeal carcinoma) or those with a mass seen on examination. Alternatively, the patient can be referred for nasal endoscopy to an otolaryngologist.

Treatment and When to Refer

Depending on the severity and location of the nasal bleed, there is a continuum of treatment options starting with direct pressure.

Direct Pressure

Initial management of all anterior nasal bleeds should include constant compression of the nostrils providing direct pressure to the septal area for 15 to 20 minutes, while the patient is sitting or standing. The patient who calls from home should be directed to hold the nose by the nostrils and to completely close their nostrils so that they cannot breathe through the nose. They should sit in front of the television with a clock nearby and instructed to switch hands if necessary. Most commonly, the patients will either get tired of holding their nose or get bored and will stop prematurely; therefore, it is necessary to ask them to entertain themselves and watch the clock to ensure the minimum of 15 minutes of pressure is held! In the office setting, strip gauze (1 inch or ½ inch) or cotton soaked in a topical decongestant (eg, oxymetazoline or phenylephrine) should be used inside the nostril and the patient should plug the affected nostril or nostrils. If available, a specialized clamp that is padded with gauze can be used to close the nostrils and apply pressure to the septum. After 20 minutes, if there is continued bleeding, the patient should be examined for possible chemical cauterization. If digital pressure stops the bleeding and the blood pressure is normal, the patient should be instructed on using saline nasal spray (3-4 puffs each nostril QID).

Cautery

Chemical cauterization using silver nitrate sticks is ideal for easily identifiable, small, discrete anterior septal bleeds. Pretreatment by spraying the nasal cavity with a topical anesthetic and vasoconstrictor (eg, lidocaine 1% with phenylephrine) is often helpful as the irritation from the cauterization will commonly cause sneezing and restart the bleeding. Gentle suctioning using a size 7 French Frazier suction can be used to clear out any bleeding or clots for enhanced visualization. Chemical cauterization using silver nitrate sticks can be performed in small unilateral bleeding from the anterior septum. The nasal septum should never be cauterized on both sides given that it can potentially result in septal perforation. If chemical cauterization is used, the patient must be given a saline nasal spray (3-4 puffs each nostril QID) to use and an over the counter lubricant gel (eg, Aquaphor® or Hydrophor® ointments) to be applied after spraying to allow the septum to stay moist. The saline spray should be used for the duration of a dry season (summer in the warm climates, winter in the cold climates). Electrocautery has been used in a surgical setting under endoscopic guidance, but is not recommended in a primary care setting given the increased chance of septal perforation.

Nasal Packing

In cases of brisk bleeding, temporary control can be attained by using devices such as a Rapid Rhino® (Applied Therapeutics, Tampla, Fla) or Merocel® nasal packs (Medtronic ENT, Jacksonville, Fla). Rapid Rhino® is an inflatable balloon device coated with a platelet aggregator (carboxymethylcellulose hydrocolloid) that is placed in the nares and consequently inflated with air to tamponade the bleeding. Merocel® nasal packs, composed of hydroxylate polyvinyl acetate material, acts as a tampon that expands when wet and has similar efficacy to traditional nasal packing. Topical decongestion and anesthesia of the nose with topical lidocaine 1% and oxymetazoline (3 drops of each per side) after removal of clots will help facilitate the placement of a nasal packing. The nasal tampon (8 cm in adult, 4 cm in child) should be lubricated at the tip with an ointment and placed along the floor of the nasal cavity (Fig 12-1) with gentle pressure until the entire packing is in the nose. Ideally, the nasal tampon should be inflated with 5 to 10 drops of oxymetazoline, penylephrine, or neosynephrine nasal drops/sprays

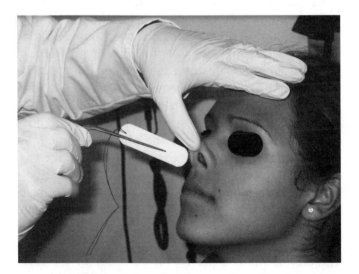

Fig 12–1. The direction in which a nasal packing should be placed. The tip of the nose should be raised with the thumb and the packing should be placed parallel and onto the floor of the nose.

after it is placed. If these medications are not available, saline may be used. The nasal packing causes increased mucous production in the nose and will cause some blood-tinged oozing. The patient should be instructed that the blood tinged oozing is normal. A constant dripping of dark blood after packing requires an otolaryngology evaluation. The nasal packing should be kept in place for 5 to 7 days and removed.

Sometimes, when a nasal tampon is not available or when a nasal tampon has failed, a traditional anterior nasal packing using antibiotic ointment-coated ribbon gauze in a systemic and stepwise fashion anteriorly in the nasal cavity to tamponade the bleeding source can be performed. The ribbon gauze is placed with a bayonette forceps and each subsequent layer is compressed onto the previous layers. The senior author (HRD) has found that formal packing is very rarely necessary as over 95% of bleeding can be controlled with nasal tampon sponges alone. If a single tampon does not control the bleeding, a second sponge can be placed on the opposite side for counter pressure. In case of failure of the two tampons, a third can be placed on the side of the bleeding. If a second packing is going to be placed on the same side, the first one should be held with a clamp so the second one does not push the first one into the pharynx. Sometimes the first packing may need to be removed and the two tampons can be placed together on the same side.

Posterior nasal packing typically consists of placing balloon devices (eg, Rapid Rhino® or Foley urethral catheters) into the posterior nasopharynx with subsequent inflation and traction. The 10 or 14 Fr Foley catheter should be placed on the floor of the nose until the tip can be seen in the pharynx. The balloon should then be inflated with 10 cc of saline and the catheter should be pulled so the balloon wedges in the posterior nasopharynx. There is significant pain associated with this maneuver. Premedication with opiates (eg, morphine) may be indicated. For Rapid Rhino® balloon device, the posterior balloon should be inflated with 10 cc and the anterior balloon should be inflated with 15 to 20 cc of saline. This is generally quite painful for the patient. A Kelley or umbilical clamp can be used to prevent the catheter from falling back into the pharynx. The clamp should be heavily padded to prevent pressure necrosis of the tip of the nose. A patient with a posterior packing should be admitted to the hospital on a monitored bed given that posterior nasal packing increases the chance of apnea or arrhythmias.

All patients with nasal packing should be treated with an anti-*Staph aureus* antibiotic while the packing is in place to prevent *S. aureus*-induced toxic shock syndrome (eg, cephalexin 500 mg po TID [children 25 mg/kg/d divided BID or TID]; penicillin allergic, clindamycin 150 mg po QID [children, 10 mg/kg/d divided Q 8hrs]). Surgical ligation or angiographic embolization is used at the discretion of the otolaryngologist when traditional packing has failed.

When to Refer

Most cases of epistaxis are self-limited and do not require a referral to an otolaryngologist. However, the following circumstances represent appropriate indications for a referral or visit to the emergency department:

- Inability to control nasal bleeding in a primary care setting
- Massive nasal bleeding associated with hypotension
- Recurrent nasal bleeds of unknown origin
- Suspected posterior nose bleed

- Bleeding associated with nasal obstruction (especially unilateral) or suspected tumor
- In general, attempts should be made using a Foley catheter for posterior bleeds or a nasal tampon for an anterior bleed before the unstable patient is transferred to an emergency department.

Referrals to an otolaryngologist is needed in cases of recurrent epistaxis or those in recurrent epistaxis, epistaxis in a peripubertal male (to rule out a juvenile nasopharyngeal angiofibroma), heavy smoker (to rule out sinonasal carcinoma), patient with a history of woodworking (increased risk of sinunasal malignancies), Asian patient (high risk of nasopharyngeal carcinoma) or those with a mass, severe septal deviation, or septal perforation seen on examination.

CHAPTER 13

Nasal Discharge

PAUL SCHALCH
QUOC A. NGUYEN
HAMID R. DJALILIAN

PAUL SCHALCH
QUOC A. NGUYEN
HAMID R. DJALILIAN

BACKGROUND

Nasal discharge, like nasal obstruction, is a very common presenting symptom in children and adults, and usually goes hand in hand with nasal obstruction and other symptoms such as sneezing. There are, however, special considerations that need to be taken into account, in order to not miss potentially life-threatening conditions that might present as innocently as a common cold. The very fact that the patient is seeking medical attention should alert the clinician that the nasal discharge may be indeed more than just a common cold. Figure 13–1 outlines the most common causes of nasal discharge.

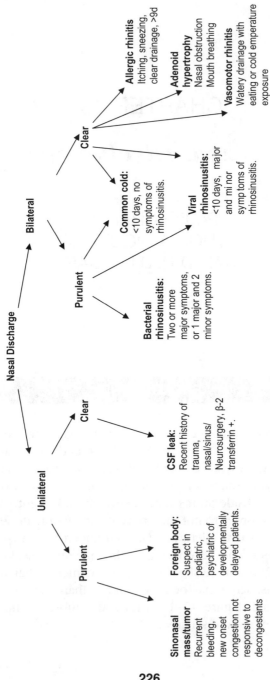

Fig 13–1. The most common causes of nasal drainage.

Nasal Discharge

Unilateral

- Purulent
  - **Sinonasal mass/tumor** Recurrent bleeding, new onset congestion not responsive to decongestants
  - **Foreign body:** Suspect in pediatric, psychiatric of developmentally delayed patients.
- Clear
  - **CSF leak:** Recent history of trauma, nasal/sinus/ Neurosurgery, β-2 transferrin +.

Bilateral

- Purulent
  - **Bacterial rhinosinusitis:** Two or more major symptoms, or 1 major and 2 minor symptoms.
  - **Viral rhinosinusitis:** <10 days, major and minor symptoms of rhinosinusitis.
- Clear
  - **Common cold:** <10 days, no symptoms of rhinosinusitis.
  - **Allergic rhinitis** Itching, sneezing, clear drainage, >9d
  - **Adenoid hypertrophy** Nasal obstruction Mouth breathing
  - **Vasomotor rhinitis** Watery drainage with eating or cold emperature exposure

EVALUATION

A careful history will help determine the nature and possible causes for nasal discharge. The elements of the history for nasal discharge are:

1. Onset.
2. Duration.
3. Constant versus intermittent.
4. Laterality
5. Triggers
6. Ameliorating and worsening factors (bending over, straining)
7. Use of medications (topical and systemic), drugs (cocaine) and tobacco
8. Previous surgery, and in particular, head trauma
9. Concurrent allergies or allergy-related conditions (asthma, conjunctivitis, eczema)
10. Nature of discharge
11. Presence of blood in the discharge, or frank epistaxis
12. Associated symptoms (loss of smell, otalgia, clogged or "popping" ears, chronic cough, headaches, vision problems, epiphora, fever, etc)
13. Associated conditions (pregnancy, rheumatologic disease, diabetes, gastroesophageal reflux, cystic fibrosis, syndromes, and congenital malformations)
14. Exposure to irritants, smoke, solvents, and so forth.

In general, rhinorrhea can be divided in purulent and nonpurulent and uni- vs. bilateral, and the diagnosis can be narrowed down once additional information is obtained, like triggering factors, history of trauma or surgery, and duration.

PURULENT RHINORRHEA, BILATERAL

Bacterial or Viral Rhinosinusitis

In general, whenever there is purulence (yellow or green discharge), bacterial infection should be suspected. Duration of purulent rhinorrhea will allow the clinician to distinguish between a common cold (or coryza), viral rhinosinusitis, or bacterial rhinosinusitis. The common cold and viral rhinosinusitis are usually self-limited and rarely last longer than 9 days, whereas bacterial rhinosinusitis might last longer if left untreated. A characteristic setting for sinusitis is when a patient reports a history of an upper respiratory infection (URI), with worsening of symptoms after 5 to 7 days. During the URI, the patient may describe yellow or green nasal discharge in the early morning, followed by clear or white nasal discharge during the day. Sinusitis is heralded by purulent nasal discharge during the whole day. Acute bacterial rhinosinusitis usually is caused by *Streptococcus pneumoniae*, *Haemophilus influenzae*, or *Moraxella catarrhalis*.

Symptoms and Signs

The usual presentation of the common cold may include persistent rhinorrhea, nasal congestion, sneezing, postnasal drip, cough, fever, watery eyes, and eustachian tube dysfunction (clogged ear sensation, inability to "pop" the ears). This clinical picture is usually self-limited and rarely lasts longer than 9 days (most commonly 7 days).

The symptoms for the definitive diagnosis of bacterial rhinosinusitis are divided into major and minor. The presence of two or more major symptoms or one major and two minor symptoms make the diagnosis or rhinosinusitis. Major symptoms include facial pain and/or pressure, facial congestion and/or fullness, nasal obstruction, nasal discharge/purulence/postnasal discharge, hyposmia/anosmia, and fever. Minor symptoms include headache, fever, halitosis, fatigue, dental pain, cough, and ear pain/pressure and/or fullness. Acute infection is defined as lasting less than 4 weeks. Viral rhinosinusitis rarely will last longer than 9 days, and it will not present with purulent (yellow or green) discharge. Examination will reveal discolored discharge in the nose, facial pain on percussion of the sinuses, or tenderness in the upper molar teeth.

Diagnosis and What Tests to Order

The common cold and acute rhinosinusitis, whether viral or bacterial, are clinical diagnoses. Bacterial rhinosinusitis is diagnosed based on the above stated criteria.

Bacterial culture of the purulence is rarely necessary and is not always accurate. Given the nasal vestibule and the vestibular hair harbor bacteria (often *Staph aureus*), the culture may grow bacteria from the vestibule. In cases of chronic bacterial rhinosinusitis (four or more episodes per year), cultures can be obtained. The best way to obtain cultures, though, is under endoscopic guidance with calcium alginate (Calgi Swabs®) swabs.

Computer tomography (CT) of the sinuses (coronal cuts without contrast) should be reserved for cases that do not respond to treatment and that present with symptoms lasting longer than 4 weeks. Ideally, CT should be obtained during asymptomatic periods and after completing a 2- to 3-week course of nasal steroid (fluticasone or mometasone 2 puffs QD each nostril) and antibiotic treatment (eg, levofloxacin 500 mg po QD, or amoxicillin clavulanate 875 mg po BID; in children, amoxicillin clavulanate ES 90 mg/kg/day divided BID × 14 days, or azithromycin 10mg/kg for 5 days). The purpose of CT imaging is not to confirm the diagnosis, but to evaluate potential anatomic problems or masses causing obstruction of the sinus outflow tracts, which may require surgical intervention.

Treatment and When to Refer

Treatment for the common cold and acute viral rhinosinusitis is symptomatic (pain medication, antipyretics) and topical nasal decongestants (eg, oxymetazoline 3 puffs BID bilateral nostrils × 5-7 days, children 1 to 2 puffs each side) as well as systemic decongestants (pseudoephedrine 60 mg po QID × 5-7 days, in children 15 mg po QID age 2-6, 30 mg po QID in age 6-12, adult dose for 12 and above). Sympathomimetic sprays such as oxymetazoline or neosynephrine should not be used for periods longer than 5 to 7 consecutive days because they may cause rebound congestion and worsening of symptoms after that point. Systemic decongestants should not be used in patients with hypertension. In addition to decongestion for viral URIs, treatment for the postnasal drainage must be given. In adults, it is beneficial to give the systemic pseudoephedrine in combination with an antihistamine (eg, loratadine/pseudoephedrine 10 mg/240 mg or desloratadine/psueudoephdrine 5 mg/240 mg QAM). In children above 12, the (des)loratadine/pseudoephedrine combination can be given, in children older than 6, loratadine 10 mg po QAM, and in children 2 to 6, loratadine 5 mg QAM can be given. Desloratadine can be given to children age 6 to 11 months (1 mg po QD), ages 1-5 years, 1.25 mg po QAM, and ages 6-11, 2.5 mg po QAM. Other treatments such as saline spray (3-4 puffs each side QID) can be used to attempt relief of persistent rhinorrhea and congestion. Alternatively, topical antihistamines (azelastine or olopatadine 2 puffs TID for 7 days) or anticholinergics such as ipratropium bromide 0.06% (2 puffs TID for 7 days) can be used for symptomatic relief. Doses are the same for both children and adults.

For treatment of bacterial sinusitis, according to the Sinus and Allergy Health Partnership, the recommendations for adult patients with mild disease who have not received antibiotics in the previous 4 to 6 weeks include: amoxicillin/clavulanate (1.75 to 4 g/250 mg/day), amoxicillin (1.5–4 g/day), cefpodoxime, cefuroxime, or cefdinir. For patients with β-lactam allergies, trimethroprim/sulfamethoxazole (TMP/SMX), doxycycline, azithromycin, clarithromycin, or erythromycin may be considered. Failure to respond to antimicrobial therapy within 72 hours should lead to either a switch to alternate antimicrobial therapy or the reevaluation of the patient. Initial therapy for previously treated adults, or with more severe disease includes a fluoroquinolone (levofloxacin 500 mg po QD for 10 days or 750 mg po QD for 5 days; or moxifloxacin 400 mg po QD × 10 days) or high dose amoxicillin/clavulanate (Augmentin XR® 2 cg/125 mg BID) for 10 days.

Initial therapy for children with mild disease who have not been previously treated includes 10 days of high dose amoxicillin/clavulanate (90 mg/6.4 mg/kg/day divided BID), amoxicillin (90 mg/kg/day divided TID), cefpodoxime (10 mg/kg/day divided BID), cefuroxime (30 mg/kg/day divided BID), or cefdinir (14 mg/kg/day divided QD or BID). The recommended initial therapy for children with more severe disease or those that have been previously treated (during the preceding 4–6 weeks) includes high-dose amoxicillin/clavulanate (90 mg/6.4 mg/kg/day). Cefpodoxime, cefuroxime or cefdinir may be considered initially for patients with penicillin intolerance (non-type-I hypersensitivity reactions (eg, rash). TMP/SMX, azithromycin, clarithromycin, or erythromycin may be used if the patient is β-lactam allergic, but they do not provide optimal coverage. Fluoroquinolones generally provide good control of bacterial rhinosinusitis and is received as second line therapy. Another consideration, particularly in patients with recurrent disease, is to consider the contribution of laryngopharyngeal reflux to the persistent inflammatory state and treatment with proton pump inhibitors.

A patient with bacterial rhinosinusitis that is chronic in nature (lasting longer than 12 weeks), recurrent rhinosinusitis (>3 times a year), those with polyps or a mass on examination, or patients presenting with other findings on CT scan such as fungal infection should be referred to an otolaryngologist for further evaluation. The presence of any complications of sinusitis, such as orbital abscess, intracranial extension, mucoceles, and in particular invasive fungal sinusitis (in immuno-compromised patients, including diabetics) should generate a prompt referral for immediate surgical treatment by the specialist.

Purulent Rhinorrhea Unilateral

Although acute bacterial rhinosinusitis could affect only one side of the patient's nose, other possible diagnoses should be ruled out before considering this diagnostic possibility. Unilateral purulent rhinorrhea combined with nasal obstruction in a child (or a developmentally delayed or psychiatric patient) should raise the suspicion of a nasal foreign body or unilateral choanal atresia. Foreign bodies can be biological in nature (beans, peanuts, popcorn), inert (plastic beads, bee bees, coins) but can also have corrosive chemicals (eg, watch batteries) that can cause severe damage to the nose in the form of scarring and septal perforation, which has significant consequences both in the short and long term.

In adults and children, unilateral purulent rhinorrhea also can herald the presence of a mass (benign or malignant) obstructing the nasal cavity, sinus drainage, or the nasopharynx on the affected side.

Symptoms and Signs

Unilateral, purulent, and occasionally foul-smelling rhinorrhea of several days' onset is characteristic of nasal foreign bodies in children. Of course, foreign bodies can be bilateral, but much less frequently. Patient might otherwise be asymptomatic. The presence of nasal pain, bloody discharge or frank epistaxis are of concern, particularly if the foreign body is thought to be an alkaline battery, like those found on watches, remote controls, or other electronic devices.

Rhinorrhea associated with unilateral nasal obstruction secondary to a tumor typically will be present over a longer period of time, and it may be purulent or bloody in nature. It may be accompanied by other symptoms suggestive of invasion or local destruction, such as epiphora, proptosis, change in facial appearance (unilateral prominence of maxilla), or cranial nerve deficits. Anterior rhinoscopy should be performed in all cases, ideally after decongesting the nasal cavities and suctioning the drainage. Foreign bodies or tumors may or may not be visible on anterior rhinoscopy. Nasal endoscopy is crucial in ruling out the presence of more posteriorly lodged foreign bodies, multiple foreign bodies, or tumors located as far back as the nasopharynx. Sensation of the face should be checked to evaluate sensation of cranial nerve V2 to ensure there is no potential tumor involvement. In a cooperative child, or a neonate, a small (7 French) suction catheter can be used to pass through each nostril to ensure that the choana are open on both sides.

Diagnosis and What Tests to Order

The diagnosis is by visualizing the foreign body. Plain x-rays, if readily available and if there is no capability to perform nasal endoscopy, should be obtained to rule out a metallic foreign body. If a foreign body is suspected, though, referral to an otolaryngologist is warranted. The diagnosis of a unilateral choanal atresia requires passing a 7 French suction catheter or an axial CT scan of the sinuses.

Imaging studies, such as CT or magnetic resonance imaging (MRI) with contrast should be obtained when a tumor is identified on nasal endoscopy or when one is suspected on clinical grounds (history of woodworking and other occupationl exposures to solvents or irritants, decreased V2 sensation, maxillary teeth falling out, or bulging of the maxilla).

Biopsy of a nasal mass should not be performed in a primary care setting given the possibility of a vascular mass, or one that is connected to the sub-arachnoid space.

Treatment and When to Refer

Retrieval of a nasal foreign body can be attempted in the office if the right instruments and equipment are present (including suction and a light source), the foreign body is readily visible, and the patient is reasonably cooperative or easily restrained. Multiple unsuccessful attempts can cause significant inflammation, which might make further attempts for removal even harder, and cause significant epistaxis or injury to the patient. Hard to remove nasal foreign bodies should be performed under endoscopic visualization in the operating room, under sedation or general anesthesia.

The patient should be referred to an otolaryngologist if the foreign body cannot be removed safely, or if there is suspicion for the foreign body to be a battery or some other corrosive foreign body, should prompt immediate referral to an otolaryngology specialist in order to minimize damage to the nose.

The presence of any mass suspected of being locally destructive or malignant should also generate a referral to an otolaryngologist for further workup and treatment. For a more detailed description of nasal masses and their implications, please refer to Chapter 11 on Nasal Obstruction.

Clear Rhinorrhea, Bilateral

Bilateral clear rhinorrhea can be approached in a similar fashion as bilateral purulent rhinorrhea, ruling out common causes first. Depending on the associated symptoms, bilateral clear rhinorrhea can also be caused by allergic rhinitis or a viral URI. The duration of this symptom determines the need for further diagnostic workup, including therapeutic trials.

Bilateral clear rhinorrhea can also be subdivided depending on the age of the patient. Aside from a possible allergic etiology, bilateral clear rhinorrhea in the pediatric population can be caused by adenoid hypertrophy. The adenoid pad, along with the palatine and lingual tonsils, is part of the lymphatic tissue in the upper aerodigestive tract. It is located in the nasopharynx and is most prominent between the ages of 2 and

5 years. In normal circumstances, it does not cause significant nasal obstruction, and it involutes progressively as the dimensions of the nasopharynx increase in size and as the child grows older. Children with significant hypertrophy of the adenoids have persistent nasal obstruction, which occasionally is accompanied with rhinorrhea (clear, unless the patient has a concurrent sinusitis, in which case it may turn purulent).

Bilateral clear rhinorrhea can also be caused by allergic rhinitis. Allergic rhinitis can present both with nasal obstruction, as well as clear rhinorrhea and sneezing. Associated symptoms can include itchy, watery eyes, irritative cough (due to postnasal drip) and even asthma. Clear rhinorrhea associated with allergies would have a more protracted course (longer than 9 days), and may be associated with specific environmental triggers.

In adults, aside from allergic rhinitis, clear rhinorrhea may be associated with either nonallergic rhinitis with eosinophilia (discussed in Chapter 11 on Nasal Obstruction) or vasomotor rhinitis, secondary to exposure to irritant fumes, solvents, exercise, cold temperatures, foods, hormonal changes and even emotional factors (discussed below).

Symptoms and Signs

Patients generally report persistent clear rhinorrhea, with or without any other symptoms of upper respiratory infection. Patients with a likely allergic cause report worsening of symptoms during certain seasons or as a result of certain exposures. Patients with perennial, nonallergic rhinitis might not report any particular inciting factors. Patients with vasomotor rhinitis most commonly will report clear watery discharge that occurs after eating or exposure to cold temperatures.

Patients with nasal obstruction and rhinorrhea secondary to adenoid hypertrophy will exhibit a so-called adenoid facies (Fig 11-3 in Chapter 11), which consists of an elongated midface, persistent open mouth breathing, high arched palate, and long incisors, with an overbite on occasion. This is a result of persistent mouth breathing that keeps the maxillary teeth away from the mandibular teeth, thus impairing the normal mechanism of growth regulation of the midface. Patients' parents may report significant snoring and restless sleep due to the persistent nasal obstruction.

Diagnosis and What Tests to Order

The diagnosis depends on the history. If adenoid hypertrophy is suspected, a lateral neck x-ray may be obtained with the head in neutral position, which allows for evaluation of the size of the adenoid pad and the degree of obstruction. If nasal endoscopy is available, the nasopharynx can be directly examined and the size of the adenoid pad documented.

Treatment and When to Refer

Treatment of allergic rhinitis is best done using topical nasal steroid sprays, topical antihistamines, or oral antihistamines. Topical nasal sprays (eg, fluticasone or mometasone) should be used 2 puffs each nostril qd [children 2-11 yo, 1 puff each nostril qd]. Fluticasone furoate is approved for ages 2 years and above, whereas fluticasone propionate is approved for ages 4 and above. Topical antihistamines (olopatadine [Patanase®] or azelastine) should be used as 2 puffs each nostril BID (patients 12 years of age and above). The patient should be instructed to spray the lateral wall of the nose and not the nasal septum. Spraying the septum is less effective. In the case of nasal steroids, spraying the septum will lead to a higher chance of epistaxis and rarely, septal perforation. Topical antihistamine, and oral antihistamines are useful when patients also suffer from other symptoms such as pruritus in the eyes or skin. The less-sedating or non-sedating oral antihistamines in order of efficacy are levocetirizine (Xyzal®) 5 mg po qd [children 6 to 11, 2.5 mg po qd], cetirizine 5–10 mg qd [children 1 to 5 yo, 2.5 mg po qd]; fexofenadine 180 mg po qd [children 2-11 yo, 30 mg po qd; children 1–2 yo; 15 mg po bid]; loratadine 10 mg po qd [children 2–5 yo, 5 mg po qd]. Cetirizine is not classified as a nonsedating oral antihistamine. Sedating oral antihistamines (eg, diphenhydramine, dimenhydrinate) are generally more effective than their nonsedating counterparts, but their duration of efficacy is shorter and due to their sedating side effects they are not used commonly. Montelukast (10 mg po QD; for children less than 15 years old, 5 mg po QD) can also be used in patients with as an adjunctive therapy or as monotherapy especially in patients with asthma and allergic rhinitis. Ocular symptoms can be treated with olopatadine one gtt BID each eye (patients aged 3 years or older).

Environmental control and avoidance of exposure to allergens is always useful in controlling symptoms and decreasing the requirements of both topical and oral medications. Simple measures such as not allowing pets (especially cats) in the bedroom, closing the bedroom windows, HEPA filters, and using mattress covers and hypoallergenic linen may, in fact, be quite effective.

The patient should be referred to an otolaryngologist if an adequate trial of nasal steroid spray and antihistamines fails to control the patient's symptoms.

More specialized immunotherapy should be reserved for severe cases that do not respond to environmental control and topical and oral medications. Patients with asthma and allergic rhinitis will require a referral to an allergist.

Adenoid hypertrophy can be managed expectantly; however, if the nasal obstruction is causing sleep apnea or other problems such as malocclusion, or deformation of the midface due to persistent mouth breathing, surgical removal of the adenoid pad is indicated.

Patients with significant adenoid hypertrophy should be referred to an otolaryngologist for adenoidectomy. Persistent rhinorrhea, not responsive to medical treatment, in the setting of allergies should prompt a referral to an otolaryngologist or allergist for formal allergy testing and initiation of immunotherapy.

Vasomotor Rhinitis

Vasomotor rhinitis is a condition characterized by clear watery bilateral nasal drainage that occurs after certain triggers. The triggers are most commonly eating, change in temperature (most commonly cold), chemical irritants (eg, smoke, pollution, perfumes), psychological stress, and even spicy foods. The rhinitis is mediated by the autonomic nervous system, which leads to the sudden start of the clear watery drainage.

Symptoms and Signs

Patients generally will complain of profuse watery nasal discharge, which on questioning will be related to certain triggers. Examination between symptoms may be normal, but the patients may have enlarged inferior turbinates on examination.

Diagnosis and What Tests to Order

The diagnosis is by history and generally no tests have to be ordered.

Treatment and When to Refer

The best treatment for vasomotor rhinitis is with ipratropium nasal sprays 0.03%, 2 puffs TID PRN bilateral nostrils. The patient should be referred to an otolaryngologist if the nasal spray is not effective or if the watery drainage is unilateral. Also, if the patient has severe nasal obstruction that does not respond to topical steroid therapy, the patient should be referred to an otolaryngologist.

Wegener's Granulomatosis

Wegener's granulomatosis is a chronic systemic disease characterized by necrotizing granulomatous vasculitis that mainly involves the small arteries and veins. Otolaryngology symptoms are presenting signs in 92% of patients.

Signs and Symptoms

The patient on the average will present at age 40. The most common symptoms are nasal obstruction, nasal drainage, sinus pain, epistaxis, hoarseness, serous otitis media, and hearing loss. Laryngeal involvement can cause hoarseness and airway obstruction symptoms. Given these symptoms are nonspecific, the diagnosis can be delayed until systemic symptoms present. Systemic symptoms include fever, malaise, night sweats, weight loss, and arthralgias. Wegener's can also involve the lungs and kidneys.

On examination the septal mucosa may be thickened or perforated. The patient may occasionally present with loss of the cartilage in the septum and a so called saddle nose deformity. The patient may have serous otitis media and hearing loss. Oral ulcers and bilateral parotid swelling may also be present.

Diagnosis and What Tests to Order

The diagnosis is made clinically and confirmed with histopathology of a nasal biopsy specimen. cANCA is a peripheral blood test that can aid in diagnosis. Its sensitivity is 66% (range: 57% to 74%), and its specificity is 98% (range: 96% to 99.5%). A screening ESR (sedimentation rate) can be a cost-effective test to obtain if suspicion is low.

Treatment and When to Refer

Treatment of Wegener's is with systemic immune suppressive agents. Wegener's isolated to the nose can be treated with nasal steroids alone. The patient should be referred to an otolaryngologist for tissue biopsy. Upon confirmation of the diagnosis, the patient will need a pulmonary and renal workup with appropriate referral.

Sarcoidosis

Sarcoidosis is an idiopathic systemic disease characterized by multisystem involvement. Sarcoidosis can uncommonly present with nasal obstruction, postnasal drainage, headache, and recurrent sinusitis. Sarcoidosis is generally very low on the differential diagnosis for patients with sinonasal complaints, but should be considered when these symptoms present in conjunction with dry mouth, dry eyes, previous facial paralysis (occasionally bilateral), or parotid gland enlargement.

On examination, the nasal mucosa can be friable with crusting and easy bleeding. Significant thickening of the nasal septum caused by granulomatous infiltration with yellowish, nodular-appearing lesions on the septum are suggestive of sarcoidosis. Crusting, and chronic low-grade local infection can ensue with secondary bacterial infection.

Diagnosis and What Tests to Order

Sinonasal sarcoidosis is established only after biopsy of granulation tissue and histopathologic examination. In most patients, the history of other areas of involvement may aid in diagnosis. A chest x-ray, serum calcium, angiotensin converting enzyme (ACE) level, and other tests will be required for further evaluation and confirmation of the diagnosis. A systemic workup will need to be pursued after diagnosis.

Treatment and When to Refer

The patient should be referred to an otolaryngologist for biopsy and nasal endoscopy. Saline irrigation of the nose (15 cc each nostril BID) should be performed in all patient with sinonasal involvement. Topical steroid nasal sprays (eg, fluticasone or mometasone 2 puffs each nostril BID) will help with the local inflammation. Treatment of isolated nasal septal sarcoid can include intralesional steroid injection. The patient should be referred to a rhinologist or an otolaryngologist for evaluation. Systemic disease will require oral immune suppressive agents and referral to other specialists. A pulmonary referral for bronchoscopy and broncho-alveolar lavage may be required.

CLEAR RHINORRHEA, UNILATERAL

Cerebrospinal Fluid Leakage

Clear, unilateral rhinorrhea, particularly in the setting of recent head trauma or nasal surgery, should alert the clinician to the possibility of cerebrospinal fluid (CSF) leakage. There are also spontaneous cerebrospinal fluid (CSF) leaks, which tend not to resolve spontaneously, as opposed to surgical or traumatic CSF leaks, which most of the time stop after 7 to 10 days. The watery rhinorrhea from CSF leaks can be profuse and tends to worsen when intracranial pressure is increased (coughing, sneezing, straining, and leaning forward).

Signs and Symptoms

A thorough history should be obtained documenting recent head/facial trauma and any nasal procedures, including septoplasty and endoscopic sinus surgery. Signs of facial and head trauma, such as periorbital ecchymoses, bruising over the mastoid tips (Battle's sign), nose fractures, hemotympanum, or bloody otorrhea may be seen. Patients might report headaches, most commonly occipital. Fever, malaise, and neck stiffness may herald meningitis, and should be documented. Patients may report clear rhinorrhea when bending over or may complain of a salty taste in the pharynx. Obesity is a risk factor for spontaneous CSF leakage, given higher CSF pressures in obese patients.

Diagnosis and What Tests to Order

Diagnosis is made by detecting β-2 transferrin, a protein highly specific for CSF, in the nasal drainage. Patients may be instructed to save the fluid in a plastic cup (eg, urine sample cup) and bring it to the office the same day to be sent to the lab for analysis. Usually 0.5 to 1 cc suffice for analysis.

Detection of glucose in the fluid with a glucose oxidase paper or the halo or target sign (a drop of clear sanguinous discharge is placed on filter paper, the blood is separated from the CSF, creating a dark dot in the center, surrounded by a clear halo of CSF) are fraught with errors. Both mucous and lacrimal gland secretions can contain glucose and can create the halo sign.

If the β-2 transferrin is positive, a high-resolution coronal CT through the skull base might diagnose the site of injury or dehiscence responsible for the CSF leak. T2-weighted MRI is another useful modality that may help in localizing the leak, although it does not define the bony anatomy. Alternatively, specialized, intrathecally administered contrast materials such as iohexol (Omnipaque™) might be used to localize the exact site of leakage. These interventions, however, usually are performed in preparation for surgical correction of CSF leaks, and usually should not be performed as a first-line diagnostic intervention.

β-2 transferrin-negative unilateral nasal discharge could represent stagnant irrigation fluid in patients with a history of prior sinus surgery or patients who use buffered saline irrigation regularly (eg, patients with chronic sinusitis). Vasomotor rhinitis can rarely cause unilateral drainage if there is severe nasal obstruction or septal deviation.

Treatment and When to Refer

If the patient has a history of a nasal trauma or surgery, then she or he should be urgently referred to an otolaryngologist for evaluation to rule out a CSF leakage. The patient can be tried on a short course of ipratropium nasal sprays 0.06%, 2 puffs TID bilateral nostrils for 1 week. If the rhinorrhea continues, the patient should be referred to an otolaryngologist for evaluation.

FURTHER READING

Anon J, Jacobs M, Poole M, Ambrose PG, Benninger MS, Hadley JA, et al. Antimicrobial treatment guidelines for acute bacterial rhinosinusitis. *Otolaryngol Head Neck Surg.* 2004;30:1–45.

Hoffman GS, Kerr GS, Leavitt RY, Hallahan CW, Lebovics RS, Travis WD, et al. Wegener granulomatosis: an analysis of 158 patients. *Ann Int Med.* 1992;116:488–498.

Lanza D, Kennedy D. Adult rhinosinusitis defined. *Otolaryngol Head Neck Surg.* 1997;117: S1–S7.

Rosenfeld R, Andes D, Bhattacharyya N, Cheung D, Eisenberg S, Ganiats TG, et al. Clinical practice guideline: adult sinusitis. *Otolaryngol Head Neck Surg.* 2007;137:S1–S31.

Vartiainen E, Nuutinen J. (1992). Head and neck manifestations of Wegener's granulomatosis. *Ear Nose Throat J.* 1992;71:423–424,427–428.

CHAPTER 14

Other Nasal and Sinus Conditions

HAMID R. DJALILIAN

DISORDERS OF SMELL

Disorders of smell can be categorized into: anosmia, the inability to smell; hyposmia, a decreased ability to smell; dysosmia, a distorted sense of smell; parosmia, an altered smell in the presence of another odor (usually unpleasant); phantosmia, perception of smell in the absence of an odor; and agnosia, inability to identify odors in the presence of the ability to detect them.

Anosmia or hyposmia are caused either by the failure of the odor to reach the olfactory neuroepithelium or from a dysfunction in the olfactory cells. The disruption in the ability of the odorant from reaching the olfactory areas of the nose are most commonly associated with acute or chronic nasal or sinus disease or nasal masses. These include upper respiratory infections, sinusitis, nasal polyposis, or various tumors of the nasal cavity. Destruction of the olfactory neuroepithelium can be caused by trauma, postviral inflammation (especially influenza virus), anterior cranial fossa surgery or tumors, or after using over-the-counter zinc nasal sprays.

Phantosmia, parosmia, and agnosia are associated with central nervous system disorders. They could be a sign of focal seizure activity, temporal lobe tumors, or as a consequence of previous nasal or intracranial surgery. History taking in the patient with smell disorders should investigate the underlying cause and associated disorders. Physical examination should concentrate on the nose

A simple test to distinguish malingerers from true anosmics is to ask the patient to smell a small vial of ammonia. If the patient states that she or he is unable to smell the ammonia, then the patient is most likely a malingerer. The stimulation from ammonia is transmitted to the brain via the trigeminal nerve and not the olfactory nerve. Patients who have true anosmia will sense the irritation/smell caused by ammonia.

Anosmia/Hyposmia

Inflammation in the nasal cavity is most often the cause of smell disorders. These processes include allergic, infectious, or vasomotor rhinitis. Long-term use of over-the-counter nasal decongestants causes rhinitis medicamentosa which leads to nasal congestions (see Chapter 11). Chronic sinus disease over time can lead to mucosal changes that can cause lowered smell sensation even after medical and surgical management.

The most common masses that cause blockage of the nose, and thus anosmia, are nasal polyps, inverting papilloma, tumors of the nasal cavity, and mass lesions of the anterior skull base such as encephaloceles, gliomas, or dermoid cysts. Finally, a lack of airflow through the nose because of a tracheotomy or laryngectomy will cause hyposmia or anosmia.

Some endocrine abnormalities, including hypothyroidism, hypoadrenalism, and diabetes mellitus, are associated with olfactory disturbances. Systemic conditions causing central dysfunction in olfactions include viral infections (most commonly influenza virus, which can damage the olfactory epithelium), Wegener's granulomatosis, sarcoidosis, as well as multiple sclerosis.

Other central causes include the natural aging process in addition to neurodegenerative disorders such as Alzheimer and Parkinson's disease, which all cause loss of olfactory cells. Any head trauma or intracranial hemorrhage can cause shearing or damage to the olfactory neuroepithelium. Uncommon central conditions include Kallman syndrome, which is an X-linked disorder with hypogonadotropic hypogonadism and anosmia due to an absence of olfactory bulbs.

What Tests to Order

All patients with a nasal mass must undergo a coronal CT scan of the sinuses with contrast. Orbital or dural involvement of a nasal mass (if discovered) is best evaluated with an MRI of the sinuses with gadolinium. Imaging studies are best done after nasal endoscopy by an otolaryngologist.

Patients suspected of having temporal lobe seizures should undergo an EEG. Patients suspected of having systemic endocrine disorders should have thyroid and adrenal function testing as well as blood glucose testing.

Treatment

Treatment of anosmia is dependent on the underlying cause. Allergic rhinitis is best treated with a combination of nasal steroid sprays (e.g., fluticasone 2 puffs each nostril qd for adults, 1 puff qd for children >4 yrs of age) and saline nasal sprays (3–4 puffs each nostril tid). Mometasone, 1 puff each nostril qd, can be used in the pediatric patient as young as 2 years of age. The patient/parent should be instructed to direct nasal sprays to the lateral wall of the nose (point the tip toward the lateral canthus of the eye on each side). Antihistamines or anti leukotrienes can be given for patients with more systemic symptoms. Decongestants are helpful when nasal steroids fail to relieve the nasal congestions, but should be avoided in patients with hypertension or cardiovascular disease.

Chronic sinusitis is treated with nasal steroid sprays and a 2-week course of antibiotics (see Chapter 13, Nasal Discharge, for more on chronic sinusitis treatment). Pediatric patients may require an adenoidectomy for chronic sinusitis management. Nasal polyps are caused by significant inflammation of the nasal mucosa and are best treated with nasal steroid sprays. If the polyps are large, surgical excision is the treatment of choice. Nasal steroid sprays are required for long-term prevention of nasal polyp recurrence. Small polyps are best treated with nasal steroid sprays.

Acute anosmia after trauma or a viral URI should be treated with a short course of oral corticosteroids (prednisone 1 mg/kg per day up to 80 mg qd for 7 days with a 7 to 8-day taper). Although there is no clinical trial to show benefit of systemic steroids, there is anecdotal evidence to support its use.

Olfactory loss from viral URIs or head trauma may recover up to 3 months postinjury. Endocrine abnormalities, for example, hypothyroidism, should be corrected if present. Counseling the patient is important so that patients utilize smoke detectors, natural gas detectors, and avoiding possible spoiled foods.

When to Refer

All patients with a nasal mass should be referred to an otolaryngologist for further evaluation. Patients who do not have resolution of their hyposmia or anosmia with medical treatment should be referred to an otolaryngologist for nasal endoscopy and for evaluation using an objective smell test such as the University of Pennsylvania Smell Identification Test (UPSIT). Dysosmia, phantosmia, parosmia, and agnosia patients should be referred to an otolaryngologist or a neurologist.

SNEEZING

Sneezing occurs when an environmental particle reaches the nasal mucosa and triggers a histamine response. Sneezing can also be triggered by stimulation of some of the branches of the trigeminal nerve such as hair removal from the face or combing of hair.

Allergic Rhinitis

Recurrent sneezing is most commonly caused by allergic rhinitis (AR). The patients' complaints may include pruritis of the nose or the eyes, postnasal drainage, or a sensation of pruritis in the nasopharynx area (caused by eustachian tube inflammation). Eustachian tube dysfunction (a feeling of plugged ears which may or may not pop intermittently) also is common in AR. Nasal examination of patients with allergic rhinitis will show inferior turbinates (lateral nasal wall), which may be swollen (boggy) and have a pale, bluishgray color and clear nasal drainage.

Treatment

Treatment of allergic rhinitis is best done using topical nasal steroid sprays, topical antihistamines, or oral antihistamines. Topical nasal sprays (eg, fluticasone or mometasone) should be used 2 puffs each nostril qd (children 2–11 yo, 1 puff each nostril qd). Fluticasone furoate is approved for ages 2 years and above, whereas fluticasone propionate is approved for ages 4 and above. Topical antihistamines (olopatadine [Patanase®] or azelastine) should be used as 2 puffs each nostril BID (patients 12 years of age and above). The patient should be instructed to spray the lateral wall of the nose and not the nasal septum. Spraying the septum is less effective. In the case of nasal steroids, spraying the septum will lead to a higher chance of epistaxis and rarely, septal perforation. Topical antihistamine, and oral antihistamines are useful when patients also suffer from other symptoms such as pruritus in the eyes or skin. The less-sedating or nonsedating oral antihistamines in order of efficacy are levocetirizine (Xyzal®) 5 mg po qd (children 6 to 11, 2.5 mg po qd), cetirizine 5–10 mg qd (children 1 to 5 yo, 2.5 mg po qd); fexofenadine 180 mg po qd (children 2–11 yo, 30 mg po qd; children 1–2 yo; 15 mg po bid); loratadine 10 mg po qd (children 2–5 yo, 5 mg po qd). Cetirizine is not classified as a non-sedating oral antihistamine. Sedating oral antihistamines (eg, diphenhydramine, dimenhydrinate) are generally more effective than their non-sedating counterparts, but their duration of efficacy is shorter and due to their sedating side effects they are not used commonly. Montelukast (10 mg po QD; for children less than 15 years old, 5 mg po QD) can also be used in patients with as an adjunctive therapy or as monotherapy especially in patients with asthma and allergic rhinitis. Ocular symptoms can be treated with olopatadine one gtt BID each eye (patients aged 3 years or older).

Environmental control and avoidance of exposure to allergens is always useful in controlling symptoms and decreasing the requirements of both topical and oral medications. Simple measures such as not allowing pets (especially cats) in the bedroom, closing the bedroom windows, HEPA filters, and using mattress covers and hypoallergenic linen may, in fact, be quite effective.

The patient should be referred to an otolaryngologist if an adequate trial of nasal steroid spray and antihistamines fails to control the patient's symptoms. More specialized immunotherapy should be reserved for severe cases that do not respond to environmental control and topical and oral medications. Patients with asthma and allergic rhinitis will require a referral to an allergist.

What Tests to Order

Allergy testing may be useful in identifying the allergen and to help with avoidance or immunotherapy. The otolaryngic allergist or general allergist may obtain in vivo or in vitro testing to help identify the most significant allergens.

When to Refer

Allergic rhinitis patients should be referred when the above described therapy is not efficacious. No referral needed for snatiation or ACHOO syndrome.

Snatiation

Snatiation is a disorder characterized by multiple sneezing that occurs after a large meal. It is thought to be an autosomal dominant trait. The term snatiation is a combination of sneeze and satiation. There is no known treatment for snatiation other than avoidance of overeating.

ACHOO Syndrome

ACHOO syndrome, Autosomal dominant Compelling Helio Ophthalmic Outburst Syndrome, is a disorder characterized by sneezing that occurs as a result of sudden exposure of a person to bright light, generally sunlight. The patient will have 2 to 3 sneezes but can be up to 40 sneezes. The syndrome is also called the photic sneeze reflex or the helio-ophthalmic outburst syndrome. The syndrome has been found to be inherited in an autosomal dominant fashion and to affect up to 23% of the population. Other than avoidance of going from a darker area into bright sunlight, there is no known treatment for ACHOO syndrome.

Vasomotor Rhinitis

See Chapter 13 on Nasal Discharge.

DRY NOSE

The mucous-producing glands in the nose and sinuses derive their stimulatory innervation from the parasympathetic branches of the facial nerve via the greater superficial petrosal nerve. Dryness in the nose will most commonly occur as anticholinergic or irritation side effect of medications. The most common medications that cause a dry nose as a side effect include antihistamines, anticholinergic topical nasal steroid sprays, or over-the-counter nasal saline sprays. In topical nasal preparations, it is often the preservative in the sprays that causes the irritation. Other causes include hot or dry climate conditions, or primary disorders of the glands such as keratoconjunctivitis sicca or Sjögren's syndrome. Interruption of the greater superficial petrosal nerve, as a result of facial paralysis, skull base fracture, or skull base surgery can also cause dryness in the nose. Occasionally, infection of the nasal vestibule (just inside the nostrils) by *Staph aureus* can cause burning and a sensation of dryness in the nose.

On examination, the nose may have some dried drainage or have an erythematous appearance to the mucosa from the irritation. Occasionally dried nasal septal mucosa or dried blood on the septum in the anterior septum (Little's area) can be seen.

Treatment

Antihistamines or nasal steroids should be reduced in dosage, changed or discontinued if their side effects are causing too much discomfort for the patient. Milder nasal steroids (eg, flunisolide or triamcinolone 1–2 puffs each nostril qd) or instructions on spraying the medication laterally will help for those who cannot discontinue the medications. Milder antihistamines (loratadine or fexofenadine) or switching to montelukast may help (see allergic rhinitis/sneezing treatment section in this chapter for dosages). For over-the-counter nasal saline users, the patient may prepare their own nasal saline by mixing 8 ounces (1 measuring cup) of boiled water that is cooled with ¼ to ½ teaspoon of pickling or kosher salt. Fresh saline should be made every 2 days. For patients with nasal dryness from climate conditions, saline nasal spray (3–4 puffs each nostril 3–4 times a day) can be used.

What Tests to Order/When to Refer

For patients with complaints of dry nose in conjunction with dry eyes and a dry mouth, anti-ssA and anti-ssB

DNA antibodies should be ordered. If suspicion for Sjögren's syndrome is high, a referral to an otolaryngologist for a lip biopsy is recommended.

VESTIBULITIS

The nasal vestibule (hairy part of inside of nostrils) harbors bacteria. Many patients have *Staph aureus* colonization of their nasal vestibule. Occasionally, due to manipulation, removal, or cutting nostril hairs, the patient may have inoculation of the vestibular skin with bacteria, which can cause a cellulitis and eventually an abscess.

Symptoms and Signs

The patient will generally present with pain and swelling of the nostril a few days after manipulation of vestibular skin/hair. On examination, the patient will have tenderness, erythema, and edema of the inside of the nostril. Occasionally, bulging from abscess formation can be seen.

Diagnosis and What Tests to Order

The diagnosis is made based on the history and physical exam findings. If purulence is seen, a culture can be obtained. In some patients, the infection can spread to the malar skin, in which case a CT of the face with contrast will help in evaluation of the extent of the infection.

Treatment and When to Refer

Given that most of these infections are caused by *S. aureus*, the treatment is best done with cephalexin (500 mg po TID × 10 days; children, 40 mg/kg/day divided TID). For penicillin allergics or those suspected of having methicillin resistant *S. aureus*, clindamycin 300 mg po QID × 10 days (children, 20 mg/kg/day divided Q 8hrs × 10 days). If methicillin-resistant *Staph aureus* is suspected, trimethoprim sulfamethoxazole 160/800 (Bactrim DS) po BID × 10 days (children, 3 mg/kg/day dosed on trimethoprim). The patient should be referred to an otolaryngologist if there is no improvement after 3 days. If there is infection involving the malar skin or there is facial abscess formation, the patient should be admitted to the hospital for intravenous antibiotic therapy.

FACIAL CELLULITIS

Facial cellulitis can occur for a variety of reasons, but generally requires a break in the skin integrity (eg, trauma, scratch, insect bite, etc) and bacterial invasion. The bacteria most commonly involved are *S. aureus* and *Streptococcus spp.* This condition is more common in diabetics or other immune-compromised patients. Recently, though, there has been an increased incidence of community acquired methicillin-resistant *S. aureus* facial cellulitis.

Symptoms and Signs

The patients generally present with erythema and edema of the face. Occasionally, an abscess pocket (fluctuance) may be palpated. There may be a surrounding area of erythema of the skin.

Diagnosis and What Tests to Order

The diagnosis is dependent on blanching erythema and tenderness of the involved area. Occasionally, desquamation of the skin with intense erythema can be seen. The patient also may have an abscess pocket that could be palpated. A fever may be present. If pus is seen, a culture should be obtained. If the patient requires admission, a CBC and blood culture should also be obtained. An HIV test should be considered if the patient has the risk factors and no other immune deficiency.

Treatment and When to Refer

A nondiabetic, immune-competent patient with a limited area of cellulitis in the face (3–4 cm diameter) can be treated with oral antibiotics as outlined under the vestibulitis section. The same referral criteria as vestibulitis should be used. The patient who is immune compromised, has an extensive cellulitis, or has abscess formation should be admitted to the hospital with IV antibiotics (vancomycin to start until culture results return) and an otolaryngology consultation.

FURTHER READING

Collie WR, Pagon PA, Hall JG, Shokeir MHK. ACHOO syndrome (helio-ophthalmic outburst syndrome). *Birth Defects Original Article Series.* 1978;114:361–363.

Leopold DA. Distorted olfactory perception. In: Doty RL, ed. *Handbook of Olfaction and Gustation.* New York: Marcel Dekker; 1995:114-115.

Teebi AS, Al-Saleh QA. Autosomal dominant sneezing disorder provoked by fullness of stomach. *J Med Genet.* 1989;126:539-540.

CHAPTER 15

Trauma to the Nose and Face

PAUL K. HOLDEN
HAMID R. DJALILIAN
BRIAN J. F. WONG

EVALUATION

Facial trauma occurs commonly in a variety of circumstances including sports, assault, motor vehicle accident, or fall. The most prominent structures in the face, that is, the nose and mandible are the areas that are most commonly affected by trauma. Nasal trauma patients typically present with pain, swelling, and/or epistaxis. More significant injuries may include altered level of consciousness, vision disturbance/orbital injuries, visible deviation/deformity, laceration, or cerebrospinal fluid rhinorrhea. Mandibular trauma patients will present with a change in the patient's bite (occlusion), trismus (inability to open mouth widely), or fractured teeth. Other areas of the face, for example, the zygoma (malar eminence) or the orbit may be fractured as well, but generally require a great amount of force and these patients present less commonly in an ambulatory setting. This chapter deals with the stable ambulatory patient. More severe injuries of the face typically are addressed in a hospital emergency room or trauma center and should be referred to such centers when encountered in the ambulatory setting.

History

In the typical ambulatory patient, one can start with a history of the traumatic event. Important considerations are:

Mechanism of injury (high/low velocity, blunt/penetrating)

Time of injury

Loss of consciousness or amnesia for the event

Change in vision (blurriness, double vision—immediate or delayed)

Amount of bleeding, if any

Nasal obstruction

Clear drainage from the nose or salty taste in the pharynx

Obvious external deformity

Change in the sense of smell

Change in how the teeth fit together

Inability to open mouth widely

Prior nasal trauma

History of nasal surgery of any kind

History of nasal recreational drug use (eg, cocaine, methamphetamine)

Past medical history

Patients who experience loss of consciousness, altered mental status, profuse bleeding that fails conservative management, or significant visual changes following the event should be referred via ambulance to the nearest hospital emergency room or trauma center for further evaluation and management. In these patients, the ABCs of emergency trauma/life support management should be followed first.

Examination

Any time a patient has suffered a trauma, a comprehensive physical examination is important to eliminate other injuries of which the patient may not be aware. The nose and face are very sensitive areas and, therefore, trauma to this location can distract the patient from noticing other sources of pain. In addition to the general physical exam, however, it is important to carry out a meticulous examination of the head and neck. Special attention should be directed toward:

Mental status or Glasgow Coma Scale (GCS)

Facial symmetry of movement and sensation

Facial, neck or scalp lacerations

Orbital Findings

Change in vision (visual acuity, light, etc)

Diplopia (especially upon range of motion)

Periorbital swelling

Ecchymosis (black eye)

Palpable inferior orbital rim step-off

Anisocoria (pupils of unequal size)

Chemosis (edema of conjunctiva)

Subconjunctival hemorrhage (red eye)

Afferent pupillary defect

Dysconjugate gaze

Epiphora (excessive tearing)

Lower eyelid laxity

Widening of the intercanthal distance (normally equal to the width of one eye)

Proptosis

Ear Findings

Swelling

Auricular hematoma

Decreased hearing

Otorrhea (drainage from the ear)

Otorrhagia (bleeding from the ear)

Battle sign (ecchymosis behind the ear, on the mastoid area)

Hemotympanum

Nasal Findings

Swelling

Crepitus

Obvious external deformity

Increase in nasal obstruction, usually unilateral

Epistaxis

Septal hematoma

Oral/Midface Findings

    Visible step-off/deformity

    Mobility of midface

    Missing/fractured teeth

    Malocclusion

    Floor of mouth hematoma/swelling

    Trismus (restriction of mandibular motion)

    Postnasal drainage of blood

Neck Findings

    Stridor

    Tracheal deviation

    Crepitus (subcutaneous emphysema)

    Collecting hematoma

    Retractions

    Voice change

During the nasal examination, a well-lit room or bright flashlight is needed to evaluate for external deformity, and anterior rhinoscopy with an otoscope or nasal speculum should be performed to rule out intranasal injuries such as septal hematoma or fracture. A driver's license photo can be a readily available reference for the patient's premorbid facial/nasal shape.

DIFFERENTIAL DIAGNOSES

More than one of the following injuries related to nasal trauma may be present at the time of presentation. Patients seen more than 14 days after the injury are considered to be delayed diagnosis. The management of delayed injuries is significantly different than in the acute setting and, therefore, should be referred nonurgently to an otolaryngologist.

EPISTAXIS

Nasal trauma frequently leads to a brief, 3- to 5-minute period of bleeding from the nose. More extensive injuries tend to bleed more. Rarely will epistaxis be excessive and persist despite conservative measures such as compression or topical vasoconstriction. In these cases, it is possible the patient has suffered an injury to a larger, deeper blood vessel or has more extensive mucosal injury intranasally. Occasionally, patients may experience brief periods of profuse bleeding that occur in a paroxysmal, delayed fashion following the trauma. This can be as long as weeks after the initial event. Persistent epistaxis requires immediate otolaryngology referral, whereas recurrent brief nosebleeds should be expedited but not urgent or emergent (unless, of course, the patient is actively bleeding). Please review Chapter 12 on epistaxis for a more in depth discussion on the management of nasal bleeding.

NASAL SEPTAL HEMATOMA

Septal hematoma should be suspected when any of the following are present on intranasal examination: swelling of the septum, purple discoloration of the septal mucosa, a ballotable/fluctuant collection on the septum, or nasal obstruction. Suspicion of septal hematoma should also be high if the patient did not have significant bleeding at the time of injury yet external evidence of injury or fracture is present.

NASAL LACERATION

Injuries can range from a superficial skin defect not requiring repair, to an extensive avulsion/laceration with exposure of intranasal anatomy. Careful visual examination should be performed to ascertain the extent of injury. When suspected, plain film x-rays may help in localizing potential foreign bodies (such as broken glass or gravel), which may be embedded in the wound. Lacerations involving cartilage should be referred to an emergency department for closure by a facial plastic surgeon or otolaryngologist.

NASAL BONE FRACTURE

The nasal bones comprise the upper one-third of the nasal dorsum. They are among the most commonly fractured bones in the body. Obvious external deformity along with crepitus upon palpation is diagnostic for fracture. In the absence of suspicion of other facial injuries, no further radiographic studies are necessary to make the diagnosis.

FRACTURE OF THE NASAL SEPTUM

Septal fracture usually accompanies nasal bone fracture. Nonetheless, it is still possible to have this injury without nasal bone fracture. This injury usually results in immediate notable obstruction of one or both nasal cavities in a patient who had normal nasal breathing prior to the injury. This injury carries a higher incidence of septal hematoma. Once visualized, further radiographic testing is not helpful unless other injuries are suspected.

MANDIBLE FRACTURE

A patient with a mandible fracture will generally present with a change in dental occlusion after trauma. The force required for a mandible fracture is very significant in a normal mandible. In an edentulous mandible, which thins because of the absence of teeth, the force required is less. The examination may show dental fractures, malocclusion, tenderness on dental percussion with a tongue depressor, a sublingual hematoma, or trismus. The best study to evaluate for a mandible fracture is a panorex x-ray of the mandible including the condyles. This will allow full visualization of the mandible. Plain x-rays (facial fracture series) may be ordered in lieu of a panorex, but are not as accurate as a panorex.

NASO-ORBITO-ETHMOID (NOE) FRACTURE

One of the more vexing injuries that can accompany nasal fracture is one that involves the NOE complex. This is because the medial canthal tendons insert on this location, which is, by definition, disrupted with this type of injury. These injuries cause widening of the intercanthal distance (which is normally about one-half of the interpupillary distance) and lower lid laxity on digital retraction (the so-called "bowstring sign"). Injuries can be unilateral or bilateral and are more commonly severe, telescoping type of nasal fracture injury (often at high velocity). Suspicion of this injury should prompt a noncontrast facial CT scan with fine cuts through the orbits for further evaluation. Radiographic evidence along with positive clinical findings will make the diagnosis of NOE fracture. An NOE fracture generally is caused by a high-velocity impact and almost never presents in an outpatient setting.

CRIBRIFORM PLATE/SKULL BASE FRACTURE

Extensive injuries to the nose can extend up into the anterior skull base or cribriform plate. Typically, these injuries are accompanied by "raccoon eyes," which is a more prominent circumorbital ecchymosis of one or both orbits. These patients may or may not present with altered mental status or a history of loss of consciousness. They may have clear rhinorrhea or salty taste in the pharynx on presentation. In the presence of this type of injury, one should have an increased alertness for delayed onset meningitis. When skull base fracture is suspected, a noncontrast high-resolution CT scan of the face with cuts through the orbits and sinuses should be obtained to make the diagnosis. If pneumocephalus is noted in the absence of an obvious fracture, a small skull base fracture is present. Rarely, CSF leak can be present without radiographic evidence of the injury. In these cases, fluid should be collected and tested for beta-2-transferrin to confirm the diagnosis. Collect the specimen in a sterile container for immediate processing. Many labs also require a tube of blood for reference. Contact your lab for specific specimen processing information prior to sending the specimen to reduce the delay in diagnosis caused by the need for multiple sampling.

SINUS FRACTURE

The paranasal sinuses can act as "crumple zones" for the eyes and brain in the presence of trauma. Nasal trauma can sometimes extend into the ethmoid, frontal or maxillary sinuses. These injuries may be visible as with a depressed frontal sinus fracture, or may have no external evidence at all, as with the majority of maxillary and ethmoid sinus fractures. When suspected, a noncontrast CT scan of the face and sinuses should be obtained. With the exception of depressed frontal sinus fractures or those extending through the posterior wall of the frontal sinus, the majority of isolated sinus fractures do not require operative intervention, but should be referred to an otolaryngologists for longitudinal observation and management.

ORBITAL FLOOR/WALL FRACTURE

The paranasal sinuses border the orbit on its medial and inferior walls. Along the medial wall lies a very thin bone, the lamina papyracea (translated: paper layer), which can easily be involved with nasal trauma. Clinical evidence suggesting this type of injury includes periorbital ecchymosis, conjunctival hemorrhage or edema, restriction/diplopia on lateral gaze of the affected eye, proptosis, or visual changes. Similarly, the orbital floor can be involved when more extensive nasal trauma is present. This injury should be suspected when periorbital swelling/ecchymosis, conjunctival hemorrhage, restriction/diplopia on upward gaze, proptosis, or enopthalmos (eye sunken into the orbit) are present. The diagnosis for either of these types of fracture is made with a noncontrast CT of the face with fine cuts through the orbits.

Precaution: Patients with possible orbital or skull base fractures should be advised against blowing the nose or sneezing through the nose. Pressurized air can track into the orbit or intracranially, which can lead to serious complications.

TREATMENT

Simple (nondisplaced fracture, without laceration or septal hematoma) nasal trauma usually requires only supportive care such as gentle icing, elevation, pain management, and abstinence from strenuous activity for a period of 1 to 2 weeks. Repeat examination after approximately 3 to 5 days is warranted to rule out a previously undetected fracture, which can be hidden by tissue edema.

Septal hematoma requires immediate drainage. Local anesthetic can be used either topically or by direct infusion into the hematoma space. A linear opening of significant enough size to allow egress of blood without reaccumulation should be created on one side of the septal mucosa only. Creating incisions on both sides increases the risk of creating a septal perforation. The blood should be "milked" out with a cotton-tipped applicator. Nasal packing has to be placed bilaterally to prevent reaccumulation of the hematoma. See Chapter 12 on Epistaxis for details on nasal packing placement.

Uncomplicated, displaced nasal fractures should be managed with supportive care and referred to a facial plastic surgeon or otolaryngologist within 3 to 5 days. The patient should be advised that immediate follow-up is important to avoid the need for more extensive surgery at a later date. Patients should bring with them photographs of themselves showing their nose (preferably at different angles) taken prior to trauma but recent enough to be accurate. Nasal fractures can only be repaired primarily in the first 14 days post-trauma. After that the bones are not usually mobile and will require surgical refracturing and reduction.

Mandibular fractures require immediate attention as they are technically open fractures with exposure to the oral bacteria. The patient with a change in his or her dental occlusion or trismus should be sent to an emergency department for evaluation and consultation with a facial plastic surgeon or otolaryngologist. Patients with mandible fractures may have undiscovered cervical spine injuries. Stabilization of the cervical spine is beneficial prior to sending the patient to the emergency department.

All other facial fractures should be referred to a facial plastic surgeon or otolaryngologist for management within 2 days of injury for surgical correction. After 14 days from the injury, correction of the fracture is significantly more difficult as some degree of callous formation has occurred. An evaluation of the cervical spine is warranted in any trauma with significant whiplash.

What Tests to Order

All patients with mandible or extensive facial fractures should have cervical spine x-rays to rule out an injury to the cervical spine. Isolated nasal fractures are made with clinical findings alone. There is no role for plain film x-rays or CT scans in these patients. Mandible fractures require a panorex of the mandible and condyles for evaluation. If a panorex is not available, four views of the mandible can be obtained. A non-contrast CT scan of the face with axial and coronal images should be obtained in patients with suspected fractures of the skull base, orbits, sinuses, mandible, or temporal bone. When suspicion of an orbital fracture is high or entrapment of an extraocular muscle is evident, include instructions to obtain fine cuts through the orbits. MRI, plain film x-rays and contrast studies have no role in any of these types of injuries. As mentioned earlier, plain film x-rays may be useful in cases where an open wound is contaminated with debris such as gravel or glass. In these special cases, x-rays can help locate foreign bodies in the wound.

When to Refer

As with most facial injuries, immediate referral to an otolaryngologist is important when concern about cosmetic or functional outcome relates to trauma. In the case of nasal trauma, special attention should be paid to the possibility of visual loss/injury, neurotrauma, significant cosmetic nasal deformity, or significant nasal obstruction.

In all cases except for contusion or minimally displaced simple nasal fractures, the otolaryngologist should be consulted early in management. Similarly, ophthalmology should be emergency consulted if concerns over vision or eye function are raised. Of course, when a significant head injury or other organ system injury is suspected, trauma surgery and any related subspecialties should be consulted quickly. Using the guide in this chapter, the appropriate study, if indicated, should already be completed (if the patient is stable) prior to contacting the consultant.

PART III

Diseases of the Mouth, Throat, and Neck

CHAPTER 16

The History and Examination of the Mouth, Throat, and Neck

EDWARD C. WU
VANESSA S. ROTHHOLTZ
HAMID R. DJALILIAN

BACKGROUND

It is often difficult to obtain a complete exam of the oral cavity, throat, and neck. The age of a patient and his or her body habitus may make a good exam more difficult to acquire, but it is important to be as thorough as possible when seeking a diagnosis. It takes time and effort to obtain an adequate examination of the oral cavity, throat and neck, but a solid knowledge of normal and abnormal findings can expedite the process. A detailed history may lead to additional findings that cannot be visualized on exam. When seeking a history and physical examination, the physician must keep in mind that all systems are connected. The oral cavity does not stop at the base of tongue, but continues to the pharynx and then down to the hypopharynx (area of the pharynx below the base of the tongue) and up to the nasopharynx. Disease that may not be seen in the oral cavity or throat may manifest itself in the neck. Maintaining a mental and physical image of the confluence of the anatomic and physiologic connections allows for a complete examination.

HISTORY

As a result of the very closely related anatomy among these structures, the presence of oral symptoms is the key indication for taking a thorough history of the mouth and throat. Likewise, the chief complaint of a new mass in the neck warrants a complete history and physical of the neck, nose, and oral cavity.

In taking a detailed history of the oral cavity, pay close attention to the deep structures as well as surface anatomy, which includes the lips, teeth, and gingival tissue. New lesions anywhere on or in the mouth, such as those acquired from trauma to the area or lesions that do not heal in 3 weeks should draw your attention, especially in patients with a history of smoking, chewing tobacco use, Betel nut users (from Southeast Asia or South Asia), or regular alcohol users. Any change in a pre-existing lesion warrants further questioning. A history of snoring or sleep apnea should be elicited and, often, additional information from the patient's partner will assist in creating a differential diagnosis. A history of dry mouth (xerostomia) in the absence of radiation therapy or medications with anticholinergic side effects may indicate a salivary gland dysfunction. Finally, the history should assess the functionality of the mouth by inquiring about swallowing difficulties, abnormal drooling, globus sensation (the feeling of something "stuck" in the throat), or alteration of taste.

A few problems of the mouth and throat that indicate a taking a specific history could be related to the teeth and gingival tissue. In many cases, the patient most likely would benefit from dental consultation, but it is the physician's duty to evaluate the problem medically in the context of the patient's complaint. Suspicion of a neck abscess warrants a good dental history and examination.

The history of the orophayrnx or throat should be composed of questions targeted toward any abnormalities in swallowing, coughing, breathing, voice, and the respective structures responsible for those functions. Questions should lead to the distinction between an infectious, obstructive, or functional cause of the patient's complaint. New onset of bad breath may alert the physician to an infectious or cancerous etiology.

When obtaining the history of the neck, it is most important to take into account the age of the patient. Whereas most pediatric neck masses are congenital or infectious/inflammatory in etiology, a neck mass in an adult over the age of 35 should be considered neoplastic until proven otherwise. The neck history should focus on duration, change in size, degree of mobility, signs of pain, swelling, and range of motion, each of which may have multiple different causes.

For many patients, especially those with oral and pharyngeal symptoms, health counseling may benefit the patient. Remind the patient of the importance of oral health and regular visits to the dentist. Important lifestyle issues such as diet, exercise, and omitting the intake of tobacco and alcohol should be addressed.

The indications and specific elements of obtaining the history are outlined in Tables 16–1 through 16–3.

Table 16–1. Indications for Taking a History of the Mouth, Throat, and Neck

---

Mouth

- Teeth and gingiva—marginal and severe gingivitis, change in color or texture of gingiva, periodontal infection, painful teeth and gingiva, bleeding gingiva, numbness to the teeth

- Lips—dryness, new or recent change in peri-oral lesion, infection (eg, herpes, syphilis), asymmetry

- Tongue—variation in tongue color and texture, glossitis, candidiasis, leukoplakia, presence of plaques on tongue, arteriovenous malformations (AVMs), canker sores/apthous ulcers, taste disturbance, change in voice, change in tongue mobility or size

- Intraoral—new and old lesions on hard/soft palate, buccal mucosa, floor of mouth

- Function—Dry mouth (xerostomia), excessive drooling, gustatory problems, dysphagia, odynophagia, apnea/snoring, bad breath

Throat

- Pain, fullness or globus sensation (feeling of something present in throat)

- Coughing—productive versus unproductive, hemoptysis

- Voice problems (eg, hoarseness, loss, change in quality and volume)

- Swallowing problems—obstructions versus mechanics

- Itchiness, constant clearing of throat

- Difficulty breathing

- Questionable foreign object

Neck

- Swelling and lumps—lymph nodes, thyroid, goiter, or masses

- Neck pain, stiffness, limitations in range of motion

- Thyroid

- Discoloration or any changes of the skin

- Tracheostomy—present or evidence of past

- Any scars noted

Table 16–2. General Questions in the History of an Oral Cavity, Pharynx, or Neck Problem

- When did the problem start?
- What is the duration of the problem?
- Is this a new, recurring or chronic problem?
  - For each case, has the patient seen a doctor about it earlier?
  - What were prior prescribed treatments?
- Do the symptoms change?
  - If so, how often do they change? Seasonally? Time of day? In different environments? For better or for worse?
- Is the problem unilateral or bilateral?
- Have any self-care tips been tried?
  - If so, how successful were they?
- How bothersome is the problem? How does it affect daily life?
- Is there bleeding or an odor?
- If there is discharge, what is the color and texture?
- If there is pain, how painful is it on a scale of 1–10, 10 being the most painful?
- If there is a foreign object within the throat, ensure that the airway is stable and then inquire about the events leading to this phenomenon
- If one of the symptoms is a painful tongue, consider systemic problems as well as those localized to the mouth
- If a thyroid dysfunction is suspected, ask questions regarding temperature tolerance and sweating

Table 16–3. Specific Questions in Obtaining a History for the Oral Cavity, Pharynx, and Neck

- Allergies
  - Has the patient ever had formal allergy testing?
  - If so, to what are they allergic?

continues

Table 16–3. *continued*

- Medication and drug use
  - Does the patient take medications (prescribed and over-the-counter) for the relief of symptoms?
  - Does the patient take medications that may be causing the symptoms? (eg, Is the dose of levothyroxine too low? Is the patient on a chemotherapeutic agent?)
  - Does the patient currently or previously use Betel nut (in south or southeast Asian patients)?

- Alcohol use
  - How many drinks per week?

- Smoking and tobacco use
  - Does the patient smoke or did she or he smoke? How long and how many cigarettes/day?
  - Is the patient frequently exposed to second-hand smoke?

- Dental history
  - When was the last time the patient went to see the dentist?
  - When will the next dental visit be?
  - Has the patient ever had any problems with his or her teeth or gingiva? How were these problems addressed?

- Occupation
  - Is there anything in the workplace that could be causing the problem(s)?
  - Is the patient exposed to any chemicals at the workplace?

- History of previous illness—Chronic health problems

- History of previous surgery
  - Has the patient undergone any head- and neck-related surgery?
  - Has the patient ever been intubated? Why? Duration? When?

- History of trauma to face, mouth, throat, neck, and surrounding areas

- Family history
  - Carcinoma, genetic disorders

- Constitutional symptoms—malaise, weight loss, bone pain, anorexia

EXAMINATION

After obtaining a thorough history of the mouth, throat, and neck, the physician should then begin the physical examination. Gloves should be worn while examining the mouth and throat, and tasks should be performed from the most comfortable to the least comfortable for the patient.

Mouth and Throat

Prior to the examination of the mouth, the patient should remove his or her dentures, retainers, or other oral prosthetics as cancers can hide under these appliances. It is important to be familiar with abnormal findings, normal findings, and variations thereof. In inspecting the mouth and throat, it is ideal to use two tongue blades simultaneously, one in each hand, with the patient's mouth illuminated from a headlight or an indirect source. The tongue blades can be used to expose difficult to access grooves in the mouth such as the gingival-buccal sulci or to push away superficial structures that may be blocking the view of a deeper structure. They can also be used to palpate structures deep in the mouth and throat that would otherwise be inaccessible by other means.

Lips

Observe the patient's lips. Note the color, pigmentation, moisture, and presence of lumps, cracking, and ulcers. Certain infectious organisms commonly manifest on the lips. If there is dark pigmentation on the lips relative to the surrounding face with similar pigmentation on the buccal mucosa, then labial lentigines and Peutz-Jeghers syndrome may be suspected. Tiny blisters or sores that are present on the lip may be attributable to herpes labialis. Carcinoma of the lip can take many forms—it is frequently crusted, ulcerated, and usually on the lower lip. If there are any darkly pigmented (purple) or reddened spots, determine if they blanch with brief pressure to ensure their benign nature.

Oral Mucosa

After examining the lips, the physician should next examine the patient's oral mucosa. At this point, it would be possible to note if the mouth is dry or wet as well as any color inconsistencies. Xerostomia, or dryness of the mouth, can be due to many different causes, ranging from a systemic disorder such as diabetes to physical sources such as trauma to the salivary glands or medications. It also may be caused by anxiety, dehydration, or drug abuse. Similarly, excessive drooling may be associated with infectious mononucleosis, tonsillitis, intraoral abscess, or more emergently, odynophagia due to epiglottitis. Any visualized ulcers or nodules should be palpated for mobility, consistency, and persistence. Determine if the abnormalities can gently and painlessly be removed with the tongue blade, and if they are removable, note the character of the mucosa underneath. If accessible, palpate any masses seen to determine if they are soft, mobile, and to gauge the depth of the lesion. A thick texture or hardness to mass or any palpated abnormal structure may suggest a malignancy.

Gingiva

After examining the oral mucosa, the physician should next look at the gingiva for color, friability, bleeding, and recession. Reddening and swelling at the edges of the gums may suggest marginal gingivitis. It would be useful to correlate this finding with a history of bleeding on irritating the gingival tissue, as in biting into hard food or brushing teeth. Deep ulcerations, bad odor, bleeding, and necrotizing tissue forming a gray membrane may indicate the presence of a carcinoma or severe infection such as trench mouth. Granulation tissue on the gingiva next to a carious tooth indicates a possible periapical abscess of the tooth.

Teeth

Upon inspection of the teeth, it is important to note their color, sensation, shape, angle, and whether any are missing. To check for looseness, gently palpate the tooth with a tongue depressor. The patient's teeth may have acquired abnormalities such as attrition due to age-related wear (often accompanied by receding gums), chipping, or other physical damage such as from trauma, or erosion due to chemical exposure. It is important to provide counseling on dental hygiene and proper care and to refer appropriately to the dentist. The patient's teeth may also have congenital or developmental abnormalities. For example, prenatal or childhood exposure to tetracycline will render the teeth with a bluish-gray stain. Bulemic patients will have erosion of the posterior aspect of the lower incisors. In Hutchinson's teeth secondary to syphilis, the sides of the teeth curve toward the biting edge and the distance between adjacent teeth are considerably greater.

Buccal Mucosa

The next part of the physical examination includes inspection of the cheek and the upper and lower gingival-buccal sulci, the region between the cheek and the gums. Note the color, texture, and presence of masses, ulcers, or other lesions. Canker sores, or aphthous ulcers, are characterized by small ulcerations surrounded by a red ring. They are commonly found throughout the mouth, but especially around the tongue and oral mucosa. Small erythematous petechiae can be due to biting, infection, trauma, or platelet deficiency. Thick, tough, nonremovable white patches in the buccal region with a history of tobacco use may suggest leukoplakia, whereas removable white patches may suggest candida infection. Lichen planus is characterized by thin, bilateral white streaks in the buccal region that are less prominent than leukoplakia but like leukoplakia is a precancerous lesion.

Palate

Inspect the hard palate by having the patient tilt his or her head back so that the hard palate behind the front teeth is fully visible. Note the color and any structural abnormalities or communication with the nasal cavity. Next, ask the patient to open his or her mouth widely and to say "ah" to check for the raising of the soft palate indicating intact glossopharyngeal and vagal nerves. A long or thick soft palate places the patient at risk for obstructive sleep apnea, which should prompt questions such as daytime sleepiness, fatigue, naps, and so forth.

Tonsils/Oropharynx

With the patient keeping his or her tongue inside the mouth, place a tongue blade to depress the tongue at most the anterior two-thirds of the tongue to assist in visualization of the soft palate, tonsils, anterior and posterior pillars, uvula, retromolar trigones, and overall condition of the pharynx. Although it is important to ask the patient to stick out the tongue to check for an intact hypoglossal nerve and other causes of decreased lingual mobility, it is easier to depress the tongue without protruding the tongue because one is not working against the muscle. Note the color, symmetry, and presence of exudate, swelling, and ulceration on the tonsils and pillars. In children, who often resist an oral cavity examination, the tongue depressor should gently be guided along the hard palate toward the pharynx. The child will then gag and allow the examiner to evaluate the pharynx. The cooperative child can be asked to look up, extend the neck, and stick out his or her tongue. Usually with that maneuver, the pharynx can be seen without the need for a tongue depressor. Tonsillar size is graded on a 1+ to 4+ system where 1+ tonsils are small and confined to the tonsillar pillars, 2+ are those that protrude beyond the pillars but are less than 50% of the way to the midline, 3+ tonsils protrude beyond the pillars and are more than 50% of the way to the midline, and 4+ tonsils touch in the midline. The tonsils should be graded without the tongue depressor too far in, which can cause a gag reflex and bring the tonsils closer. Being mindful not to gag the patient, palpate the tonsils for tenderness or hardness. When observing for symmetry, note any deviation of the uvula to the right or left that may indicate a defect in the glossopharyngeal nerve of the opposite side. Red, swollen tonsils with white exudate and tender anterior cervical lymph nodes may suggest a bacterial infection or mononucleosis. A protruding bony growth at the midline of the palate is known as torus palatinus, which is a relatively common feature with no adverse effect.

Tongue

When initially evaluating the tongue, request that the patient protrude the tongue. Ask the patient to move the tongue all the way to the left and then right. This allows inspection of the lateral and the undersurface of the tongue, which are the most common areas for carcinoma development. It is critical to look at the most posterior portion of the lateral tongue. Following antibiotic therapy, it is possible to acquire extended yellow papillae at the dorsum of the tongue. In glossitis, the tongue becomes dark red. The retromolar trigone, which is the area of the mandible behind the third molar, is a relatively common site of carcinoma development and should be inspected and palpated with extra care and detail.

On the floor of the mouth, arteriovenous malformations (AVMs) may develop. The severity of AVMs varies from minor (eg, varicose veins that develop with age) to severe (necessitates resection). Torus mandibularis, much like torus palatinus, is a protruding bony growth from the mandible extending from the floor of the mouth. It also is a common polymorphism that is harmless. Cancer should be suspected if there is a soft tissue mass or an ulcer that has been present for more than 3 weeks on the floor of the mouth. Look at the undersurface and sides of the patient's tongue for any irregularities as those are the most common sites of carcinomas.

Floor of Mouth/Base of Tongue

Palpate the floor of the patient's mouth bimanually by placing the index and middle fingers of the dominant hand on the patient's floor of mouth and the fingers of the nondominant hand under the patient's chin. This will allow the physician to palpate any abnormalities on the floor of the mouth as well as evaluate the submandibular glands. Bilateral swelling, pain, and hardness on the floor of the mouth associated with difficulty breathing and swallowing and an abnormally elevated tongue may suggest Ludwig's angina, and the patient should be immediately directed to the nearest emergency room for possible airway management. Palpation of the base of the tongue for risk of tongue cancer is very important, especially in patients who smoke, chew tobacco or Betel nut, or use alcohol.

Voice/Dysphagia

If the patient has chronic breathing or vocal problems such as voice loss, hoarseness, or changes in voice quality or volume, a deeper look into the larynx may be desired. Have the patient protrude his or her tongue and gently grasp it with a piece of gauze, pulling it slightly outward so that the pharynx is exposed. Insert a sterilized warm mirror into the back of the patient's mouth and carefully push the uvula and soft palate superiorly. The warming will prevent fogging of the mirror. With a headlight, adjust the light until the inner portions of the pharynx are visible. Inspect the vocal folds and surrounding cartilage and the visible portions of the superior trachea. Note the color of the vocal folds (normally white) and the presence of any inflammation, lesions, masses, nodules, or asymmetry. Ask the patient to breathe deeply through the mouth and say "eee" or "ha ha ha" to check for any abnormal movement of the vocal folds. For a complete examination in a patient with voice or swallowing abnormality, or if the physician is inexperienced in the examination of the glottis, referral to an otolaryngologist is imperative.

Neck

When beginning to examine the neck, completely expose the patient's neck. If the patient is wearing a collared shirt, a scarf, or any clothing that would obscure the neck, ask the patient to remove it. On first inspection, note the symmetry and the presence of masses, swelling, enlarged lymph nodes, or scars indicating prior tracheostomy, neck dissection, or thryoidectomy. Ask the patient to move the head vertically and horizontally noting any limitations in the range of motion of the neck. Ask if the patient has any pain or discomfort associated with rotating, flexing, or extending the neck in any direction. Bimanually palpate the parotid and submandibular salivary glands as described above. Note the symmetry and whether there is swelling, pain, abnormal discharge from the intraoral ducts, or tenderness in each gland.

Place the patient's head and neck in a neutral position. Bimanually palpate the lymph nodes in the neck using the undersurface of the index and middle fingers of both hands in a symmetric fashion. During the lymph node examination, it may be helpful to flex the patient's neck slightly. For each lymph node, note the size, shape, boundaries, mobility, consistency, and tenderness. Normal lymph nodes are small, less than one centimeter, mobile, discrete, and not tender to the touch.

The suggested order of lymph node palpation is:

a. In front of the ears (preauricular and parotid)
b. Superficial to the mastoid process (posterior auricular)
c. Posteriorly at the base of the skull (occipital)
d. At the posterior angle of the mandible (jugulodigastric)
e. Halfway between the angle of the mandible and the chin (submandibular)
f. At midline a short distance behind the chin (submental)—may be done bimanually
g. Superficial to sternocleidomastoid muscle, along the anterior and posterior edges (anterior cervical)

h. Along anterior edge of trapezius muscle (posterior cervical)

i. Deep to the sternocleidomastoid muscle (deep cervical chain)

j. Deep in angle formed by clavicle and sternocleidomastoid muscle (supraclavicular)

See Figure 16–1 for the location of the lymph nodes of the head and neck.

It may be difficult to distinguish a palpated lymph node from a vessel or a muscle. If this is the case, remember that a lymph node can be moved up and

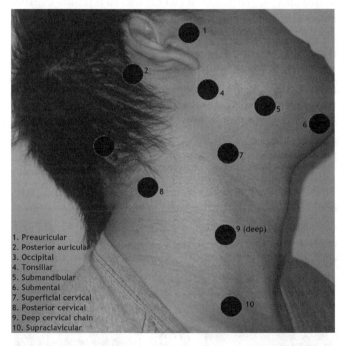

1. Preauricular
2. Posterior auricular
3. Occipital
4. Tonsillar
5. Submandibular
6. Submental
7. Superficial cervical
8. Posterior cervical
9. Deep cervical chain
10. Supraclavicular

Fig 16–1. Cervical lymph node chains as shown on a patient. All nodal areas (anterior, posterior cervical, submandibular, postauricular, submental, and parotid) should be palpated.

down and side to side, whereas the carotid pulsates. There are four symmetric masses in the neck that may be palpated: (1) lateral processes of C1; (2) the ptotic (droopy, descended) submandibular glands; (3) the greater cornu of the hyoid; and (4) the carotid bulbs. The lateral processes of C1 will be hard, nonmobile, symmetric, and palpable in some patients just deep to the angle of the mandible. The ptotic submandibular glands will be most commonly seen in the elderly and will be protruding below the mandible and have a soft grainy sensation. The greater cornu of the hyoid will be palpable anterior to the sternocleidomastoid muscle (SCM) and superior to the thyroid cartilage. The hyoid can be palpated between the two hands on the two sides of the neck and its mobility can be appreciated. The carotid bulbs will be symmetrically located in the upper neck anterior to the SCM and will pulsate.

After examining the lymph nodes in the neck, the physician should inspect the surface anatomy of the trachea and observe for any deviations in shape and symmetry. Following identification of the thyroid gland's location, attempt to bimanually palpate each lobe of the thyroid gland. This can be accomplished either facing the patient or from behind the patient. The thyroid gland is normally very difficult to palpate if it is not enlarged. If palpable, note the size, shape, consistency, and presence of nodules or tenderness of each lobe. The patient should be asked to swallow, which will elevate the trachea and allow the thyroid gland to roll under the fingers of the examiner.

IMAGING

Radiographic imaging of the neck is typically used for visualizing soft tissue detail (epiglottitis, retropharyngeal abscess/hematoma), foreign bodies (eg, fish bone) or for cervical spine evaluation. The soft tissue width anterior to the cervical spine is approximately 7 mm at C2 and 22 mm at C7. The critical views in this series include the AP and lateral views. A plain film can visualize evidence of airway narrowing, for example, the steeple sign in the presence of croup or the thumb sign in epiglottitis.

To work up a neck mass or head and neck tumor, a CT scan of the neck with contrast must be obtained. In the case of cancer of the neck region, otolaryngologists typically order CT, MRI scans, or rarely both, stating specifically that there is suspicion of a cancerous mass. In addition to CT and MRI, radioactive fluorodeoxyglucose positron emission tomography (FDG-PET) has recently been demonstrated to be an effective locator of metastatic primary cancers in the head and neck. To assess the mandible, radiologic mandible series or mandibular panoramic (panorex) imaging can be obtained. Use of ultrasound generally is limited to imaging the thyroid gland, cystic neck masses, and the carotid arteries.

CHAPTER 17

Lesions of the Oral Cavity

AARON G. BENSON
RYAN LEONARD
HAMID R. DJALILIAN

BACKGROUND

Patients frequently present with an oral cavity lesion. The differential diagnosis of these lesions is long and complex and entire books have been dedicated to this subject. In this chapter, we attempt to describe the most common of these lesions (Fig 17-1). Due to limitation in space, we refer the reader to an online atlas of oral lesions at the University of Iowa Oral Pathology at http://www.uiowa.edu/~oprm/AtlasWIN/AtlasFrame .html

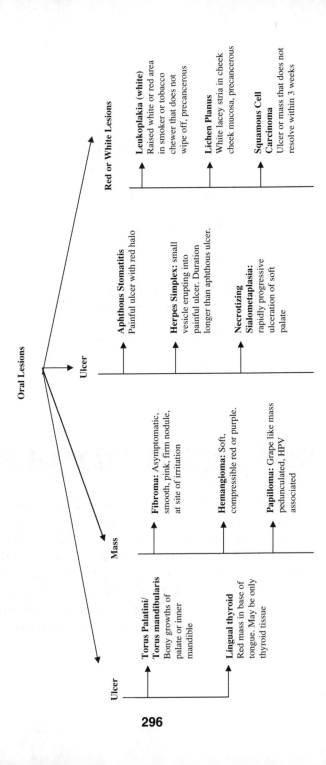

Oral Lesions

Ulcer

- **Torus Palatini/ Torus mandibularis** Bony growths of palate or inner mandible
- **Lingual thyroid** Red mass in base of tongue. May be only thyroid tissue

Mass

- **Fibroma:** Asymptomatic, smooth, pink, firm nodule, at site of irritation
- **Hemangioma:** Soft, compressible red or purple.
- **Papilloma:** Grape like mass pedunculated, HPV associated

Ulcer

- **Aphthous Stomatitis** Painful ulcer with red halo
- **Herpes Simplex:** small vesicle erupting into painful ulcer. Duration longer than aphthous ulcer.
- **Necrotizing Sialometaplasia:** rapidly progressive ulceration of soft palate

Red or White Lesions

- **Leukoplakia (white)** Raised white or red area in smoker or tobacco chewer that does not wipe off, precancerous
- **Lichen Planus** White lacey stria in cheek cheek mucosa, precancerous
- **Squamous Cell Carcinoma** Ulcer or mass that does not resolve within 3 weeks

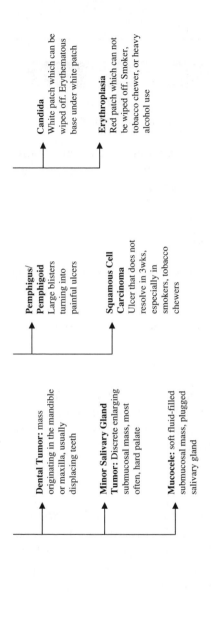

Fig 17–1. The most common oral lesions.

CONGENITAL

Torus Palatinus and Torus Mandibularis

Torus palatinus and torus mandibularis are benign bony growths on the hard palate and/or the lingual surface of the mandible. Malignant degeneration has not been reported.

Symptoms and Signs

Tori are always firm and have a bony consistency. These growths are painless, and often grow so slowly that they often go unnoticed by the patient. These lesions can be pedunculated or contain multiple lobes.

Diagnosis and Tests to Order

The diagnosis typically is made by examination. Their location on the midline palate or the inner surface of the mandible along with the characteristic bony consistency is usually sufficient.

When to Refer

Generally these lesions do not require treatment. However, if the bony growth interferes with dentures or affects the patient's ability to eat, then the patient should be referred to an otolaryngologist or an oral surgeon for surgical resection.

Lingual Thyroid

During normal embryonic development, the thyroid tissue descends from the base of the tongue and into the neck as the branchial arches fuse around it. The foramen cecum on the tongue base is the remnant from this descent. Not surprisingly, nearly 90% of ectopic thyroid tissue is found within the dorsum of the tongue and involves the foramen cecum.

Symptoms and Signs

It is assumed that the majority of these lesions go undetected and are asymptomatic. However, at puberty the increased metabolic demand and the gland's inability to increase thyroid hormone secretion leads to an increase in TSH and stimulation of the gland. This enlargement can cause a fullness or foreign body sensation, dysphagia, or worse, airway obstruction from the mass affect on the pharynx. There is also a high incidence of developing hypothyroidism especially if the lingual thyroid tissue represents the body's entire available thyroid.

Diagnosis and Tests to Order

Thyroid function studies should be conducted due to the risk of developing hypothyroidism. The diagnosis is usually made by seeing a hyperdense mass in the tongue on CT of the neck with contrast. In approximately 70% of cases of lingual thyroid there is no other thyroid tissue present.

Treatment and When to Refer

As lingual thyroid often goes unnoticed, it can also be managed conservatively. Often exogenous thyroid supplementation will suppress hormonal activities and thus shrink the thyroid tissue. Symptoms of dysphagia, bleeding, or upper airway obstruction warrant a referral to an endocrinologist and an otolaryngologist.

Developmental Cysts

Developmental cysts of the oral cavity are rare in occurrence, but there are several areas of the oral cavity in which they can occur. Types of developmental cysts found in the oral cavity are dermoid cysts, nasoalveolar cysts, and duplication cysts. Dermoid cysts often form at embryonic fusion lines. The most common oral cavity site for oral dermoid cyst is the floor of the mouth. Dermoid cysts usually contain keratin debris and can also contain hair follicles, sweat glands etc. Duplication cysts can occur anywhere throughout the alimentary tract including the floor of mouth and tongue. Nasoalveolar cysts develop between the maxillary prominences and therefore are manifest in the gingivolabial sulcus.

Symptoms and Signs

Dermoid cysts and duplication cysts that can cause problems with speaking, mastication, respiration, and/or swallowing as they enlarge. Nasoalveolar cysts present as smooth, tender, edematous areas of the nasolabial fold. The ala is often elevated as well.

Diagnosis and Tests to Order

The diagnosis can often be made by examination. Imaging is useful in determining the extent of the lesion and its relation to other structures. CT will generally show a cystic mass with contents similar to fat density. MRI is the test of choice in evaluating the soft tissue planes and involved structures.

Treatment and When to Refer

The recommended treatment of a developmental cyst is complete excision. A referral is warranted to an otolaryngologist once the diagnosis is made. If the cystic tissue is completely removed, then the rate of recurrence is low.

ULCERS

Aphthous Stomatitis

Aphthous stomatitis is the most common mucosal ulceration of the oral cavity. It affects approximately 20% of the population. Although the exact pathogenesis is not entirely known, several factors including stress, local trauma, and allergy are generally implicated as exacerbative agents. There is a higher incidence of apthous stomatitis for professionals, nonsmokers, and higher socioeconomic class. Apthous stomatitis ulcers are classified as minor, major, or herpetiform based on the severity and duration of symptoms.

Symptoms and Signs

Apthous stomatitis typically presents as painful ulcers up to 10mm with a surrounding erythematous halo on nonkeratinizing mucosal surfaces (labial, buccal, ventral and lateral tongue, floor of the mouth, soft palate, tonsillar pillars). The lesions most commonly are self-limiting, resolving within 10 days without scarring. Major lesions usually occur on the palate and may coalesce to become larger, and deeper and take months to heal.

Diagnosis and Tests to Order

Patients with recurrent symptoms should be considered for workup for nutritional deficiencies such as iron, vitamin B, and folic acid. Also, there is a higher incidence of autoimmune disorders and immunodeficiency. Behcet's disease (oral and genital ulcers, ophthalmic inflammation, dermatologic lesions), Crohn's disease, gluten sensitivity enteropathy, and HIV should all be considered. Complete blood count, erythrocyte sedimentation rate, potassium hydroxide test, viral cultures to rule out other entity, and tissue sample for biopsy all may be part of the workup.

Treatment and When to Refer

Treatment is often not necessary. Symptomatic improvement can be seen with use of topical corticosteroids (triamcinolone 0.1% ointment), or Magic Mouthwash (diphenhydramine, viscous lidocaine 4%, and aluminum hydroxide/magnesium hydroxide/simethicone), or topical anesthetics (benzocaine 20% gel) applied to the lesion(s) QID for 1 week. Lesions present for greater than 2 weeks, deeply ulcerated or nonhealing areas should have a biopsy for histologic diagnosis to rule out malignancy. The biopsy should be taken from the periphery of the lesion and include some normal tissue. A biopsy of the central part of an ulcer generally will show just necrotic tissue. A patient with an ulcer that has not resolved after 3 weeks should be referred to an otolaryngologist.

Herpes Simplex Infection

Herpes related lesions also commonly affect the oral cavity and lips. It is often a diagnostic challenge to differentiate apthous ulcers from viral entities. As herpes simplex virus 1 (HSV1) affects 60 to 90% of the population, HSV-related mucosal lesions are quite common. Primary infection tends to occur through contact and saliva in younger population, but asymptomatic viral shedding in infected individuals provides a constant source for infection.

Symptoms and Signs

Approximately 5 to 7 days after exposure from an infected person, a viral prodrome usually presents with mucosal tenderness for 24 to 48 hours. Small vesicles erupt and quickly develop into ulcerated lesions on both keratinized and nonkeratinized surfaces. Lesions can be present for up to 2 weeks and are generally self-limited. Reactivation of the dormant HSV can occur during adulthood, especially during psychologically stressful situations.

Diagnosis and What Tests to Order

The key differences in HSV infection versus apthous ulcers are the presence of vesicles, ulcers involving the gingival and viral prodrome. Other entities that should be in the differential are herpangina, hand-foot-mouth disease, and fifth disease. Laboratory tests are not usually needed for diagnosis but may include viral antibody titers, culture of vesicle fluid, and viral isolates in an immune compromised patient.

Treatment and When to Refer

Antiviral treatment (acyclovir 400 mg po TID × 7 days; in children dosage should not exceed 80 mg/kg/d) reduces the duration of the symptoms if given within the first 3 days of onset. Topical acyclovir ointment can be applied 6×/day for 7 days. Referral should be made to an otolaryngologist if the ulcer does not resolve within 3 weeks.

Necrotizing Sialometaplasia

Necrotizing sialometaplasia is a benign disorder involving the salivary glands. It most commonly affects the minor salivary glands on the posterior palate. An inflammatory process leads to ischemia and infarction of the salivary vessels with subsequent coagulative necrosis. The key aspect of this disorder is correct diagnosis as it closely mimics features of a malignant process including erosion of mucosa and possibly bone.

Symptoms and Signs

Affected areas tend to be painless, but may have some associated tenderness or numbness. The ulcers tend be 1 to 3 cm and craterlike in appearance. There is often local edema as well. Palatal ulcers are usually unilateral, but may be bilateral. The differential includes squamous cell carcinoma, mucoepidermoid carcinoma, and lymphoma. The distinguishing factor is its rapid onset. Necrotizing sialometaplasia ulcer will occur over a span of 3 to 14 days, compared to a few weeks to months for cancerous lesions.

Diagnosis and What Tests to Order

The diagnosis is clinical. Further testing is rarely needed once the diagnosis has been made. If an otolaryngologist is not available, the biopsy should be done to include some of the normal tissue surrounding the ulcer.

Treatment and When to Refer

Referral for biopsy is warranted. Inadequate tissue sample may lead to inaccurate diagnosis due to the extent of necrotic tissue. These lesions are self-limiting, often with full regression in up to 5 weeks.

Pemphigus Vulgaris/Cicatricial Pemphigoid

Pemphigus is a group of autoimmune disorders affecting the desmosomes in the skin and mucosa. Pemphigus vulgaris is the most common of the group and tends to affect first the mucosa of the upper respiratory tract and continuing to the skin up to years later. Mucous membrane (cicatricial) pemphigoid primarily affects the mucosa of the upper aerodigestive tract and ocular region. Cicatricial pemphigoid also has characteristic deposits of IgG and C3 in the basement membrane. These disorders are chronic in nature with a continuous course of forming blisters, sloughing to form ulcers, and then reforming new vesicles. The differential diagnosis includes other autoimmune disorders such as Behcet's and lupus, epidermolysis bullosa, HSV, apthous stomatitis, Stevens-Johnson syndrome, linear IgA disease, erythema multiforme, and bullous lichen planus.

Symptoms and Signs

The typical course for pemphigus vulgaris is the formation of the bullae, erosion of tissue, forming a painful ulcer followed by the formation of a new vesicle or bulla. The oral cavity, the oropharynx, soft palate, buccal mucosa, and labial mucosa most commonly are affected. Scarring does not typically take place and the lesions heal quickly. Cicatricial pemphigoid more commonly affects minimally keratinized surfaces like the gingiva and palate. Scarring due to the deposits do not usually occur in the oral cavity, but frequently are seen in the eye, nasopharynx, larynx, and so forth.

Diagnosis and What Tests to Order

Diagnosis is made by examination based on the mucosal patterns, denuding superficial layers of uninvolved adjacent mucosa (Nikolsky's sign), biopsy, and immuno-fluorescence specifically for pemphigus/pemphigoid.

Treatment and When to Refer

The treatment for both disorders usually includes systemic immunosupression. Pemphigus vulgaris was once fatal and still carries a 5% mortality rate with the associated morbidities with immunosuppressive treatment. Corticosteroids, cyclophosphamide, and non-steroidals are part of the treatment. Dapsone therapy along with topical high-potency topical steroids can be used for cicatricial pemphigoid. The patients should be referred to an otolaryngologist for biopsy if not possible at a primary care setting. The long-term management is best done by a dermatologist. If a biopsy is obtained in the primary care setting, the specimen should be placed in saline and delivered to the pathologist the same day. Pemphigus or pemphigoid should be mentioned to the pathologist as a possible diagnosis so immunofluorescence is performed.

Glossitis/Burning Mouth

Inflammation of the tongue can occur for a variety of reasons including candidal infections, vitamin B deficiency, postradiation xerostomia, and benign migratory glossitis (geographic tongue). Burning mouth can have multiple etiologies but the aforementioned problems are generally the culprit. Candidal infections (thrush) most commonly occur in neonates and the elderly or those with diabetes or immune-suppression. Geographic tongue is a common condition that affects up to 3% of the general population. It presents with sensitivity of the tongue to hot or spicy foods. The tongue will have an area of erythema where atrophy of the papilla has occurred. Surrounding that area will be a white hyperkeratotic border. The red area resembles a geographic map. The lesion will generally resolve spontaneously and the normal papilla will return. The cause is unknown.

Treatment and When to Refer

Treatment of glossitis consists of supportive care. Magic Mouthwash (diphenhydramine 12.5 mg/5 mL, 240 mL; hydrocortisone 60 mg; nystatin powder 6 million units, tetracycline 1.5 g) swish and spit 5 mL QID can be used. Magic Mouthwash has different formulas and the formula should be stated for the pharmacist. Triamcinolone acetonide dental paste (brand names, Kenalog in Orabase®, Oralone®) peanut-sized on the lesion can be used QID for 2 weeks to help with the patients' symptoms. Thrush should be treated with nystatin swish and spit 5 to 10 cc QID in adults and 0.5 cc in each cheek QID in children. If there is no resolution of the symptoms after 2 weeks, the patient should be referred to an otolaryngologist.

MASSES

Fibromas

Fibromas are common growths or masses of the oral cavity that usually arise due to a source of chronic irritation or injury. They are the most common tumor-like growth found in the oral cavity. These lesions generally arise quickly and are most commonly found on the buccal mucosa near the point of dental occlusion although they can arise anywhere in the oral cavity, including the tongue. There are many unusual subtypes of oral fibromas and they are generally classified based on location and histologic characteristics. Pyogenic granuloma is a similar entity and is generally included in this group as well. The most common location for pyogenic granuloma is on the buccal gingiva between teeth. Other lesions in the differential include giant cell fibroma, neurofibroma, salivary gland tumor, giant cell granuloma, and mucocele.

Symptoms and Signs

Fibromas usually present as asymptomatic, smooth, pink, firm nodules up to 2 cm in size. The source of irritation should be investigated and is often found near the lesion. Pyogenic granulomas present as rapidly growing smooth-surfaced mass. It is most common in pregnant patients.

Diagnosis and What Tests to Order

Diagnosis is made by examination and biopsy.

Treatment and When to Refer

As many concerning lesions can arise with the same presentation, a persisting lesion longer than 2 weeks should be referred for biopsy. The diagnosis is made by histology, and the treatment is simple excision. Recurrence rates are low if the irritant is discovered and removed. The most common irritants are dentures or rough edges to teeth.

Papilloma

Squamous papillomas frequently occur in the oral cavity. These lesions are benign and are usually associated with human papilloma virus (HPV) 6 or HPV 11.

Degeneration of papilloma to carcinoma or verrucous leukoplakia is possible but uncommon. In HIV patients, multiple papillomas can be present.

Symptoms and Signs

These lesions present as a painless, solitary pedunculated mass that is warty or with small grapelike extensions on a narrow stalk. The most common oral sites are the buccal, lingual, labial, and soft palatal mucosa.

Diagnosis and What Tests to Order

The warty projection appearance of the lesion is usually sufficient for diagnosis. A comprehensive exam should be done to ensure other sites such as the larynx are clear.

Treatment and When to Refer

Management of papillomas is excision. Except for HIV patients, oral papillomas have a much lower recurrence rate than genital or laryngeal sites.

Minor Salivary Gland Tumors

Tumors of minor salivary glands comprise less than 10% of salivary tumors. Statistically, at least 60% of minor salivary tumors will be malignant. The most common malignancy is adenoid cystic carcinoma. The most common benign tumor of the minor glands is pleomorphic adenoma. As there are many salivary glands in the head and neck, these tumors can arise from many areas from the nasopharynx to the larynx. The most common areas, however, are the hard palate and floor of mouth.

Symptoms and Signs

Minor salivary tumors usually present as a discrete, enlarging, and painless submucosal mass.

Diagnosis and What Tests to Order

Diagnosis is made with biopsy after comprehensive exam and cranial nerve testing. CT may be beneficial if invasion of local structures is suspected.

Treatment/When to Refer

Treatment of minor salivary gland tumors is surgical. Recurrences are fairly common as these tumors tend to have pseudopodia that may project in different directions, which complicate the excision. Treatment of malignant tumors generally involves excision with possible radiation and chemotherapy based on the tumor grade and extent of invasion. The patient should be referred to an otolaryngologist for evaluation and treatment.

Hemangiomas

Oral hemangiomas are not very commonly encountered. They typically follow the similar phases as true hemangiomas being not present at birth, undergoing a rapid proliferation, and then slowly involuting. Hemangiomas of the oral cavity do not solely affect the mucous membranes. They may also involve the oral musculature and bone. The mandible is affected twice as often as the maxilla, and the muscle most commonly invaded is the masseter muscle.

Symptoms and Signs

Mucosal malformations are usually readily identified. Examination of the oral cavity reveals a soft, compressible mucosa with a blue or purple hue. Intramuscular and intraosseous lesions are more difficult to recognize. Intramuscular lesions may not be noticed or discovered on imaging, finding the lesion to be more invasive than suspected. Intraosseous malformations tend to present with loosening teeth, root resorption, bleeding gingiva, or even hemorrhage following dental extraction. The differential for an osseous lesion should also include ameloblastoma or giant cell tumor.

Diagnosis and What Tests to Order

A comprehensive exam should be performed if oral or cutaneous hemangiomas are noted, as they may be present in other areas such as the subglottic region. If evaluation of the oral cavity raises suspicion, MRI of the neck with gadolinium should be the initial test. This should give details regarding the depth of the lesion. Malformations involving bone would be best examined with CT of the neck with contrast including bone windows.

Treatment and When to Refer

The proliferative phase is mainly managed be observation or corticosteroids. Lesions in the involuting phase are observed. Incomplete involution occurs in about 20% of cases and these can be managed via simple excision. Other options include sclerosing agents, laser therapy, or cryotherapy depending on the accessibility of the lesion. Urgent treatment is necessary if the lesion involves the oropharynx or subglottic areas.

Mucocele

Mucoceles or mucous retention cysts are commonly found in the oral cavity. They can be formed from either major or minor salivary glands. A history of trauma (eg, biting, chewing, manual compression) is common. Children and young adults are more commonly affected. Differential diagnosis includes hemangioma, lymphangioma, minor salivary tumor, lipoma, and pyogenic granuloma.

Symptoms and Signs

Mucoceles initially present as small mucus-filled vesicles that are dome shaped and compressible. As the lesion matures, scarring and fibrosis of the lesion may occur and its spontaneous regression decreases. A ranula is a mucocele of the sublingual gland that presents either beneath the tongue as a thin, bulging, transparent structure (like a frog's neck), or as a painless cervical mass.

Diagnosis and What Tests to Order

Diagnosis is made by exam and confirmed on excision. Other testing is generally not necessary unless other lesions in the differential are suspected.

Treatment and When to Refer

Definitive treatment involves excision or marsupialization (opening the cortex of the cyst to allow drainage) of the mucocele. If resection is undertaken, fibrotic portions as well as the involved salivary glands must be removed as well.

Lipoma

Lipomas of the oral cavity are uncommon. They are benign in nature, and are usually found in adults.

Symptoms and Signs

Oral lipomas present as soft, painless, submucosal lesions that are slowly enlarging in the buccal or lingual mucosa, or in the floor of mouth. The differential could include mucocele or neurofibroma.

Diagnosis, Treatment, and When to Refer

Definitive diagnosis and treatment are with simple excision. Recurrence rate is low. A referral to an otolaryngologist for removal is warranted.

Dental Tumors

A variety of dental masses and tumors exist. They are mentioned but not discussed in the context of this text. They include ameloblastoma, odontogenic keratocyst, cementoblastomas, and various bone cysts. These tumors are best treated by oral surgeons.

PRECANCEROUS AND SUSPICIOUS FOR CANCER

Discolorations of oral mucosa are often clinically evident, many of which raise concern for cancer of the oral cavity either due to their appearance or their malignant potential.

Leukoedema

Leukoedema presents as diffuse whitening or clouding of the superficial buccal (cheek) mucosa. It represents a normal variant of tissue chiefly in those with increased pigmentation.

Leukoplakia

Leukoplakia is a term referring to a white superficial plaque on the mucosal surface. Its simple presence does not always signify precancerous potential although it is considered a precursor to cancer. The incidence of developing a cancerous lesion from leukoplakia ranges from 10 to 25% and is related to the degree of dysplasia of the mucosa. The chief risk factor for developing leukoplakia is tobacco in all of its forms. This is not the most common factor for white plaque formation in the mouth, however. Trauma from biting, chewing, or chronic irritation causes a hyperkeratosis that appears as a white plaque more frequently. Frictional trauma is not associated with dysplasia and therefore is not a cancerous precursor. Leukoplakia can appear as a discrete, raised, plaque. Other variants present as an ulcer, erosion, nodular, or verrucous lesion. These characteristics along with site and the degree of dysplasia dictate management options. For example, verrucous leukoplakia has a much higher incidence of degenerating into squamous cell carcinoma. The tongue, floor of mouth, and retromolar trigone are more likely sites to develop carcinoma when leukoplakia is present.

Diagnosis and Treatment

Leukoplakia is classified on biopsy. Once the characteristics are defined as benign, precancerous, or malignant the proper treatment algorithm is prescribed. Benign lesions are observed, and rebiopsied only if changes occur. Premalignant lesions need to be removed. The techniques available include surgery, laser, cryotherapy, and cautery. The patient should be referred to an otolaryngologist for evaluation and treatment.

Erythroplakia

Erythroplakia presents as a red patch on the oral mucosa. It is a precancerous lesion with a higher rate of developing squamous cell carcinoma than leukoplakia. These red plaques or patches are often found along with leukoplakic patches and are usually classified together. They have a much higher incidence of malignant degeneration. The patient should be referred to an otolaryngologist for evaluation and treatment.

Lichen Planus

Lichen planus represents a T-cell mediated inflammatory condition. The chronic inflammatory process forms stria over the buccal mucosa (inside the cheek), tongue, or gingiva. As there is an inflammatory process involved. Lichen planus is present in other inflammatory disorders like lupus, Sjögren's disease, and primary sclerosing cholangitis. Malignancy develops in 5% of affected individuals of the erosive form of lichen planus.

Symptoms and Signs

Lichen planus can present as asymptomatic erythematous stria, or painful erosive ulcerations with fibrinous exudates often with bilateral or multifocal mucosal involvement.

Diagnosis

Reticular lichen planus or the white stria can be diagnosed on examination. For ulcerative, erosive lesions, definitive diagnosis is made on histopathologic examination and immunofluorescence.

Treatment

For asymptomatic lesions, no treatment is necessary and observation is acceptable. Medical therapy can range from topical steroids or tacrolimus, intralesional, or systemic steroids, or immunosuppressive medications. The patient should be referred to an otolaryngologist or oral pathologist for evaluation.

Candida

Candidiasis is a relatively common infection of the mouth and can affect the oral cavity, oropharynx, and oral commissure. Although often part of the body's normal flora, it can arise as an opportunistic infection. Conditions like diabetes mellitus, immunosupression, corticosteroid therapy, antibiotic therapy, denture use, and xerostomia can promote conditions for candidal growth.

Symptoms and Signs

The most recognizable form of oral candida is in multiple pseudomembranes that typically remove easily with scraping. Other signs include a generalized erythema or atrophic appearing mucosa that is tender and may have a burning sensation. Deeply ulcerated areas can be present in immunosupressed individuals. A hyperkeratosis or leukoplakic lesion along the occlusal line may also represent candida. Differential diagnosis of hyperkeratotic lesion includes vitamin deficiency, erythroplakia, leukoplakia, squamous cell carcinoma, and lichen planus.

Diagnosis and Tests to Order

In most candidal lesions, the clinical presentation is sufficient for diagnosis. Potassium hydroxide (KOH) smear or periodic acid-Schiff may confirm suspicions. For more difficult hyperkeratotic lesions, biopsy may be required to rule out other pathology. Fungal cultures can be obtained with the understanding that a positive culture can be present in 50% of normal adults.

Treatment and When to Refer

Medical therapy includes topical and or systemic anti-fungal agents. Topical forms are commonly sufficient for treatment, reserving the systemic treatments for the more severe forms of the disease. Nystatin swish and spit 5cc QID (in children 1-2 cc QID) should be used for 5 to 10 days (48 hours after symptom resolution). If the patient wears dentures, the dentures need to be cleaned using nystatin and a toothbrush to prevent reinoculation.

Squamous Cell Carcinoma

Squamous cell carcinoma (SCC) of the oral cavity can develop from a variety of genetic and environmental factors. The genetic capability to react to alterations in the cell cycle have a known component in developing carcinoma placing the oral cavity at risk with its continually dividing cells. Carcinogenic toxins like tobacco, betel nuts (used in south and southeast Asian countries), and alcohol have known roles as well. Other risk factors include poor dentition, lower socioeconomic status and chronic inflammation. Keys to a good prognosis for oral carcinoma hinge on early detection. The most common oral cavity sites are lower lip, lateral tongue, and floor of mouth.

Symptoms and Signs

SCC can present as a red or white plaque, ulcer, erosion, mass, or exophitic lesion. Symptoms can vary from asymptomatic to extreme pain. Lymph node involvement is of importance to note as there is generally an increased mortality of 50% when nodes are positive.

Diagnosis and What Tests to Order

Malignancy is confirmed on biopsy of the lesion. Once performed, additional workup should include a complete blood count, and comprehensive metabolic profile. Imaging should include a photograph of the lesion if possible, CT to analyze the degree of spread, and a chest radiograph. Panorex may be needed for possible mandibular invasion. Other portions of the metastatic workup may include MRI or FDG-PET scan.

Treatment and When to Refer

Referral should be made to an otolaryngologist and ideally a head and neck cancer specialist at a head and neck cancer center where treatment can be coordinated with radiation and medical oncologists when indicated. Multimodality treatment is necessary for advanced disease. For local disease only, treatment may include surgical excision or radiation.

Black/Pigmented

Black or dark pigmented lesions of the oral cavity exist from many different etiologies. Some are associated with syndromes or medications, and others may be from implanted materials such as dental amalgam. The major concern of pigmented lesions is the aggressiveness and prognosis of mucosal melanoma even though its incidence is less than 1% of melanoma cases. Medications commonly associated with mucosal pigmentation include quinine, minocycline, estrogen, 5-fluorouracil, and doxorubicin.

Melanotic macules are discrete and uniformly pigmented with defined margins. They generally occur along the vermilion border. They are not considered to have malignant potential. Macules are often associated with syndromes such as Peutz-Jegher's syndrome and can be present in systemic disorders like Addison's disease. Melanotic nevi are rare in the oral cavity and occur twice as often in females. They are considered to be a precursor to melanoma as they arise from altered melanocytes. Nevi are found along the buccal mucosa, labial mucosa, gingiva, and alveolus.

Mucosal melanoma tends to occur more often in African-American and Asian populations although rare even in them. Those that arise from a precursor lesion become flat with variations in borders and pigments. Nodular lesions can present de novo and tend to grow rapidly. Sites most commonly involved in melanoma are hard and soft palate, and the gingiva. Most melanomas are treated with excision. The remainder of treatment varies based on depth, sites, invasion, and so forth. As previously mentioned, prognosis is generally poor regardless of site.

DRY MOUTH

Dry mouth can be caused by side effects of certain medications, nasal obstruction (chronic mouth breathing), systemic disease (eg, Sjögren's, diabetes mellitus, etc), loss of salivary gland mass (secondary to radiation), smoking, or dehydration (Table 17–1). The treatment is dependent on the cause. For medications, changing the regimen will generally help. In disorders such as Sjögren's and postradiation dry mouth, salivation stimulants (eg, pilocarpine 5 mg po QD, or cevimeline 30 mg PO tid) or the use of artificial saliva may help. Depending on the etiology, the patient may need referral if the systemic disease is uncontrolled or if medical management does not improve symptoms.

DROOLING

Drooling generally is not caused by hypersalivation, but rather poor control of normal salivation. It is generally normal up to the age of 6. Drooling after the age of 6 years is generally seen in patients with neuromuscular disorders such as cerebral palsy (CP), amyotrophic lateral sclerosis (ALS), Parkinson's disease, trauma, stroke, facial paralysis, severe mental retardation, seizures, encephalopathy, or encephalitis. Because of the difficulty in coordinating the oral phase of swallow, the patients will develop salivary pooling and spillage. Drooling can be seen as a side effect of some

Table 17–1. Differential Diagnosis of Dry Mouth

Nasal obstruction

Smoking

Diabetes mellitus

Sjögren's syndrome

Postradiation to the upper aerodigestive tract

Drugs

Anticholinergic agents: atropine, atropinics, and hyoscine

Proton-pump inhibitors (eg, omeprazole)

Antidepressants, including tricyclic compounds

Phenothiazines

Benzodiazepines

Antihistamines

Bupropion

Opioids

Antihypertensives: alpha-1 antagonists (eg, terazosin and prazosin); alpha-2 agonists (eg, clonidine); beta-blockers (eg, atenolol, propanolol), which also alter salivary protein levels

Diuretics

medications including clozapine, lithium, and parasympathetics (cholinergics and anticholinesterases). The treatment consists of oral motor therapy (by a speech pathologist), anticholinergics (eg, glycopyrrolate 1–2 mg po BID-TID, children, 0.05 mg/kg po Q4-8hrs), or surgical therapy. The pediatric patient should be referred to a pediatric otolaryngologist for evaluation and treatment. The adult patient rarely will require surgical treatment and changing medications or speech therapy generally will suffice.

HALITOSIS

Halitosis is a symptom rather than a disease. It can be caused by multiple problems including chronic sinusitis, dental caries, dorsal tongue bacterial infestation, chronic tonsillitis, tonsillith, laryngopharyngeal reflux, or an upper aerodigestive tract malignancy. It is most commonly caused by overgrowth of anaerobic bacteria in the upper aerodigestive tract.

Symptoms and Signs

The patients will complain of a foul odor to their breath. A history of post-nasal drainage, sour taste in the pharynx, dental caries, sore throat, swallowing or voice disturbance, or foul smelling white foreign bodies from the tonsils should be obtained. If a heavy tobacco or alcohol history is present, a malignant tumor of the upper aerodigestive tract should be on the differential diagnosis. A complete examination of the teeth, tongue, pharynx, and nose should be performed.

Diagnosis and What Tests to Order

The diagnosis is dependent on the etiologic factor and will be based on the history and examination.

Treatment and When to Refer

Dental caries should be referred to a dentist. If an acute abscess (granulation tissue or swelling on the gingival) is seen, clindamycin 300 mg po QID (in children, 20 mg/kg/d divided TID or QID) for 7 days will help relieve the acute infection until the patient sees the dentist. If the dorsal tongue does not have the normal red or pink appearance to it (eg, brown, white, or black), the patients should be instructed to use their tooth brush to brush the dorsal tongue.

Patients with chronic tonsillitis should be treated with a 2 week course of clindamycin 300 mg po QID (in children, 20 mg/kg/d divided TID or QID). Chronic sinusitis can be treated with a 2 to 3 week course of nasal steroid (eg, fluticasone or mometasone) 2 puffs (one puff in children) each nostril QD and amoxicillin/clavulonate 875 mg BID (in children, 40 mg/kg/d divided TID). A referral to an otolaryngologist for nasal endoscopy is warranted if the symptom continues despite the above measures. Laryngopharyngeal reflux treatment is outlined in Chapter 18, Sore Throat. Treatment of tonsilliths is outlined in Chapter 20 on swallowing problems. If there is no improvement of the symptoms within 3 weeks, the patient should be referred to an otolaryngologist for laryngoscopy to rule out a malignancy.

FURTHER READING

Gupta A, Epstein JB, Sroussi H. Hyposalivation in elderly patients. *J Can Dent Assoc.* 2006;72:841–846.

Lal D, Hotaling AJ. Drooling. *Curr Opin Otolaryngol Head Neck Surg.* 2006;14:381–386.

CHAPTER 18

Sore Throat

MEHDI SINA-KHADIV
PAUL SCHALCH
VICTOR PASSY
HAMID R. DJALILIAN

BACKGROUND

The pain and discomfort associated with a sore throat drive millions of children and adults to seek medical attention in emergency departments[1] and from their primary care physicians annually, accounting for up to 2% of such visits, yet most sore throats are self-limited. The most common causes of sore throats are viruses, including the ones responsible for the common cold or influenza (Fig 18–1). The most important bacterial cause of sore throat is group A beta-hemolytic *Streptococcus* (GAS), accounting for about 10 to 30% of cases —it is also the major treatable cause of sore throat. The most common microbial causes of sore throat are listed in Table 18–1. One of the major challenges physicians face when dealing with sore throat is identifying those patients who require specific antimicrobial agents

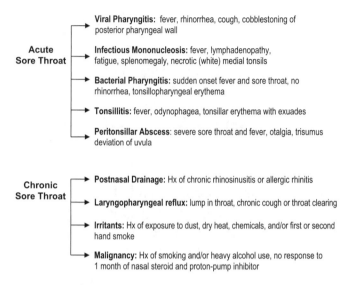

Acute Sore Throat

Viral Pharyngitis: fever, rhinorrhea, cough, cobblestoning of posterior pharyngeal wall

Infectious Mononucleosis: fever, lymphadenopathy, fatigue, splenomegaly, necrotic (white) medial tonsils

Bacterial Pharyngitis: sudden onset fever and sore throat, no rhinorrhea, tonsillopharyngeal erythema

Tonsillitis: fever, odynophagea, tonsillar erythema with exuades

Peritonsillar Abscess: severe sore throat and fever, otalgia, trisumus deviation of uvula

Chronic Sore Throat

Postnasal Drainage: Hx of chronic rhinosinusitis or allergic rhinitis

Laryngopharyngeal reflux: lump in throat, chronic cough or throat clearing

Irritants: Hx of exposure to dust, dry heat, chemicals, and/or first or second hand smoke

Malignancy: Hx of smoking and/or heavy alcohol use, no response to 1 month of nasal steroid and proton-pump inhibitor

Fig 18–1. The most common causes of sore throat.

and attempting to minimize the unnecessary use of these agents in patients who will not benefit from such therapy. With rare exception, GAS is the only treatable cause of sore throat; however, 75% of patients seen by physicians receive antibiotic therapy. The discussion in this section focuses on acute versus chronic causes of sore throat as well as adult versus pediatric causes of sore throat.

ADULT ACUTE SORE THROAT

Viral Pharyngitis

Viruses are responsible for 85 to 95% of sore throats in adults.[2] The major causes of viral pharyngitis include influenza, parainfluenza, coronavirus, rhinovirus, adenovirus, enterovirus, herpes simplex virus (HSV), Epstein-

Table 18–1. Microbial Causes of Acute Pharyngitis

	Pathogen
Bacterial	Streptococcus, group A
	Streptococcus, groups C, G
	Mixed anaerobes
	Neisseria gonorrhoeae
	Corynebacterium diphtheriae
Viral	Rhinovirus
	Coronavirus
	Adenovirus
	Herpes simplex type 1 & 2
	Parainfluenza
	Coxsackie A
	Epstein-Barr virus
	Cytomegalovirus
	Human immunodeficiency virus
	Influenza A, B

Barr virus (EBV), and the human immunodeficiency virus (HIV). None of these organisms presents a unique clinical picture which complicates the ability of physicians to distinguish among the pathogens. The major goal of the physician is to identify patients with GAS pharyngitis in order to prescribe antibiotics to these patients and to avoid treating viral causes of sore throat with antibiotics. The discussion here concentrates on the common viruses that cause pharyngitis (coronavirus, rhinovirus, and adenovirus).

Symptoms and Signs

Symptoms and signs of viral pharyngitis include sore throat, discomfort or difficulty in swallowing, fever, tender and enlarged lymph nodes in the neck, and joint pain or muscle aches. The patients will commonly have postnasal drainage or nasal congestion. The examination shows mild to moderate erythema of the pharynx with cobblestoning of the posterior pharyngeal wall. This cobblestoning represents hypertrophy of pharyngeal lymphoid tissue.

Diagnosis and What Tests to Order

Several formulae incorporating epidemiologic and clinical factors of sore throat have been devised which improve diagnostic accuracy primarily by identifying patients with a very low risk of GAS infection. Factors indicating low risk include the absence of fever and pharyngeal erythema, and the presence of obvious signs and symptoms of a viral upper respiratory infection (URI)—nasal congestion and drainage, cough. Unless the clinician can rule out streptococcal infection with great confidence on the basis of clinical and epidemiologic evidence, patients with acute pharyngitis should be tested for the presence of GAS. This can be done with either a throat culture or a Rapid Streptococcal Antigen Test (RSAT). A negative RSAT and the presence of signs and symptoms of a viral URI allow for the diagnosis of viral pharyngitis. Occasionally in the early stage of strep pharyngitis, the RSAT may not be positive but the culture examination will show GAS growth. Therefore, it is recommended that a culture of the pharynx be obtained when signs and symptoms of a URI are absent and RSAT is negative.

Treatment and When to Refer

Symptomatic patients will benefit from rest, maintenance of adequate oral hydration, acetaminophen and nonsteroidal anti-inflammatory drugs (NSAIDs) if fever and pain are present, and gargling with warm salt water. Over-the-counter lozenges containing menthol and mild local anesthetics also provide temporary relief from severe throat pain. Topical lidocaine spray can be used for symptomatic relief as well. For a great majority of cases of viral pharyngitis, no further therapy is necessary; however, if patients encounter difficulty breathing, or have sore throat for greater than two weeks, they should be referred to an otolaryngologist for further workup.

Infectious Mononucleosis

Infectious mononucleosis (IM) is an illness caused by the Epstein-Barr virus. EBV is transmitted by intimate contact with body secretions, primarily oropharyngeal secretions such as saliva. Coughing, kissing, and sharing utensils all contribute to EBV transmission.

Symptoms and Signs

The classic features of IM include the triad of fever, sore throat, and lymphadenopathy in the presence of fatigue. Occasionally, splenomegaly, palatal petechiae, and rash (following ampicillin or amoxicillin administration) are seen. The fever is usually low grade and chills are uncommon. A history of sore throat frequently is accompanied by pharyngeal inflammation and tonsillar exudates which can appear white, gray-green, or even necrotic (The classical appearance of the tonsils in IM is that of medial necrosis on both tonsils). Additionally, palatal petechiae with streaky hemorrhages and blotchy red macules can be present, although this finding has also been seen in patients with streptococcal pharyngitis. Characteristically, the lymphadenopathy is symmetric and more typically involves the anterior and posterior cervical chains with large and moderately tender nodes. Also, a distinguishing feature of sore throat caused by IM is that the lymphadenopathy may become more generalized. Lastly, the lymphadenopathy peaks in the first week and then gradually subsides over 2 to 3 weeks. Recent studies have shown that in patients with IM, lymphadenopathy was present in all patients, fever in 98%, and pharyngitis in 85% of patients.[3] IM typically presents with a prodrome of malaise, headache, and low-grade fever before development of these more specific signs.

Diagnosis and What Tests to Order

In young adults with the classic triad of fever, sore throat, and lymphadenopaty, EBV-induced IM should be suspected. The necrotic appearance of the medial aspect of the tonsils is a characteristic finding. To confirm clinical suspicion, a test for heterophile antibodies (Mono spot test) and a peripheral blood smear can be ordered—patients positive for heterophile antibodies are diagnosed with IM. Furthermore, a peripheral blood smear with atypical lymphocytosis in heterophile-positive patients more sensitively diagnoses IM. Lastly, in patients with early signs and symptoms of IM, a negative heterophile antibody test should not rule out EBV infection, as the rates of false negative tests can reach up to 25% in the first week of infection. A repeat heterophile antibody test or tests for specific EBV antibodies should be performed.

Treatment and When to Refer

The standard approach to treating individuals with IM is supportive care. Acetaminophen (500 Q 6hrs) and NSAIDs reduce or entirely alleviate the fever, sore throat, and malaise that plague infected persons. Adequate oral hydration and nutrition are also important. Finally, adequate rest is important; however, complete bed rest is both unnecessary and discouraged. Referral to an otolaryngologist is warranted if the clinical picture and laboratory are conflicted.

The use of corticosteroids in the treatment of EBV-induced IM has not been demonstrated to be effective. A meta-analysis of seven studies did not find sufficient evidence to recommend steroid treatment for symptom relief; moreover, two studies reported severe complications in patients receiving corticosteroid compared to placebo.[4] Therefore, corticosteroid therapy is not recommended for routine cases of IM as it is generally a self-limited illness. Patients with IM should be seen by a specialist if symptoms persist beyond 3 to 4 weeks or signs or symptoms of airway obstruction or splenic rupture become apparent. The patient should be advised against participating in activities that involve contact to the abdomen (eg, sports, etc) to prevent the possibility of a splenic rupture.

Bacterial Pharyngitis

There are a number of bacterial organisms that can cause sore throat—including group A *Streptococcus*, non-group A *Streptococcus*, mixed anaerobes, and *Neisseria gonorrhoeae*. Of these organisms, GAS is the major treatable cause of sore throat.

Group A Beta-Hemolytic Streptococcus

GAS accounts for approximately 5 to 10% of cases of sore throat in adults.

Symptoms and Signs. The characteristic clinical findings suggestive of GAS pharyngitis include a sudden

onset of sore throat and fever, tonsillopharyngeal exudates, anterior cervical lymphadenitis, and leukocytosis.
It is important to note that if cough and rhinorrhea are
present, a viral cause of sore throat is more likely.

Diagnosis and What Tests to Order. It is of utmost
importance for the physician to determine if a case of
sore throat is caused by GAS versus other microbial
causes; in such a case, the Centor criteria may be useful. The Centor criteria call for evaluation of patients
with sore throat for, (1) tonsillar exudates, (2) tender
cervical adenopathy, (3) fever, and (4) lack of cough.
The more criteria that are met, the higher the likelihood of GAS infection and thus the need to perform
either a RSAT or pharyngeal culture to confirm the
diagnosis. The presence of three or four of the criteria
indicates that the chance of GAS is approximately 40
to 60%. The absence of three or four of the criteria
indicates a 20% chance of GAS infection.

Treatment and When to Refer. The treatment of choice
for group A streptococcal pharyngitis is a 10-day course
of oral penicillin (Pen VK 500 mg po QID, in children
amoxicillin 90 mg/kg/d divided TID) because this agent
has proven efficacy, a narrow spectrum, safety, and
low cost. In cases of penicillin allergy, erythromycin
(400 mg po QID, in children 40 mg/kg/d divided TID)
or azithromycin (500 mg po QD for 3 days, in children
10 mg/kg/d divided QD for 3 days) can be used. When
treating GAS pharyngitis, the objectives are to prevent
supportive complications such as peritonsillar or retropharyngeal abscess, cervical lymphadenitis, and renal
or cardiac valvular involvement. Treating GAS will prevent rheumatic fever and decrease infectivity. The
patients generally will not spread the infection after
72 hours of antibiotic therapy and may return to work/
school at that point. Typically, antibiotics do not shorten

the clinical course of the disease significantly as the great majority of patients with sore throat caused by GAS will have resolution of symptoms within 3 to 4 days even without therapy. The antibiotics will help reduce the chance of complications of GAS including rheumatic heart disease, and so forth. If there is no resolution of symptoms after treatment, or patients begin to complain for difficulty breathing or "hot potato" voice, or on examination there is medial displacement of the tonsils, lateral displacement of the uvula, or trismus, the patients should be referred to an otolaryngologist for evaluation of a peritonsillar abscess. Patients with more than 6 GAS infection in a year will benefit from tonsillectomy as the tonsils are colonized by GAS and cause the recurrent infection.

Neiserria gonorrhoeae

Neisseria gonorrhoeae is a rare, sexually transmitted cause of acute pharyngitis seen in some patients. Although colonization of the pharynx with *N. gonorrhoeae* is usually asymptomatic, clinically apparent pharyngitis sometimes develops, and pharyngeal colonization may be associated with disseminated disease.

Symptoms and Signs. When symptomatic oral infections occur, pharyngitis is the most common manifestation. Most commonly these patients will present after 10 days of penicillin therapy for a presumed strep pharyngitis with continued symptoms. Signs to look for on exam include an erythematous pharynx, bilateral tonsillar enlargement, significant exudates, and other signs of *N. gonorrhoeae* infection such as urethral discharge and dysuria.

Diagnosis and What Tests to Order. The diagnosis should be confirmed by throat culture on Thayer-Martin medium.

Treatment and When to Refer. If the case is uncomplicated, treatment consists of a single 125-mg dose of
intramuscular ceftriaxone. Cefixime 400 mg orally in
a single dose can be given. Consideration should be
given to treatment of possible concomitant chlamydial
urethritis infection as the two tend to occur together
commonly. If the above treatment fails, the patient
should be referred to an otolaryngologist.

Tonsillitis

The tonsils are lymphoid tissues that act as part of the
immune system to clear bacteria and other microorganisms from the oropharynx. When foreign matter
enters the body through the mouth, the tonsils act as
a filter—trapping microorganisms and setting off the
immune response to attack the invading particles. The
resulting immune reaction is a kind of low-grade infection in the tonsils. Tonsillitis occurs when the infection
gets more serious, and the tonsils become painful and
inflamed. Like other causes of sore throat, most cases
of tonsillitis are viral and less often caused by bacteria.

Symptoms and Signs

The typical features of tonsillitis include red, inflamed
tonsils, white or yellow tonsillar crypts or exudates,
sore throat with painful swallowing, fever, and enlarged
lymph nodes in the neck.

Diagnosis and What Tests to Order

The diagnosis of tonsillitis involves clinical suspicion,
a thorough physical examination, and laboratory tests
including throat culture or RSAT, a CBC to rule out a

more serious infection, or a heterophile antibody test to determine if the sore throat is caused by IM.

Treatment and When to Refer

If the rapid strep test is positive or the throat culture grows streptococcus, a 10-day course of oral penicillin (Pen VK 500 mg QID) should be prescribed. If the cause of tonsillitis is determined to be viral, supportive care with acetaminophen and NSAIDs for fever and pain, adequate oral hydration, gargling with salt water, and lozenges containing menthol and local anesthetics (eg, lidocaine spray) are enough to provide symptomatic relief until the tonsillitis resolves. Recurrent tonsillitis (more than 6 per year) warrants a referral to an otolaryngologist for a tonsillectomy. Other reasons for referral include asymmetric tonsils, tonsillar hypertrophy in a post-transplant patient, or infection spread beyond tonsils (eg, peritonsillar abscess).

Peritonsillar Abscess

Peritonsillar abscesses are the most common deep infections of the head and neck in adults with the highest incidence between the ages of 20 to 40 years. Traditionally, peritonsillar abscesses have been regarded as the endpoint of a spectrum that begins as acute tonsillitis, progresses to cellulitis, and eventually forms an abscess in the capsule that attaches the tonsil to the pharyngeal wall. A group of 20 to 25 mucous salivary glands, called Weber's glands, located in the space just superior to the tonsil in the soft palate, have been implicated in the formation of peritonsillar abscesses.[5] Weber's glands function to clear the tonsillar area of any trapped debris and if they become inflamed, local cellulitis can develop—the resulting scarring and obstruction of the ducts that drain these glands may progress to abscess formation. A peritonsillar abscess can progress into a parapharyngeal space abscess. A parapharyngeal space abscess will then progress inferiorly and compromise the airway at the hypopharyngeal level.

Symptoms and Signs

Patients with peritonsillar or parapharyngeal space abscess present with severe sore throat (that can be unilateral), fever, malaise, odynophagia, and otalgia. The throat pain is significantly worse on the affected side and is often referred to the ear on the same side (because of the irritation of the glossopharyngeal nerve that travels behind the tonsil). On physical examination trismus (inability to open the mouth) is a common finding and may complicate the examination. With a clear view of the oropharynx, there may be an obvious abscess at the superior pole of the affected tonsil and markedly tender cervical lymphadenitis may be palpated on the affected side. Alternatively, instead of seeing the exudate, the affected tonsil may be extremely swollen with contralateral deviation of the uvula. Swallowing is also highly painful, resulting in pooling of saliva or drooling. Patients often speak in a muffled or "hot potato voice."

Diagnosis and What Tests to Order

Peritonsillar abscesses are almost always first encountered by primary care or emergency department physicians, and those with appropriate training and experience can diagnose and treat most patients. The diagnosis of peritonsillar abscess frequently is made based on a thorough history and physical examination. The differential diagnosis is lengthy and includes infectious mononucleosis, peritonsillar cellulitis, and parapharyngeal abscess. In cases when the diagnosis of peritonsillar abscess is in question, radiographic imaging or the finding of pus on needle aspiration above the tonsils may help confirm the diagnosis. Ultrasonography, either transcutaneous or intraoral, can be helpful in identifying an abscess and in distinguishing peritonsillar abscess from peritonsillar cellulitis. If it is suspected that the infection has spread beyond the peritonsillar space or some complication involving the lateral neck space is suspected, a computed tomography (CT) scan with contrast is needed.

Treatment and When to Refer

The keys to effectively treating peritonsillar abscesses are to adequately drain the abscess and start antibiotic therapy—this combination results in resolution of the abscess in 90% of cases. The main procedures for the drainage of peritonsillar abscesses are needle aspiration, incision and drainage, and immediate tonsillectomy. In the absence of a previous history of recurrent pharyngitis, a needle aspiration or incision and drainage above the tonsil are preferred to tonsillectomy. Needle aspiration or incision should be made after topical and injected lidocaine, though lidocaine generally does not work well in an infected area. The patient should be given a Yankauer suction to hold in their mouth to help with clearing saliva and any pus. A 16-g needle attached to a 10-cc syringe should be inserted above the tonsil where the greatest bulge exists. The needle should never be inserted lateral to the tonsil to avoid the external carotid artery. If the bulging area above the tonsil is pulsatile, otolaryngology consultation should be obtained prior to insertion of a needle due to the rare possibility of aberrant carotid artery course.

Initial empiric antibiotic therapy should include antimicrobials effective against group A *Streptococcus* and oral anaerobes. The favored regimens include oral amoxicillin-clavulanate (875 mg po BID × 10 days, children 40 mg/kg/d divided BID) or clindamycin (300 mg po QID for 10 days, children 20 mg/kg/d divided po QID × 10 days). The patient should be asked to eat some yogurt daily to prevent diarrhea. In emergency cases or if oral therapy cannot be used, parenteral ampicillin-sulbactam (1.5 g IV Q 6hrs, children 200 mg/kg divided Q 6hrs) or clindamycin (900 mg IV Q 8hrs, children 30 mg/kg/d divided Q 8hrs) can be used with equal success. Abscess pockets discovered on CT imaging that are less than 1 cm are generally treated with antibiotics and do not require drainage. The indications for admission include inability to drink with signs of dehydration and spread of infection beyond the peritonsillar area (see below). A parapharyngeal space abscess requires drainage through the neck and should be admitted to the hospital with an otolaryngology consultation for urgent management.

The complications of peritonsillar abscess are numerous and potentially fatal; they include airway obstruction, hemorrhage from erosion of the carotid sheath, thrombosis of the internal jugular vein, aspiration pneumonitis or lung abscess from ruptured peritonsillar abscess, mediastinitis, jugular vein suppurative thrombophlebitis—or Lemierre's syndrome. If any of these complications are suspected the patient should immediately be admitted to the hospital and otolaryngology consultation should be obtained.

Postnasal Drainage

Postnasal drainage at the onset of a viral URI can cause a sore throat. For detailed information on treatment, see Chapter 13 on nasal discharge.

ADULT CHRONIC SORE THROAT

Chronic sore throat in an adult is most commonly due to postnasal drainage or laryngopharyngeal reflux disease. Empiric treatment with a nasal steroid spray (eg, fluticasone or mometasone 2 puffs QD) and a proton-pump inhibitor (eg, omeprazole 40 mg po QAM 1 hour before breakfast) can be tried for 1 month in a patient with no smoking or heavy alcohol use. A patient with a smoking history or heavy alcohol use and chronic sore throat will need to be referred to an otolaryngologist for laryngoscopy to rule out a malignancy of the upper respiratory tract.

Laryngopharyngeal Reflux

Laryngopharyngeal reflux (LPR) is an entity distinct from gastroesophageal reflux disease (GERD). Whereas retrograde movement of gastric contents into the esophagus is defined as GERD, LPR is the backflow of stomach contents into the laryngopharynx. The incidence of heartburn in LPR is <40%, whereas the incidence of esophagitis in LPR is 25%. Therefore, the majority of patients with LPR do not have esophagitis, the diagnostic sine qua non of GERD. The major differences in LPR and GERD are outlined in Table 18–2.

Symptoms and Signs

Patients with LPR will present with a variety of complaints as outlined in Table 18–3. Examination may show erythema and cobblestoning of the posterior pharyngeal wall. The laryngeal mirror examination will show erythema of the vocal folds and the posterior

Table 18–2. Differences Between GERD and LPR

Laryngopharyngeal Reflux	Gastroesophageal Reflux
Upright (daytime) or supine refluxers	Supine (nocturnal) refluxers
Short duration of acid exposure	Prolonged periods of acid exposure
Normal esophageal motility and acid clearance	Dysmotility and prolonged esophageal acid clearance
Heartburn uncommon	Heartburn present in nearly all
Upper esophageal sphincter dysfunction.	Lower esophageal sphincter dysfunction

Table 18–3. Presenting Symptoms of Patients LPR Patients

Chronic sore throat	Chronic dysphonia
"Postnasal drip"/"chronic phlegm"	Intermittent dysphonia
Chronic cough	Vocal fatigue
Dysphagia	Voice breaks
Globus	Chronic throat clearing
Intermittent airway obstruction	Excessive throat mucus
Wheezing	Chronic airway obstruction

aspect of the larynx (arytenoids and postcricoid region) at the opening of the esophagus.

Diagnosis and What Tests to Order

The diagnosis of LPR generally is clinical and dependent on history and laryngeal exam findings. If the larynx cannot be visualized in the primary care setting, a trial of empiric therapy with proton-pump inhibitors (PPI) can be given. Dual-pH probe (one probe below the upper esophageal sphincter and one above the lower esophageal sphincter) testing over 24 hours can help with the diagnosis, but is only necessary if a trial of PPI fails and all symptoms and signs point to LPR.

Treatment and When to Refer

The first line of treatment for LPR is PPI therapy (eg, omeprazole 40 mg po QAM 1 hour before breakfast). The patients should be instructed on the importance of reflux precautions (Table 18–4). Sometimes twice-a-day therapy must be used if the patient continues to have symptoms at night. The nightly dose has to be given 1 hour before breakfast. Esomeprazole has the longest half-life of all the PPIs currently available on the market in the United States. The patient should be referred to an otolaryngologist if symptoms are not significantly improved after 1 month of therapy. A chronic

Table 18–4. Reflux Precautions Instructions for Patients

Dietary

Foods to avoid: citrus, tomato, vinegar, high fat foods (fried, etc), coffee and caffeinated beverages, alcohol, and peppermint

Behavioral

Avoid eating 3 to 4 hours prior sleeping

No smoking

Eat smaller meals

Avoid exercising after eating

Avoid wearing garment with a tight waist (eg, pants, etc)

sore throat which does not improve with PPI therapy, especially in a patient who has a history of heavy alcohol usage or smoking, can represent a first sign of an upper aerodigestive tract malignancy.

Carcinoma of the Upper Aerodigestive Tract

Carcinoma of the tonsil, base of tongue, oropharynx, hypopharynx, or larynx can present with a chronic sore throat, dysphagia, odynophagia, or a chronic otalgia (referred pain from irritation of cranial nerve IX or X). These cancers, most commonly squamous cell carcinomas, generally will present in patients with a history of heavy smoking (present or past) or a heavy alcohol use.

Symptoms and Signs

The patients most commonly will present with a chronic sore throat. The patient may also have symptoms described above. The examination may show a mass or ulcer in the pharynx or tonsillar area or may be normal. A normal examination does not rule out an occult carcinoma submucosally located in the base of the tongue or one located in the larynx or hypopharynx which will not be seen on a routine oropharyngeal examination.

Diagnosis and What Tests to Order

The diagnosis depends on tissue biopsy. However, a chronic sore throat (>3 weeks) in a smoker or alcohol abuser with an ulcer in conjunction with an ulcer or mass in the upper aerodigestive tract should make the physician highly suspicious of cancer. A biopsy of the lesion or ulcer should be performed if easily accessible. Otherwise, the patient should be referred to an otolaryngologist for biopsy. A CT scan of the neck with contrast is obtained to evaluate for metastasis to the neck.

Treatment and When to Refer

The treatment of carcinoma of the upper aerodigestive tract involves multidisciplinary treatment by a head and neck cancer team.

Irritants

Throat irritation from dust, low humidity and dry heat, chemicals, first or secondhand smoke, and air pollution can all lead to chronic sore throat. Avoidance is the best treatment. Referral to an otolaryngologist for laryngoscopy is warranted if avoidance does not improve the symptoms within a month.

PEDIATRIC ACUTE SORE THROAT

Viral Pharyngitis

Viruses are the most common cause of acute pharyngitis in children. Respiratory viruses, such as influenza virus, parainfluenza virus, coronavirus, rhinovirus, and adenovirus are frequent causes of acute pharyngitis. Other viral causes of acute pharyngitis include coxsackievirus, echovirus, and herpes simplex virus. Most cases of pharyngitis occur during the winter and early spring, when respiratory viruses are most prevalent.

Symptoms and Signs

Some general features of viral causes of sore throat include coryza, cough, diarrhea, and characteristic exanthems. The sore throat caused by adenovirus may be associated with conjunctivitis and fever—referred to as pharyngoconjunctival fever; the pharyngitis and the conjunctivitis can persist for 7 and 14 days, respectively. Herpangina, characterized by fever and painful, discrete, gray-white papulovesicular lesions on an erythematous base on the soft palate, is a specific syndrome caused by coxsackievirus or echoviruses. These lesions become ulcerative and usually resolve within 7 days. Finally, a specific syndrome caused by coxsackievirus A16, hand-foot-mouth disease, is characterized by painful vesicles and ulcers throughout the oropharynx associated with vesicles on the palms, soles, and sometimes on the trunk or extremities. These lesions usually resolve within 7 days.

Diagnosis and What Tests to Order

Diagnosing viral pharyngitis is based on clinical and epidemiologic factors, the Centor criteria (see beginning of chapter) can be employed to assess the risk of GAS pharyngitis—patients with high risk of GAS infection can get a RSAT and/or throat cultures, whereas those at low risk can receive supportive care.

Treatment and When to Refer

Viral causes of sore throat are usually benign and self-limiting. Supportive care with acetaminophen and NSAIDs, oral hydration, gargling with salt water, and topical anesthetic spray (eg, lidocaine) are enough to ameliorate the symptoms until the viral infection resolves. Stridor, signs of respiratory distress, drooling, and changes in the voice could signify serious and life-threatening infections and require immediate evaluation by an otolaryngologist.

Infectious Mononucleosis

See adult section above.

Bacterial Pharyngitis

See adult section above.

Group A Beta-Hemolytic Streptococcus

See adult section above. The only difference between adults and children with GAS is that in children younger than 3 years of age, symptoms are atypical and include nasal congestion and discharge, low-grade fever, and anterior cervical adenopathy. In such cases, patients typically have contacts that are infected with GAS. Treatment in children is with amoxicillin 80 mg/kg divided TID (penicillin allergics, erythromycin ES 40 mg/kg divided 2 to 4 times a day) for 10 days.

Epiglottitis

See Chapter 21, Airway Obstruction.

Tonsillitis

See adult section above.

Peritonsillar Abscess

See adult section above.

CHRONIC PEDIATRIC SORE THROAT

Chronic Rhinosinusitis with Postnasal Drip

Chronic rhinosinusitis is defined as inflammation of the mucosa of the nose and paranasal sinuses lasting for at least 12 consecutive weeks. It is the most commonly diagnosed chronic illness in the United States. Postnasal discharge can be a cause of chronic sore throat in children as well. The most common cause of chronic sinusitis in children beyond allergy treatment is adenoid hypertrophy. The best first line of treatment of chronic sinusitis in children is adenoidectomy. The patient should be referred to an otolaryngologist for evaluation. Treatment with nasal steroids (eg, mometasone 1 puff QD each nostril) can be given for parents who are reluctant for their children to undergo surgery. If symptoms do not improve significantly with nasal steroids, a referral to an otolaryngologist is warranted.

Irritants

See adult section above.

Miscellaneous Causes

Chronic causes of sore throat in children include laryngopharyngeal reflux, chronic mouth breathing (secondary to adenoid hyperplasia), voice abuse, and connective tissue disorders and malignancy. If the patient's symptoms do not fit the disorders described above, the patient should be referred to a pediatric otolaryngologist for further evaluation.

REFERENCES

1. Armstrong GL, Pinner RW. Outpatient visits for infectious diseases in the United States, 1980 through 1996. *Arch Intern Med.* 1999;159(21):2531-2536.
2. Worrall GJ. Acute sore throat. *Can Fam Physician.* 2007;53(11):1961-1962.
3. Rea TD, Russo JE, Katon W, Ashley RL, Buchwald DS. Prospective study of the natural history of infectious mononucleosis caused by Epstein-Barr virus. *J Am Board Fam Pract.* 2001;14(4):234-242.
4. Candy B, Hotopf M. Steroids for symptom control in infectious mononucleosis. *Cochrane Database Syst Rev.* 2006;3:CD004402.
5. Passy V. Pathogenesis of peritonsillar abscess. *Laryngoscope.* 1994;104:185-190.

CHAPTER 19

Hoarseness

ESTHER L. FINE
ROGER L. CRUMLEY

BACKGROUND

Hoarseness broadly describes any abnormality in the voice quality, volume, or endurance. Normal phonation depends on the controlled expulsion of air via functioning lungs and diaphragm, passage of the air through the vocal tract resulting in vibration and a mucosal wave, and proper resonance of the sound throughout the oropharynx and nasopharynx. Formation of vowels and consonants occurs in the oropharynx, nasopharynx, and oral cavity. This chapter focuses on disorders affecting only the vocal tract, but the astute physician should keep in mind that changes in the voice can occur in patients with an entirely normal and functioning glottis (vocal cords/folds) (Fig 19–1).

The glottis (true vocal folds) opens during respiration and closes during phonation and swallowing to prevent aspiration. Thus a patient with hoarseness

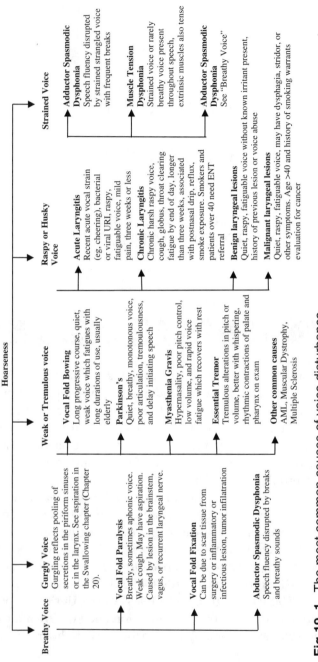

Hoarseness

Breathy Voice

Gurgly Voice
Gurgling reflects pooling of secretions in the piriform sinuses or in the larynx. See aspiration in the Swallowing chapter (Chapter 20).

Vocal Fold Paralysis
Breathy, sometimes aphonic voice. Weak cough. May have aspiration. Caused by lesion in the brainstem, vagus, or recurrent laryngeal nerve.

Vocal Fold Fixation
Can be due to scar tissue from surgery or inflammatory or infectious lesion, tumor infiltratation

Abductor Spasmodic Dysphonia
Speech fluency disrupted by breaks and breathy sounds

Weak or Tremulous voice

Vocal Fold Bowing
Long progressive course, quiet, weak voice which fatigues with long durations of use, usually elderly

Parkinson's
Quiet, breathy, monotonous voice, poor articulation, tremoulousness, and delay initiating speech

Myasthenia Gravis
Hypernasality, poor pitch control, low volume, and rapid voice fatigue which recovers with rest

Essential Tremor
Tremulous alterations in pitch or volume, better with whispering, rhythmic contractions of palate and pharynx on exam

Other common causes
AML, Muscular Dystrophy, Multiple Sclerosis

Raspy or Husky Voice

Acute Laryngitis
Recent acute vocal strain (eg. cheering), bacterial or viral URI, raspy, fatiguable voice, mild pain, three weeks or less

Chronic Laryngitis
Chronic harsh raspy voice, cough, globus, throat clearing fatigue by end of day, longer than three weeks, associated with postnasal drip, reflux, smoke exposure. Smokers and patients over 40 need ENT referral

Benign laryngeal lesions
Quiet, raspy, fatiguable voice without known irritant present, history of previous lesion or voice abuse

Malignant laryngeal lesions
Quiet, raspy, fatiguable voice, may have dysphagia, stridor, or other symptoms. Age >40 and history of smoking warrants evaluation for cancer

Strained Voice

Adductor Spasmodic Dysphonia
Speech fluency disrupted by strained strangled voice with frequent breaks

Muscle Tension Dysphonia
Strained voice or rarely breathy voice present throughout speech, extrinsic muscles also tense

Abductor Spasmodic Dysphonia
See "Breathy Voice"

Fig 19–1. The most common causes of voice disturbance.

may also have respiratory insufficiency or aspiration, which should be assessed during the history and physical. These findings can be subtle, for example, the long-term smoker with emphysema and undiagnosed laryngeal cancer may be sedentary enough not to notice any change in his respiratory effort.

TAKING A HISTORY IN A PATIENT WITH HOARSENESS

The patient should be asked to specifically describe the problem. Is the problem voice fatigue, change in quality, poor projection, change in range, or a spastic sound? As always, duration, severity, exacerbating and alleviating factors, and concurrent events (such as recent colds, stressful events) are relevant components of the history. Ask about breathing, swallowing, and signs of aspiration, such as coughing or choking while eating, or pneumonias. Elicit other ongoing problems such as cough, congestion, postnasal drip, reflux, weakness, muscle spasm, and weight loss. Neurologic disorders, cancer, trauma (such as seatbelt pressure on the neck or choking), cardiac disorders (such as enlarged right atrium, thoracic aneurysm, or risk factors for such), pulmonary disorders, reflux, thyroid problems, metabolic disorders, allergy, and psychiatric history are all potential contributing factors in the past medical history. Family history of any of the above may also direct the workup. Past surgical history is particularly important because many common procedures have been implicated in recurrent laryngeal nerve injury including carotid endarterectomy, thyroidectomy, cardiac surgery (in particular aortic arch and patent ductus arteriosus), anterior spine approaches, and thoracic surgery. The use of tobacco and alcohol are critical to assess. Hoarseness in a smoker over 40 is considered cancer until proven otherwise, and referral to an otolaryngologist is recommended.

EXAMINATION OF THE HOARSE PATIENT

The examination begins during the history taking, during which careful assessment of voice quality can be made. Evaluate the quality, strength, and fluency of the voice. Is the voice raspy but normal volume? Is it breathy? Does it have a strained quality? Is it lower or higher than seems appropriate? Look for accessory (neck) muscle use while the patient speaks. Determine whether the voice becomes weaker over time.

A complete head and neck examination should be performed. The eyes should be assessed for extraocular movements and signs of Horner's syndrome (involvement of the sympathetic chain or carotid artery). Findings in the nose, oral cavity, and oropharynx can suggest pathology in the vocal tract. Signs of allergy include blue boggy turbinates and congested mucosa. Reflux and postnasal drip both cause a cobblestone appearance (raised lymphoid tissue in the back of the pharynx) in the pharynx. Nasal papillomata should spark concern for the same in the larynx. Cranial nerve function, especially IX, X, and XI should be evaluated. A mirror laryngoscopy should be performed to evaluate vocal fold movement. The neck should be palpated to look for neck masses or thyroid tumors. The patient's overall neuromuscular function should be assessed.

ACUTE HOARSENESS

Most commonly, acute hoarseness will occur during or after a viral upper respiratory tract infection (URI), or after loud screaming (eg, after sports or entertainment event).

Symptoms and Signs

The patient will present with a sudden onset of loss of voice or hoarseness. The patient can commonly have a cough and post-nasal drainage. The examination will show changes consistent with a URI including nasal congestion, a cobblestone appearance in the posterior pharynx, and mild edema of the vocal folds in patients with URI. Patients with hoarseness after loud screaming will have a normal exam with the exception vocal fold edema or erythema.

Diagnosis and What Tests to Order

The diagnosis is generally by history. An acute loss of voice with an antecedent URI or loud screaming is diagnostic. Generally no tests need to be ordered.

Treatment and When to Refer

The first line of treatment for patients with acute hoarseness is an intramuscular injection of 10 mg of dexamethasone (0.1 mg/kg in children). The dexamethasone can be repeated in 2 to 3 days if the symptoms have not resolved and the patient has an event at which they must speak. If not available, prednisone 1 mg/kg for 5 days can be given. The patient should be asked to stop smoking, stop antihistamines, and to stop drinking caffeine. The patient should be encouraged to drink more water. In dry climates or in the winter, a humidifier at bedside will be helpful. Antireflux medications (omeprazole 40 mg po QAM before breakfast, in children, 0.5 mg/kg/d) and nasal anticholinergics to stop the postnasal drainage (ipratropium 0.06%, 2 puffs each nostrils TID, 1 puff children) should also be given. Antibiotics are not generally needed as this represents a viral disorder. The patient with hoarseness after loud screaming should be treated with corticosteroids and proton-pump inhibitors (PPIs). The patient should be referred to an otolaryngologist if there is persistent hoarseness beyond 3 weeks.

CHRONIC HOARSENESS

Chronic hoarseness (over 3 weeks) can occur for a variety of reasons including laryngopharyngeal reflux, smoking, benign or cancerous lesions of the vocal folds, as well as neuromuscular problems such as vocal fold paralysis, parkinsonism, amyotropic lateral sclerosis, and so forth. The most common of these is laryngopharyngeal reflux.

Symptoms and Signs

The patient will generally present with a few week history of hoarseness. There may or may not be an inciting event. If mirror laryngoscopy can be performed, it is invaluable.

Diagnosis, Treatment, and When to Refer

The diagnosis of hoarseness generally requires laryngoscopy and sometimes laryngeal stroboscopy. If the primary care physician is unable to perform laryngoscopy, an empiric treatment with omeprazole 40 mg po QAM before breakfast, in children, 0.5 mg/kg/d for 1 month can be given to see if there is relief of symptoms. If symptoms continue beyond a month, the patient should be referred to an otolaryngologist for laryngoscopy and definitive diagnosis. Professional singers should be referred to laryngologists for stroboscopic examination.

CHAPTER 20

Swallowing Problems

ESTHER L. FINE
HAMID R. DJALILIAN

BACKGROUND

Normal swallowing is a complex process requiring the coordination of the oral cavity, pharynx, larynx, and esophagus. Accurate evaluation and diagnosis of swallowing disorders depends on the understanding of the basic process of swallowing, which is divided into four phases:

Oral preparatory—This is the manipulation of the food to prepare it for swallowing. Ideally, lips close completely after the food is introduced, and the buccal and labial muscles tense to keep food out of the sulci. The tongue rolls laterally to position food for mastication.

Oral—The tongue lifts and propels the bolus back into the pharynx along the hard palate. Cranial nerves V, VII, and XII are important for these first two phases.

Pharyngeal—An involuntary portion of the swallow mediated by the brainstem with some cortical input. The tongue base pushes the bolus into the pharynx while the soft palate elevates to cause velopharyngeal closure and prevent reflux into the nose, and the larynx elevates and closes. The pharynx contracts to propel the bolus, making contact with the tongue base. The cricopharyngeus muscle relaxes to allow the food to pass into the esophagus. Cranial nerves IX and X are involved.

Esophageal—Coordinated contraction of the esophagus propels the bolus downward. Relaxation of the lower esophageal sphincter allows for the bolus to enter the stomach. This is mediated by the medulla. Figure 20–1 outlines the most common causes of swallowing problems.

TAKING A HISTORY ON A PATIENT WITH SWALLOWING PROBLEMS

Begin with the standard history relating to onset, duration, severity, timing, and alleviating and exacerbating factors. Ask the patient to describe exactly where anatomically and at what point in the swallow they are having trouble, and with what specific textures the problem occurs. Have the patient point to the site that seems problematic. Is the swallow painful? Does the food stick and where? Does regurgitation or vomiting occur and, if so, is it during the swallow, immediately after, or delayed? When it occurs, is the food partially digested or completely undigested? Are there voice problems as well? Is the patient aspirating and, if so, how many pneumonias if any have occurred?

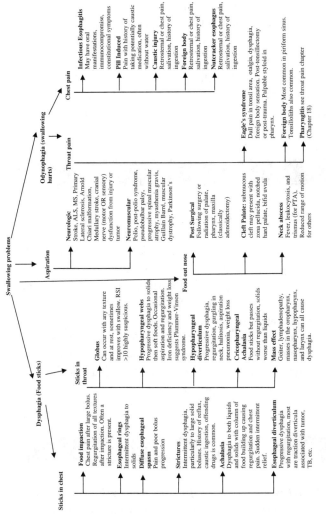

Fig 20–1. The most common causes of swallowing problems.

Swallowing problems

Dysphagia (Food sticks) — **Odynophagia (swallowing hurts)**

Sticks in chest

Food impaction Chest pain after large bolus. Regurgitation of all textures after impaction. Often a stricture is present.

Esophageal rings Intermittent dysphagia to solids

Diffuse esophageal spasm Pain and poor bolus progression

Strictures Intermittent dysphagia, particularly to large solid boluses. History of reflux, caustic ingestion, offending drugs is common.

Achalasia Dysphagia to both liquids and solids with column of food building up causing regurgitation and chest pain. Sudden intermittent relief.

Esophageal diverticulum Progressive dysphagia with regurgitation, most are traction diverticula associated with tumor, TB, etc.

Sticks in throat

Globus Can occur with any texture and at rest, sometimes improves with swallow. RSI >10 highly suspicious.

Hypopharyngeal webs Progressive dysphagia to solids then soft foods. Occasional aspiration and regurgitation. Iron deficiency and weight loss suggests Plummer-Vinson syndrome.

Hypopharyngeal diverticulum Progressive dysphagia, regurgitation, gurgling in neck, halitosis, aspiration pneumonia, weight loss

Cricopharyngeal Achalasia Food sticks but passes without regurgitation, solids worse than liquids

Mass effect Goiter, lymphadenopathy, masses in the oropharynx, nasopharynx, hypopharynx, and larynx can all cause dysphagia.

Aspiration

Neurologic Stroke, ALS, MS, Primary Lateral sclerosis, Arnold Chiari malformation, Medullary stroke, cranial nerve (motor OR sensory) dysfunction from injury or tumor

Neuromuscular Polio, post-polio syndrome, pseudobulbar palsy, progressive spinal muscular atrophy, myasthenia gravis, Guillain Barré, muscular dystrophy, Parkinson's

Food out nose

Post Surgical Following surgery or radiation of palate, pharynx, maxilla (classically adenoidectomy)

Cleft Palate: submucous cleft may present with zona pellucida, notched hard palate, bifid uvula

Throat pain

Neck abscess Fever, leukocytosis, and trismus (for PTA), Reduced range of motion for others

Eagle's syndrome Dull pain in tonsil area, otalgia, dysphagia, foreign body sensation. Post-tonsillectomy or post-trauma. Palpable styloid in pharynx.

Foreign body Most common in piriform sinus. Tonsilloliths also common.

Pharyngitis see throat pain chapter (Chapter 18)

Chest pain

Infectious Esophagitis May have oral manifestations, immunocompromise, constitutional symptoms

Pill Induced Pain with history of taking potentially caustic medication, often without water

Caustic injury Retrosternal or chest pain, salivation, history of ingestion

Foreign body Retrosternal or chest pain, salivation, history of ingestion

Nutcracker esophagus Retrosternal or chest pain, salivation, history of ingestion

Is the patient losing weight and, if so, how much? Assess for other symptoms suggesting neurologic or neuromuscular dysfunction.

The past medical history should focus on potential neurologic and neuromuscular disorders and history of trauma. Past surgical history should include head and neck, cardiovascular, thoracic, and gastric surgery. Medications that cause tardive dyskinesia and extrapyramidal effects are important to be aware of.

EXAMINATION OF THE PATIENT

Perform a complete head and neck evaluation including evaluation of the voice quality and cough. Pay particular attention to the tongue, palate, and oropharynx. Neurologic evaluation should include cranial nerves, gross motor strength, and cerebellar testing. Observe the patient swallowing. Place a finger above the thyroid cartilage to confirm the elevation of the larynx. Chest can be examined for signs of COPD from chronic aspiration. The abdomen should be examined for organomegaly. Hemoccult testing may be positive with a neoplasm or esophagitis.

COMMONLY ORDERED TESTS

Bedside swallow evaluation by trained speech pathologist: This is most commonly ordered on inpatients to evaluate their safety for oral intake following an event likely to adversely affect the swallow, such as a stroke, brain injury, or surgery.

Videofluoroscopy (modified barium swallow): The patient is initially seated in the upright position and asked to swallow barium with a variety of textures. The timing, speed, and effectiveness of the swallow with different consistencies of foods all can be assessed. The swallow in different positions and using treatment strategies can also be evaluated. This will not capture the esophageal phase of the swallow. This test helps to assess the oral and pharyngeal phases of swallow, and is different from the barium swallow in that a speech pathologist is present when the test is performed.

Esophageal manometry: The patient swallows a probe containing three pressure sensors. This is positioned such that pressure is measured at the upper esophageal sphincter, esophageal body, and lower esophageal sphincter. Alternatively, the tube can be positioned to measure the pharynx, upper esophageal sphincter, and esophageal body. This test helps to test for esophageal achalasia.

Esophagram (barium swallow): The patient is positioned prone and asked to swallow barium of various textures (unless a perforation is suspected, in which water soluble contrast is used). Intrinsic and extrinsic anatomic defects can be identified. The advantage over the modified barium swallow is dilation of the esophagus occurs allowing for contours to be seen well. The entire pharynx and esophagus can be imaged, although this is institution dependent and you should indicate specifically if you suspect a pharyngeal or hypopharyngeal defect.

Esophagoscopy: This can be performed under conscious sedation with a flexible endoscope, typically by a gastroenterologist, or in the operating room under general anesthesia with a rigid esophagoscope by an ENT. This test is performed by some otolaryngologists transnasally without sedation in the office.

pH monitoring: A probe is inserted transnasally into the esophagus and pH is monitored for 24 hours. This test is useful for checking for gastroesophageal reflux disease (GERD), especially proton-pump inhibitor resistant GERD.

Flexible laryngoscopy: A flexible fiberoptic scope is passed through the nostril and advanced to the level of the soft palate to evaluate the larynx.

Flexible Endoscopic Evaluation of Swallowing (FEES): This test is performed at the bedside of hospitalized patients to evaluate the oral and pharyngeal phases of the swallow. It is performed using different consistencies of food mixed with food coloring by an otolaryngologist and a speech pathologist.

ASPIRATION

Aspiration can occur during any of the first three phases of the swallow. During the voluntary phases, the airway remains open, so poor bolus control can result in spillage into the larynx. A delayed pharyngeal phase will also allow food to spill into the vallecula, or piriform sinuses, or enter the airway. If the swallow is sequentially normal but weak, material can remain in the pharynx and fall into the airway during normal respiration. Many patients with these problems also have diminished or absent laryngospasm, further predisposing to aspiration and pneumonia.

Most causes of aspiration are neurologic and degenerative affecting motor coordination and/or affecting sensory function. Below is a brief list of common disorders causing dysphagia.

Medullary (brainstem) causes: ALS, primary lateral sclerosis, postpolio syndrome, Arnold-Chiari malformation, medullary strokes.

Lower motor neuron disorders: progressive spinal muscular atrophy, psuedobulbar palsy, polio, postpolio syndrome.

Neuromuscular: Myasthenia gravis, Guillain-Barré syndrome, muscular dystrophy

Myopathies: Dermatomyositis, metabolic

Extrapyramidal: Parkinson's, tardive dyskinesia

What Tests to Order

Speech therapy evaluation and modified barium swallow are the best starting tests for aspiration. The problem in these patients generally is in the pharyngeal phase of swallow.

Treatment

Treat the underlying cause of the disease (specifics are beyond the scope of this chapter), and offer speech therapy for compensatory strategies. Stop any offending medications. Patients with severe symptoms resulting in weakness, weight loss, electrolyte abnormalities, or aspiration pneumonia in the short term should have a nasogastric feeding tube placed, and in the long term be considered for gastrostomy tube placement, requiring referral to gastroenterology, interventional radiology, or general surgery.

When to Refer

Most patients do not require otolaryngology referral. Patients with a known neurologic or neuromuscular disorder require otolaryngology referral only if the cough is weak or absent, or if the voice is hoarse, suggesting insufficient laryngeal closure that may be amenable to surgical improvement by vocal fold augmentation. Patients without a known disorder who are aspirating should be referred to otolaryngology for a full head and neck examination including inspection of the hypopharynx and larynx. This is particularly important in patients over 40 with smoking and drinking habits.

PAIN IN THROAT WITH SWALLOWING

Pharyngitis

See Pharygitis in Chapter 18.

Foreign Body

Other common foreign bodies of the throat are fish bones and seeds, which often lodge in the piriform sinus. Children may have impaling of the palate or tonsil due to running with an object in their mouths. This puts them at risk of carotid artery injury and foreign bodies in these areas should only be removed by a specialist after appropriate imaging studies (CT with contrast of the neck).

What Tests to Order and When

AP and lateral soft tissue neck x-rays will help identify any radiopaque foreign bodies such as fish bones. Any penetrating injury to the lateral soft palate or tonsil should be evaluated with a CT-angiogram of the neck to determine if carotid injury is present. The clinician should be aware of the calcification of the thyroid cartilage and cricoid cartilage which starts in the 3rd or 4th decade of life (Fig 20–2).

When to Refer

Patients should be made NPO in case operative intervention is needed, and should be seen urgently by an otolaryngologist if a pharyngeal foreign body is suspected. All penetrating injuries to the lateral palate or tonsil (eg, falling with pencil in mouth) should be sent to the emergency department for imaging to rule out a carotid injury and pseudoaneurysm formation.

Tonsillith

Tonsilliths are foul smelling white concretion that occur in tonsillar crypts. Food that gets trapped in tonsillar crypts gathers bacteria and forms a foul smelling concretion that the patient coughs up or removes with manipulation. They can present when the patient complains of a foreign body sensation in the pharynx. The patient often first has the foreign body sensation while eating something hard and may even gag, and thus will present complaining specifically of a foreign body.

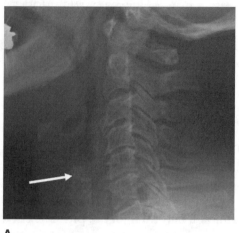

A

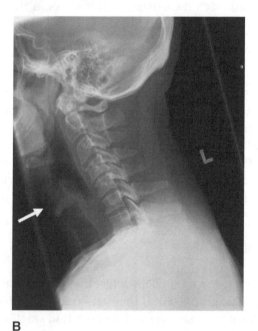

B

Fig 20–2. A. Lateral neck x-ray in a patient showing a calcified thyroid cartilage (*arrow*). **B.** Lateral neck x-ray in a patient showing a normal thyroid cartilage shadow without calcification (*arrow*).

Treatment and When to Refer

Tonsilliths can be teased out with a blunt instrument, and patients can gargle saline or use a water pik after eating to keep them from forming in the future. If they continue to be a problem chronically and cause significant halitosis (bad odor to breath) the patient should be referred to an otolaryngologist for tonsillectomy. Other foreign bodies will require removal by an otolaryngologist.

Eagle's Syndrome

Eagle's syndrome is a condition characterized by persistent dull pharyngeal pain in the tonsil area, otalgia, dysphagia, odynophagia, and sometimes a foreign body sensation, when swallowing which is caused by an excessively long styloid process or a calcified stylohyoid ligament. Three muscles and two ligaments attach to the styloid process, all of which are involved in swallowing. Because the styloid is located between the external and internal carotid artery, deviation of the styloid can cause pain in the areas supplied by that vessel. Most cases present in on examination, the styloid process can be palpated behind the tonsillar fossa as a dull hard process. Palpation of the area will duplicate the patient's pain.

Diagnosis and What Tests to Order

The diagnosis is by history and the characteristic physical examination. A lateral soft tissue x-ray will show an elongated styloid process or a calcified stylohyoid ligament.

Treatment and When to Refer

The patient should be referred to an otolaryngologist for confirmation of diagnosis and treatment if desired by the patient. Treatment consists of removal of part of the styloid process.

PAIN IN CHEST WITH SWALLOWING

Infectious Esophagitis

Infectious esophagitis is a disorder that generally affects patients who are immunocompromised due to chemotherapy, human immunodeficiency virus (HIV), transplantation, or poorly controlled diabetes.

Symptoms and Signs

The patients generally present with severe odynophagia. The infection will often manifest in the mouth and pharynx as well. *Candida* is the most common organism in both HIV and non-HIV infected patients, followed by cytomegalovirus (CMV) and herpes simplex virus (HSV). Candidal esophagitis is an AIDS-defining illness.

Diagnosis and What Tests to Order

If the patient is not systemically ill, suspected candidal infection can be managed empirically. HSV and CMV can be diagnosed endoscopically, although if esophagoscopy is not easily available, a barium esophogram can be helpful. If oral lesions are present as well, they can be scraped with a slide or tongue depressor and a KOH preparation can be made to observe if hyphae are present.

Treatment and When to Refer

Candidal esophagitis is treated with fluconazole 200 mg loading dose followed by 100 mg orally daily for 14 to 21 days. If no response is seen after 72 hours, endoscopy should be ordered for definitive diagnosis. Patients who do not respond to fluconazole can be treated with voriconazole orally, or one of the echinocandins (such as caspofungin) intravenously. HSV and CMV esophagitis resolve spontaneously in immunocompetent hosts. For immunocompromised patients, use acyclovir 400 mg po five times daily for 14 to 21 days. The patient should be referred to a gastroenterologist if symptoms fail to improve with systemic treatment for endoscopy and biopsy.

Pill-Induced Esophagitis

Pill-induced esophagitis generally presents with a sudden onset of odynophagia, chest pain or retrosternal pain with a history of taking a possible offending medication, often without water and/or before sleep. Medications include alendronate, emepronium bromide, tetracycline, KCl, quinidine, beta-blockers, nonsteroidal anti-inflammatory drugs (NSAIDs), calcium channel blockers, and iron. The diagnosis is by history.

Tests to Order

If clinical suspicion is high, diagnosis can be presumptively made. Endoscopy should be ordered if the presentation is severe or unusual. An air-contrast barium esophagram can be ordered if endoscopy is not available.

Treatment

If possible, stop the offending drug. If the medication is essential, use a liquid form. For future prevention patients should be counseled to take the pill with 8 oz of water, remain upright for 30 minutes and, if possible, eat a meal afterward. Patients with an enlarged right atrium or who have undergone cardiac surgery are at increased risk of pill-induced esophagitis, and should always be counseled to use these precautions. Acutely, the patient can be treated with proton-pump inhibitors (eg, omeprazole 40 mg po) to reduce any further esophagitis from reflux.

When to Refer

The patient should be referred to a gastroenterologist if endoscopy deemed necessary (eg, recurrent problem). If there is bleeding or excessive vomiting, the patients should be admitted to the hospital for urgent esophagoscopy and intravenous fluids.

Caustic Injury

Caustic injury is generally found in toddlers or adults who attempt suicide. Typically, the history of ingestion is known but the offending material (solid or liquid) should be identified. Alkali such as lye (eg, drain openers) cause liquefaction necrosis and deeper burns than acidic liquids (eg, bleach). Symptoms vary and include epigastric and retrosternal pain and salivation. Be aware that the severity of symptoms does not always correlate with the degree of injury. Strictures can later form, particularly at the areas of anatomic narrowing: the cricopharyngeus, the aortic arch, and the lower esophageal sphincter. There is also an increased risk of squamous cell carcinoma in this population.

Treatment and When to Refer

Patients should be sent to the emergency department with otolaryngology evaluation. Pediatric patients should be sent to a center with pediatric otolaryngologists if available. Intubation may be necessary and endoscopy should be performed within 48 hours.

Nutcracker Esophagus

Nutcracker esophagus is caused by high amplitude contractions of the distal esophagus with normal propagation. The patients present with chest pain without dysphagia.

Diagnosis and What Tests to Order

The diagnosis is by esophageal manometry. Manometry will show distal esophageal pressures above 220 mm Hg after swallowing.

Treatment and When to Refer

Controlled studies on the treatment of this disorder are limited and small. Diltiazem 180 to 240 mg/day has been found to help these patients. Tricyclic antidepressants, botox, isosorbide, and sildenafil have also demonstrated efficacy in small studies. Referral can be made on a nonurgent basis to a gastroenterologist after more concerning causes of chest pain are ruled out.

Esophageal Foreign Body

Esophageal foreign bodies generally occur either in toddlers (eg, foreign objects, coins, etc) or in the elderly (eg, poorly chewed meat due to poor dentition). The patient usually has a clear history of swallowing a foreign body, which may include a choking event and vomiting. Pediatric patients may present after an unwitnessed event, and the diagnosis is presumptive. It is important to try to assess what type of object was swallowed and the timing of the ingestion. Button batteries are an emergency regardless of location of impaction, as they cause a chemical burn. Sharp objects raise a concern for possible perforation.

What Tests to Order

An antero-posterior and lateral x-rays of the neck and chest will identify radiopaque foreign bodies. Also, attention should be given to free air under the diaphragm or in the neck in case of a perforation.

When to Refer

Patients should be sent to the emergency department, where they can undergo an otolaryngology consultation. If the foreign body is in the stomach, general surgery or gastroenterology consultation should be obtained. If a foreign body passes into the duodenum, then it will traverse the gastrointestinal tract. In general, patients who are obstructed above the cricopharyngeus muscle, or who have swallowed a sharp object, should be referred to an otolaryngologist for rigid endoscopy.

FOOD STICKS IN THROAT

Globus

Occasionally, patients will present with a sense of food sticking in the throat. This can occur with any texture, and may be made better or worse by the swallow itself. The globus sensation reflects inflammation of the pharynx, and the most common cause is reflux disease. Previously thought to be psychogenic, globus now is attributed to inflammation of the esophageal opening due to reflux of gastric content. Laryngoscopy will show postcricoid edema and erythema.

Diagnosis and What Tests to Order

The reflux symptoms index has been shown to correlate well with a positive pH probe study when the score is greater than 10. This index asks the patient to score from 0 to 5 (with 5 being severe): hoarseness, throat clearing, postnasal drip, dysphagia, breathing difficulty, cough, globus, and heartburn/reflux. Dual-probe pH study is the gold standard for diagnosis, however, it is reasonable to initiate therapy without the study if suspicion is high.

Treatment and When to Refer

Medical management consists of lifestyle management (Table 18–4 in Chapter 18) proton-pump inhibitor (PPI) (eg, omeprazole 40 mg po QAM ideally an hour before breakfast) for 2 months. Sometimes, twice-daily PPI is given if the diagnosis is made by laryngoscopy and no response is found with once-daily PPI. If there is no significant improvement of symptoms after 1 month of therapy, the patient should be referred to an otolaryngologist for laryngoscopy. The patient should be referred to an otolaryngologist right away if a heavy smoking (>20 pack years) or a heavy alcohol consumption history of if the patient is losing weight due to the dysphagia. For other patients, refer if twice-daily proton-pump inhibition and behavioral management of reflux fails to alleviate symptoms in 4 months, or if concern exists for another process causing the dysphagia.

Hypopharyngeal Webs

Patients with hypopharyngeal or upper esophageal webs generally present with intermittent dysphagia to solids, with food sticking in the neck or chest, and sometimes aspiration and regurgitation. Webs can be independent of other problems, or can be a part of Plummer-Vinson syndrome. This is a triad of hypopharyngeal and proximal esophageal webs, iron deficiency anemia, and weight loss; 85% of patients are women. Symptoms are progressive, initially dysphagia is present intermittently only with solid foods, and then to soft foods. Webs and strictures arise as a result of chronic inflammation. Patients with Plummer-Vinson syndrome may have signs of iron deficiency including glossitis and chelosis.

Diagnosis and What Tests to Order

Barium esophagram will show a hypopharygeal web. These typically are anterior initially, then become circumferential as the disease progresses. An iron panel will confirm iron deficiency. After referral, esophagoscopy should be performed.

Treatment and When to Refer

Mechanical disruption of webs with dilation techniques under an otolaryngologist or gastroenterologist's guidance is the treatment of choice. The patient should be referred to an otolaryngologist for esophagoscopy and esophageal dilation after diagnosis. Iron and vitamin B replacement should be done if a deficiency is present.

Cricopharyngeal Achalasia

Cricopharyngeal achalasia is characterized by restricted upper esophageal sphincter opening and increased resistance to bolus passage. The patients will present with a complaint of food sticking in the neck.

Diagnosis and What Tests to Order

The diagnosis is by barium esophagram or esophageal manometry. Esophagram may show a cricopharyngeal bar. Esophageal manometry will show the increased pressure at the level of the upper esophageal sphincter (cricopharyngeus muscle).

Treatment and When to Refer

Laryngopharyngeal reflux is thought to be a causative factor in the development of cricopharyngeal achalasia and twice a day PPI (eg, omeprazole 40 mg po BID for 2 months) should be started. If conservative medical therapy fails, the patient should be referred to an otolaryngologist for treatment. Most treatment strategies beyond PPI therapy attempt to relax the cricopharyngeus muscle. Options include botulinum toxin (Botox®) injection, cricopharygeal myotomy, and dilation.

Hypopharyngeal Diverticulum

If an anatomic or physiologic obstruction of the esophagus is present, the pressure created above the obstruction can cause an outpouching (diverticulum) in the area immediately above the obstruction. These pulsion diverticula are often associated with a motility disorder such as cricopharyngeal achalasia. Zenker's diverticulum is the most common diverticulum and is most often seen in patients in the 7th decade, with males being more commonly affected than females.

Symptoms and Signs

The patients generally present with dysphagia with food sticking in the throat, regurgitation of nondigested food, cough, halitosis, gurgling in the neck, and in severe cases, aspiration and pneumonia. Other diverticuli occur in nearby areas of weakness and cause similar symptoms.

Diagnosis and What Tests to Order

A barium esophagram will generally show a diverticulum immediately above the upper esophageal sphincter (cricopharyngeus muscle).

Treatment and When to Refer

The patients should be referred to an otolaryngologist for surgical treatment if the symptoms are causing aspiration, malnutrition, or a quality of life problem for the patient. Prior to surgery nutritional supplementation may be necessary as these patients can be malnourished.

Mass Effect

Masses outside of the hypopharynx or proximal esophagus can cause dysphagia from extrinsic pressure. Neck masses such as goiters, tumors, lymphadenopathy, and even cervical osteophytes can cause dysphagia and the sense of food sticking in the throat.

Diagnosis and What Tests to Order

If an extrinsic mass is large enough to cause dysphagia, it will generally be palpable on physical examination. A CT scan of the neck with contrast will help clearly delineate the mass. A fine needle aspiration is needed as a starting point for tissue identification.

Treatment When to Refer

Immediate referral to the emergency department is needed if the patient also has severe or acute airway compromise. If signs of an acute infection exist (eg, tenderness, acute onset, skin erythema) a 10-day course of antibiotics (cephalexin 500 mg po TID, in children 10 mg/kg TID; for penicillin allergics, clindamycin 300 mg po QID, for children, 15 mg/kg/d divided TID or QID). If there is no airway compromise or signs of acute infection, the patient should be referred to an otolaryngologist for evaluation including nasopharyngoscopy, laryngoscopy, and fine needle aspiration. If after resolution of the infection, a mass is still present, the patient should be referred to an otolaryngologist to rule out a malignancy in the upper aerodigestive tract. A CT scan of the neck with contrast should be obtained prior to referral to expedite the patient's care.

FOOD STICKS IN CHEST

Food Impaction

Food impaction in the esophagus will most commonly occur in the elderly due to their poor dentition or their inability to chew the food well with dentures. The patient will present with sudden onset of chest pain and dysphagia after eating a large bite of dense food, often meat. The patient often will be unable to swallow liquids after the impaction occurs, and will regurgitate after attempts.

Diagnosis and What Tests to Order

Anteroposterior and lateral chest x-ray may identify the site of impaction, and can identify free air if perforation has occurred.

Treatment and When to Refer

The patient should be referred to an emergency department for management. Intravenous glucagon (1–2 mg) can be given to relax the lower esophageal sphincter and can sometimes relieve the obstruction. An otolaryngologist consultation for endoscopy and disimpaction will be necessary. If an otolaryngologist is not available, gastroenterologists can also perform the procedure as well.

Esophageal Rings

Patients with esophageal rings generally present with intermittent dysphagia to solid foods. Schatzki's ring is a ring at the gastroesophageal junction and is the most common location for an esophageal ring.

Diagnosis and What Tests to Order

A barium esophagram should be ordered which is diagnostic. The patient should be referred to an otolaryngologist or gastroenterologist for dilation upon diagnosis to prevent food impaction problems.

Strictures

Dysphagia occurs when the esophageal lumen is less than 15 mm. Strictures arise in response to inflammation and/or injury, with acid (ie, peptic stricture) being the most common cause. Other etiologies include medication, caustic injury, radiation, tumor, infection, iatrogenic, autoimmune disorders, and congenital. Patients present with intermittent dysphagia and odynophagia with solids, often separated from previous events by months or years. Impaction, regurgitation, vomiting, and weight loss can result. Extrinsic masses, though not causing stricture, will cause similar symptoms and should be excluded in the workup.

Diagnosis and What Tests to Order

A barium esophagram generally will aid in identifying the stricture and its cause. Many times, though, an esophagoscopy needs to be performed for diagnosis.

Treatment and When to Refer

PPI therapy (eg, omeprazole 40 mg po BID) is needed when signs of reflux are present. This will help prevent the progression of the stricture by continued acid exposure. NSAIDs and other potentially aggravating medications should be stopped if possible. The patient should be referred to an otolaryngologist or gastroenterologist for evaluation. If dysphagia is present to soft foods, the patient is losing weight or nutritionally compromised, or if a food impaction has occurred, dilation may be necessary.

Diffuse Esophageal Spasm

This is caused by intermittent uncoordinated contractions of the esophagus, resulting in dysphagia, chest pain, and regurgitation of undigested food.

Diagnosis and What Tests to Order

Esoghageal manometry is diagnostic. Barium esophagram will show a "corkscrew esophagus." A cardiac workup starting with an EKG and possibly stress testing must be performed to rule out a concurrent cardiac ischemia.

Treatment and When to Refer

Nitrates (eg, isosorbide dinitrate 5 mg PO before a meal or 2.5 mg sublingual after a meal) and calcium channel blockers (eg, diltiazem 120 mg po QD) have been used in randomized controlled studies and found to be successful. More invasive treatments including botulinum toxin injection and esophageal dilation are used in severe cases that do not respond to medical management. The patients should be referred to a gastroenterologist for evaluation and treatment if medical therapy fails.

Esophageal Achalasia

Esophageal achalasia is caused by high pressure from muscular contraction in the lower esophageal sphincter and defective peristalsis. This results in a column of undigested material backing up in the esophagus. The patients will have dysphagia to both liquids and solids, regurgitation of undigested material, coughing or choking during sleep, chest pain, and weight loss. Patients may compensate with physical maneuvers or drinking carbonated beverages.

Diagnosis and What Tests to Order

Barium esophagram will show a classic "bird's beak tapering."

Treatment and When to Refer

The patient should be referred to a gastroenterologist for further workup including esophageal manometry or esophagoscopy. Treatment options are pharmacologic therapy with calcium channel blockers or nitrates (see diffuse esophageal spasm above for dosage), Botox® injection, dilations, or myotomy.

FOOD COMES OUT NOSE

This occurs during the pharyngeal phase due to insufficient closure of the velopharynx. The velopharynx is defined as the area in the nasopharynx where the soft palate closes during swallowing. Velopharyngeal insufficiency occurs when the area is not closed and food is propelled into the nose during swallow. The palate must make complete contact with the posterior pharyngeal wall to prevent this problem, thus, a defect in either structure (palate or nasopharynx) can result in nasal regurgitation. These patients will have a hypernasal speech (air escaping through nose while talking).

Postadenotonsillectomy Velopharyngeal Insufficiency (VPI)

This is a common early complication of adenoidectomy, or adenotonsillectomy. A patient with an enlarged adenoid is used to not raising the palate as much during swallow (due to the apposition of the large adenoid). Once the adenoid is removed, for the first 1 to 2 weeks, the patient may have some regurgitation of food into the nose after swallowing because the palate is not completely closing the nasopharynx.

Diagnosis

The diagnosis is clinical and no tests are required in the setting of a postadenoidectomy patient.

Treatment and When to Refer

Generally, the problem resolves over the first 2 to 3 weeks postadenoidectomy. If it does not resolve, speech therapy is tried for 1 year before undertaking any further treatment. The patient should be seen by the otolaryngologist who performed the surgery. Surgical treatment is considered if the problem persists more than 1 year.

Surgical and Postradiation Velopharyngeal Insufficiency

Patients who have had surgery or radiation of the palate or pharynx may experience nasal regurgitation.

What Tests to Order and When

The diagnosis is clinical, however nasopharyngoscopy will be performed by the otolaryngologist to confirm the diagnosis and to determine the exact area of insufficiency.

Treatment and When to Refer

Patients with a history of head and neck cancer should already be under the care of an otolaryngologist, but should make an earlier visit if new symptoms arise, including regurgitation. Patients without cancer should be referred for further evaluation.

Cleft Palate

A patient with a cleft palate or a history of a repaired cleft palate can commonly have nasal regurgitation. The diagnosis is based on the history. Patients with a submucous cleft (clefting of the underlying palatal muscle or bone with an intact mucosa) are also prone to this condition. These patients will have notching of the posterior hard palate on palpation at the junction between the hard and soft palate. The patient also may have a bifid uvula.

When to Refer

Cleft palate patients are best served by referral to a craniofacial team, as a multidisciplinary approach is often necessary for treatment, as well as evaluation for other organ system defects associated with clefts.

FURTHER READING

Cockeram A. Canadian Association of Gastroenterology Practice Guidelines: evaluation of dysphagia. *Can J Gastroenterol.* 1998;12:409–413.

Pappas PG, Rex JH, Sobel JD, et al. Infectious Diseases Society of America. Guidelines for treatment of candidiasis. *Clin Infect Dis.* 2004;38:161–180.

Spechler SJ. AGA Guidelines on the management of patients with dysphagia caused by benign disorders of the distal esophagus. *Gastroenterology.* 1999;117:233–254.

Tutuian R, Castell D. Esophageal motility disorders (distal esophageal spasm, nutcracker esophagus, and hypertensive lower esophageal sphincter): modern management. *Curr Treat Options Gastroenterol.* 2006;9:283–294.

Wo JM, Frist WJ, Gussack G, Delgaudio JM, Waring JP. Empiric trial of high-dose omeprazole in patients with posterior laryngitis: a prospective study. *Am J Gastroenterol.* 1997;92:2160–2165.

CHAPTER 21

Airway Obstruction

GURPREET S. AHUJA
HAMID R. DJALILIAN

WORKUP OF THE COMPROMISED PEDIATRIC AIRWAY

Airway obstruction, in adults or children, may be associated with stridor. Stridor is essentially a harsh respiratory noise which results from turbulence generated by air flow past a partially obstructed airway. It must be emphasized that stridor is a clinical sign and not a diagnosis. Its presence warrants need for further work to determine the cause of the airway compromise.

Like the workup for any other entity, workup of a child with stridor involves procuring a comprehensive history. A thorough examination of the head and neck may include a flexible endoscopic evaluation of the upper airway. Radiographic studies may be indicated under specific circumstances. Finally, some patients may need to be taken to the operating room for a direct laryngoscopy and bronchoscopy under general anesthesia for diagnostic and therapeutic purposes. The most common causes of airway obstruction in children is outlined in Figure 21-1.

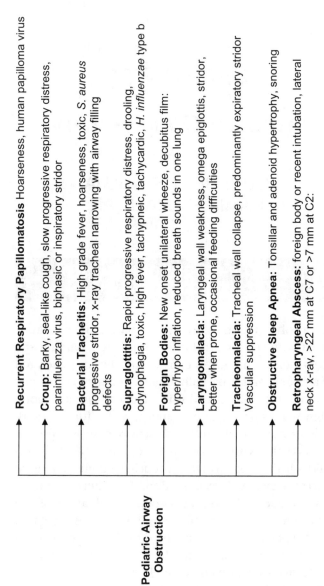

Pediatric Airway Obstruction

- **Recurrent Respiratory Papillomatosis** Hoarseness, human papilloma virus

- **Croup:** Barky, seal-like cough, slow progressive respiratory distress, parainfluenza virus, biphasic or inspiratory stridor

- **Bacterial Tracheitis:** High grade fever, hoarseness, toxic, *S. aureus* progressive stridor, x-ray tracheal narrowing with airway filling defects

- **Supraglottitis:** Rapid progressive respiratory distress, drooling, odynophagia, toxic, high fever, tachypneic, tachycardic, *H. influenzae* type b

- **Foreign Bodies:** New onset unilateral wheeze, decubitus film: hyper/hypo inflation, reduced breath sounds in one lung

- **Laryngomalacia:** Laryngeal wall weakness, omega epiglottis, stridor, better when prone, occasional feeding difficulties

- **Tracheomalacia:** Tracheal wall collapse, predominantly expiratory stridor Vascular suppression

- **Obstructive Sleep Apnea:** Tonsillar and adenoid hypertrophy, snoring

- **Retropharyngeal Abscess:** foreign body or recent intubation, lateral neck x-ray, >22 mm at C7 or >7 mm at C2:

Fig 21–1. The most common causes of pediatric airway obstruction.

HISTORY

In procuring the history about an infant or child with stridor, it is important to establish if the stridor was present at birth or developed at a later point. Stridor relating to laryngomalacia may be apparent within days to weeks after birth, but stridor associated with a subglottic hemangioma may not present until several weeks to a few months later. Determine the severity of the stridor—whether it is persistent at rest or only when the patient is active or crying; if it is associated with apneic episodes, or accompanied by any periods of duskiness or cyanosis. Check if the stridor changes with alteration in position, as in laryngomalacia, where the stridor may be less pronounced with the baby is prone. Also, check if the child's cry or voice has changed since the onset of the stridor. Ask for any history of difficulty feeding, new onset of drooling, or associated fever. Also, ask for any history of intubation in the past. One must maintain a high index of suspicion for foreign body aspiration, and ask for history that might suggest aspiration including any history of choking, gagging, or sudden onset of coughing.

PHYSICAL EXAM

A quick assessment of the patient will allow you to determine if you are dealing with mild, moderate or severe respiratory compromise. With mild airway compromise, the patient may exhibit stridor, but without associated nasal flaring or retraction. With moderate compromise, the stridor will be louder, and may be associated with nasal flaring, substernal or intercostals retractions, or circumoral cyanosis. The child may appear anxious, as well. With severe airway compromise, the stridor may either be louder, or actually decrease in amplitude as air exchange diminishes. The child will exhibit nasal flaring, tachypnea, and/or cyanosis; the child may appear restless and anxious, with signs of air hunger, and eventually may even start appearing lethargic.

Based on that quick assessment, you will be able to determine if you are dealing with an airway emergency—prompting you to move quickly, or if the child appears stable, you will have the option to systematically establish the etiology of the patient's stridor. In performing your exam, it is important to distinguish stridor from stertor. Stertor is a lower pitched snoring sound generated typically in the pharynx from obstruction in the nose or pharynx. Determine if the stridor is inspiratory, expiratory or biphasic. Inspiratory stridor suggests obstruction at the level of the glottis or above. Biphasic stridor accompanies glottis or subglottic obstruction whereas expiratory stridor is associated with mid- to distal tracheal obstruction.

Examination involves a comprehensive head-and-neck assessment including evaluation for neck masses and a good intraoral exam looking for floor of mouth or tongue swelling, tonsillar hypertrophy, salivary pooling in the pharynx, and intraoral or pharyngeal foreign bodies. Look for skin hemangiomas, and for any impairment in neurologic status (eg, cerebral palsy).

ENDOSCOPY

Flexible fiberoptic laryngoscopy allows a bedside dynamic, awake evaluation of the proximal airway including the nasal passages, the pharynx, the supraglottis, and the glottis, at the bedside. It does not allow bedside evaluation of the subglottis or tracheobronchial airway. Rigid laryngoscopy/tracheobronchoscopy under general anesthesia is the modality of choice for diagnostic evaluation and therapeutic interventions involving the airway, particularly in the pediatric population.

Compared to flexible bronchoscopy, rigid bronchoscopy in the operating room allows a much better diagnostic evaluation of the subglottic and tracheobronchial airway because of superior optics, while also allowing the option to ventilate the patient during the assessment. Rigid endoscopy also serves as a therapeutic tool in the removal of foreign bodies of the aerodigestive tract, ablation of airway papillomas, excision of cysts in the valleculae or subglottis, management of hemangiomas or select subglottic stenoses, among others.

RADIOGRAPHIC STUDIES

Plain Films

Anteroposterior and lateral views of the neck and chest sometimes may provide useful information. In infants and toddlers, the lateral view must be obtained with the neck extended in inspiration. If a foreign body is suspected, inspiratory/expiratory views (or decubitus views in younger children), may reveal air-trapping and hyperinflation of the lung from partial obstruction. Total opacification of the lung can also be seen, but hyperinflation tends to be more common.

Fluoroscopy

Fluoroscopy allows for dynamic evaluation of the airway as in tracheomalacia, extramural vascular compression, or in foreign body aspiration.

Esophagogram and Modified Barium Swallow

Esophagogram can be a useful study when looking for vascular anomalies including vascular rings. A radiolucent foreign body may appear as a filling defect in the study. Occasionally, gastroesophageal reflux will be identified on an esophagram, though the incidence of a false negative reading is high. Aspiration as a primary entity, or associated with a laryngeal cleft or rarely with a tracheoesophageal fistula may be detected with a modified barium swallow.

CT/MRI

CT or MRI may be necessary in evaluating for vascular anomalies of the chest, or for soft tissue masses of the neck or mediastinum that may compromise the airway.

DIFFERENTIAL DIAGNOSIS

Based on the age of the child with stridor, the differential diagnosis will vary.

In neonates, the most common cause of stridor is laryngomalacia, accounting for two-thirds of the neonates with stridor. It is followed by bilateral vocal fold paralysis in 10% and congenital subglottic stenosis in 5%. Other entities to be considered in the differential include laryngeal webs, cysts, clefts, masses, or vascular rings. In an infant, the differential should include acquired subglottic stenosis, vascular rings, cysts, posterior laryngeal cleft, hemangioma, tracheomalacia, or foreign body aspiration. In older children, inflammatory conditions can occur more commonly (eg, supraglottitis, croup, and bacterial tracheitis). Other conditions in this age group that case respiratory compromise include recurrent respiratory papillomatosis, foreign bodies, or mass lesions.

LARYNGOMALACIA

Laryngomalacia is the commonest cause of stridor in neonates, accounting for nearly two-thirds of newborn and early infants with stridor. The course is generally self-limiting, with nearly 85% of patients undergoing resolution within 12 and 24 months of age. The patients have abnormal flaccidity of the supraglottic tissues with no pathognomonic histologic finding. Delayed neuromuscular control has been postulated as a cause. Babies with laryngomalacia manifest inspiratory stridor, which may be accompanied by increase in work of breathing associated with tachypnea, retractions, and nasal flaring. The baby may also exhibit feeding difficulty. More severe cases may have periods of apnea or cyanosis. Flexible laryngoscopy usually reveals an omega-shaped epiglottis which prolapses posteriorly, short aryepiglottic folds, and bulky arytenoids that prolapse anteriorly. Airway films may be considered to look for concomitant distal airway anomalies. Management consists of close observation of the patient's feeding and weight gain. Surgery may be indicated in a small minority if the patient exhibits feeding difficulties, failure to thrive, apnea, or cyanotic events. Surgical options include supraglottoplasty in the absence of other airway anomalies, or tracheostomy if the laryngomalacia is associated with other airway conditions.

TRACHEOMALACIA

Tracheomalacia is distinct from laryngomalacia, and the terms must not be used interchangeably. Tracheomalcia suggests collapse of the tracheal walls. It is associated with predominantly expiratory stridor. Tracheomalacia may be primary or may occur secondary to vascular compression, tracheoesophageal fistula, relapsing polychondritis or Ehlers-Danlos syndrome. Secondary tracheomalacia may also be iatrogenically induced by prolonged intubation or following a tracheostomy. Diagnosis may be made by fluoroscopy but must be confirmed with airway endoscopy. Depending on its severity, surgical intervention may be warranted. This may include surgical correction of a vascular ring, or aortopexy and innominate artery suspension in the presence of compression by an aberrant innominate artery. Other causes may necessitate a tracheostomy to maintain the airway.

CROUP

Common in children between 6 months and 2 years of age, croup is most frequent in the spring and fall, and typically is preceded by symptoms of an upper respiratory infection (URI). The barky, seal-like cough may be accompanied by gradually progressive respiratory distress. The most common causative organisms are the parainfluenza and influenza viruses. The patients may exhibit low-grade fever, and may have a biphasic or inspiratory stridor associated with a hoarse voice or cry. They have no drooling, and can comfortably lie on their back or side. Chest x-ray may show the steeple sign with narrowing of the subglottis (Fig 21-2). Treat-

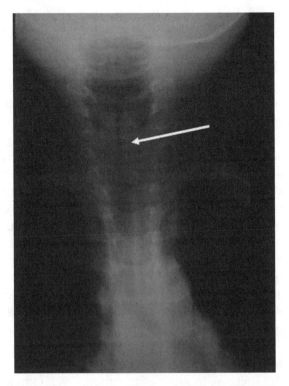

Fig 21–2. The classic steeple sign (*arrow*) seen on a chest radiograph seen in a child with croup. The swelling in the area below the larynx causes the narrowing which is a characteristic finding.

ment includes humidification and hydration. They may respond to racemic epinephrine. Consider admitting the patient for observation if she exhibits increasing respiratory difficulty with tachypnea, restlessness, retractions, or stridor at rest. A minority of the patients may need endoscopic evaluation in the OR, with intubation considered if they are manifesting cyanosis or significant increase in work of breathing. Role of steroids in the management of croup is debatable though they are used rather frequently.

SUPRAGLOTTITIS

Although most physicians may use the term epiglottitis, supraglottitis is the preferred term as it more accurately describes the disease entity given the more diffuse nature of the infection. Supraglottitis is most commonly caused by *Haemophilus influenzae* type B. Less commonly, it can be as a result of *Staphylococcus aureus* or beta-hemolytic *Streptococcus*. Its incidence has diminished considerably since the introduction of the *Haemophilus influenzae* type b (Hib) vaccine. However, it can still sporadically be encountered in children, and must be considered especially in nonvaccinated patients with acute respiratory distress. Supraglottitis tends to occur more commonly in the winter, and more often in children between 2 and 6 years of age. Typically, children with supraglottitis may complain of odynophagia or difficulty breathing. They may appear toxic, have high fever, are tachypneic and tachycardic, may be drooling, and manifest inspiratory stridor. They may exhibit increase in work of breathing, even exhibiting air hunger. They may appear anxious. They will usually be unwilling to lie down, and will prefer to sit in the upright position with the chin thrust forward, the neck hyperextended, and their tongue protruding to maintain their airway. Their voice may sound muffled. Eventually they may become exhausted from their respiratory effort, leading to rapid deterioration in their airway. Supraglottitis is a true airway emergency due to the potential for precipitous airway compromise.

If you suspect supraglottitis in a child, be very careful to avoid any manipulation. Do not draw blood or start an IV. Keep the child as calm as possible. Exciting the child may precipitate airway obstruction. Immediately alert the otolaryngologist and the anesthesiologist on call, and make arrangements immediately to bring the patient to the operating room. A lateral neck radiograph of the airway should be performed in the ER, and will reveal supraglottic swelling (the so-called thumb sign—see the adult section below). Airway in these patients needs to be secured in the operating room. The parent should be allowed to accompany the child to the OR, where the child may be breathed down with an inhalation anesthetic while maintaining spontaneous ventilation. These patients should not be paralyzed, as loss of spontaneous respiratory drive may prove catastrophic. The otolaryngologist will perform the laryngoscopy/bronchoscopy, confirming the diagnosis and securing the airway either with an endotracheal tube (ETT) or the ventilating bronchoscope. The patient can be maintained intubated in the pediatric intensive care unit (PICU) until an air leak is detected around the ETT and flexible pharyngoscopy suggests decreased supraglottic edema. The patient is kept sedated to avoid accidental extubation, while intravenous antibiotic therapy (eg, cefuroxime 30 mg/kg divided Q 12hrs) is initiated. Extubation is usually possible between 24 and 72 hours. If, however, the institution lacks a PICU, it would be more prudent to perform a tracheostomy before transferring the patient to a facility with a PICU, as it makes for safer transportation. Antibiotic therapy should be continued for 14 days.

BACTERIAL TRACHEITIS

Another potential cause of acute airway compromise that usually afflicts older children is bacterial tracheitis. Patients usually present with high-grade fever and hoarseness, appear toxic, and have progressive stridor. X-rays show a normal supraglottis, and may suggest subglottic and tracheal narrowing with airway filling defects in some patients. Direct laryngoscopy and bronchoscopy, in the OR are diagnostic, revealing a normal supraglottis, and subglottic as well as tracheal mucosal edema with purulent secretions in the airway. The endoscopy also allows lavage of the airway to evacuate the purulent secretions. *Staphylococcus aureus* is the most common culprit. The patient is intubated following the endoscopy enabling continuing pulmonary toilet, while appropriate antibiotic therapy is instituted. Extubation usually is possible when the child is nontoxic and afebrile.

FOREIGN BODIES

Most foreign body aspirations occur in children 15 and younger, with the 1- to 3-year-olds being the most susceptible. Vegetable matter (ie, food) tends to be the most commonly aspirated item in these toddlers. Older kids tend to aspirate nonorganic material including buttons, balloons, parts of toys, erasers, and so forth. Foreign body aspiration is a serious matter. The National Safety Council estimates that there are 2,900 deaths each year in the United States because of foreign body aspiration. Many others suffer brain injury from prolonged periods of oxygen deprivation when the airway gets blocked by a foreign body. Death from choking occurs most commonly in children under 5, with two-thirds of those being less than a year old. Successful identification of an aspirated foreign body often requires a high index of suspicion. It is important to gather the history carefully. The aspiration may be witnessed or unwitnessed. The classic history of a body aspiration may include only a severe coughing episode with a brief cyanotic phase. Examine the child and listen for any noisy breathing (including any evidence of wheezing), hoarseness, or impairment in chest movement. Wheezing of new onset, especially if it is heard only on one side of the chest, is strongly suspicious for the presence of a foreign body. Decreased breath sounds in one lung raise the possibility of foreign body aspiration. X-rays of the neck and/or chest may reveal a metallic foreign body or lead-containing glass. Most often, no object is visualized on x-ray. That is because most aspirated foreign bodies (including vegetable matter, ie, food, as well as plastics) are not visible on radiographs. There are some indirect markers of foreign body inhalation on chest x-ray. Inspiratory/expiratory films or decubitus films may suggest partial or complete obstruction (Fig 21–3). Fluoroscopy may reveal impaired diaphragmatic movement with a differential in lung volumes.

Management of suspected airway foreign body involves a pediatric otolaryngology consultation and a prompt trip to the operating room for airway endoscopy to remove the foreign body. Tracheotomy or thoracotomy may be rarely necessary to enable successful retrieval.

RECURRENT RESPIRATORY PAPILLOMATOSIS

Recurrent respiratory papillomatosis (RRP) is the most common benign neoplasm of the larynx in children and the second most common cause of hoarseness in the pediatric age group. Two distinct forms of RRP have been identified. The juvenile form is more aggressive and usually occurs in children, but occasionally in adults as well. The adult form is less aggressive. RRP is generally diagnosed between 2 and 3 years of age with

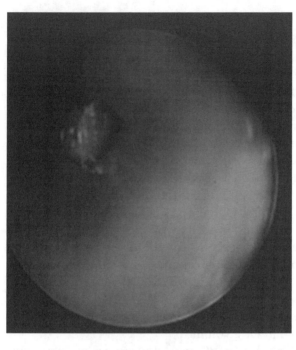

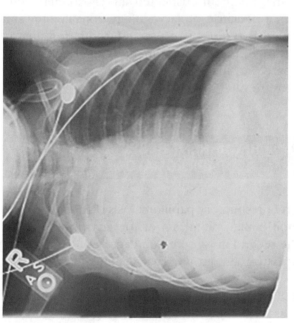

Fig 21–3. A peanut obstructing the right mainstem bronchus (*right*) causing complete obstruction and complete opacification of the right lung in a child (*left*).

75% of the patients being diagnosed by age 5. There is typically a 1-year delay in diagnosis following the onset of symptoms; 1,500 to 2,500 new pediatric cases of RRP are annually identified in the United States. Incidence of RRP is reported to be 4.3 per 100,000 children with 15,000 estimated surgical cases per year. The disease is transmitted from the infected mother's birth canal. The causative organism is the human papilloma virus (HPV). HPV types 6 and 11 are most commonly associated with RRP. Types 16 and 18, whereas less common, have the greatest malignant potential. HPV Type 11 and initial presentation before age 3 are associated with more aggressive disease with need for more frequent debridement and higher likelihood of tracheal involvement by the papillomas or need for tracheotomy.

Patients with RRP usually present with hoarseness. Stridor, inspiratory or biphasic, may be observed. The patient may also present with respiratory difficulty, chronic cough, recurrent pneumonias, failure to thrive, dysphagia, or acute life-threatening events. Surgical debridement is the mainstay of management of RRP with the objectives including reduction of tumor burden, establishment of a safe airway, improvement of voice, reduction of interval between surgeries, and limitation of spread of the disease. Surgery primarily involves either debridement of the papillomas with a microdebrider or ablation of the lesions with a laser. Adjuvant treatments include intralesional injection of cidofovir or mumps vaccine. Other treatment options have included use of photodynamic therapy to support laser ablation, oral administration of indole-3-carbanol, or subcutaneous administration of interferon-alpha. These adjuvant treatment modalities have exhibited variable results. The introduction of the human papilloma virus vaccine may carry some promise in reducing the incidence of RRP in future generations.

OBSTRUCTIVE SLEEP APNEA (OSA)

See section under adult airway obstruction.

INFECTIOUS MONONUCLEOSIS (IM)

IM can cause airway obstruction in the pediatric or adult patients. See Chapter 18 on sore throat for more information on diagnosis and treatment of IM.

ADULT AIRWAY OBSTRUCTION

Upper airway obstruction in the adult can have multiple etiologies including traumatic, infectious, mechanical, neoplastic, or allergic. The patients generally will present with shortness of breath. It is critical to note that normal pulse oximetry does not indicate that the patient's airway is not obstructed. A drop in peripheral oxygenation is often the last indicator of airway obstruction. The patients generally will be tachypneic, possibly retracting suprasternally or in the chest wall, and be tachycardic. As always, airway assessment should be done immediately. The most common causes of adult airway obstruction are noted in Figure 21–4.

TRAUMATIC AIRWAY OBSTRUCTION

See Trauma to the Neck, Chapter 26.

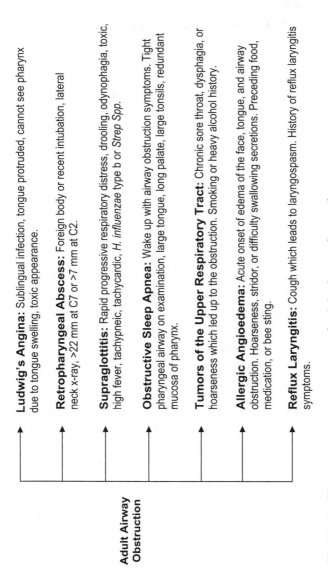

Adult Airway Obstruction

Ludwig's Angina: Sublingual infection, tongue protruded, cannot see pharynx due to tongue swelling, toxic appearance.

Retropharyngeal Abscess: Foreign body or recent intubation, lateral neck x-ray, >22 mm at C7 or >7 mm at C2.

Supraglottitis: Rapid progressive respiratory distress, drooling, odynophagia, toxic, high fever, tachypneic, tachycardic, *H. influenzae* type b or *Strep Spp.*

Obstructive Sleep Apnea: Wake up with airway obstruction symptoms. Tight pharyngeal airway on examination, large tongue, long palate, large tonsils, redundant mucosa of pharynx.

Tumors of the Upper Respiratory Tract: Chronic sore throat, dysphagia, or hoarseness which led up to the obstruction. Smoking or heavy alcohol history.

Allergic Angioedema: Acute onset of edema of the face, tongue, and airway obstruction. Hoarseness, stridor, or difficulty swallowing secretions. Preceding food, medication, or bee sting.

Reflux Laryngitis: Cough which leads to laryngospasm. History of reflux laryngitis symptoms.

Fig 21–4. The most common causes of adult airway obstruction.

INFECTIOUS AIRWAY OBSTRUCTION

All fascial spaces of the neck are connected and their connection allows infections to spread from one space to another. Infections can involve these spaces starting from the pharynx, a lymph node (eg, lymphadenitis), a dental infection, or after dental work. It is most commonly caused by gram-positive and anaerobic bacteria.

Ludwig's Angina

Ludwig's angina is an infection of the sublingual fascia space. This infection generally starts at a dental root that spreads beyond the mandible and involves the sublingual space. The bacteria that cause this infection are gram positives and anaerobes. As a result of the edema from the infection the tongue gets pushed up and back and eventually causes obstruction of the airway from the closure of the pharynx.

Symptoms and Signs

The patient will present with difficulty breathing swallowing and pain in the mouth and tongue. On examination, the patient generally will be in distress with a fever and may be drooling. The patient's floor of mouth and submental area will be edematous and the tongue will be sitting close to the palate and sometimes can be protruding. Even with the examiner's greatest effort with a tongue depressor, the pharynx cannot be seen.

Diagnosis and What Tests to Order

The diagnosis is made by the characteristic edema of the tongue and the patient's difficulty swallowing.

These patients can rapidly progress to an airway obstruction and will need urgent treatment. In an outpatient setting, it is best to have the patient transported to the nearest emergency department via an ambulance. In a hospital setting, first, the airway must be secured if there is any doubt on its stability using fiberoptic nasal intubation or an emergency tracheostomy. After airway management, a CBC and a CT of the neck with contrast should be obtained to evaluate the extent of the infection. Rarely, these patients will present early enough to not require emergency airway management.

Treatment and When to Refer

Treatment of Ludwig's angina is with clindamycin 900 mg q8hrs (children, 30 mg/kg/day IV divided q8hrs). An otolaryngology and dentistry/oral surgery consultation must be obtained urgently for the drainage of the infection and for a dental evaluation, respectively. Otolaryngology consultation is critical for early management of the airway.

Peritonsillar Abscess/Parapharyngeal Space Abscess

See Sore Throat, Chapter 18.

Retropharyngeal Abscess

Retropharyngeal abscess is an infection in the retropharyngeal space which occurs as a result of spread from a pharyngeal bacterial infection or from trauma to the posterior pharyngeal wall. Trauma can occur as a result of a foreign body (eg, bone in food, or pencil in mouth), intubation, or endoscopy. This infection can be fatal if there is airway obstruction or spread to the mediastinum. It is most commonly caused by gram-positive and anaerobic bacteria.

Symptoms and Signs

The patients generally will present with a sore throat, odynophagia, dyspnea, and neck rigidity. On examination, the patients will have edema of the posterior pharyngeal wall, fever, lymphadenopathy, drooling, and possibly stridor.

Diagnosis and What Tests to Order

The findings on the examination, a recent history of trauma to the pharynx, and a lateral soft tissue neck x-ray will help in the diagnosis. The normal lateral soft tissue neck x-ray should have less than 7 mm of soft tissue anterior to C2 and less than 22 mm at C7, the so called "7 at 2, 22 at 7" rule (Fig 21–5). A CT scan of the neck with contrast after airway assessment and management will establish the extent of the abscess.

Treatment and When to Refer

The treatment is with clindamycin 900 mg q8hrs (children, 30 mg/kg/day IV divided q8hrs). An otolaryngology consultation must be obtained for airway management and drainage of the infection.

Infectious Mononucleosis

See Sore Throat, Chapter 18.

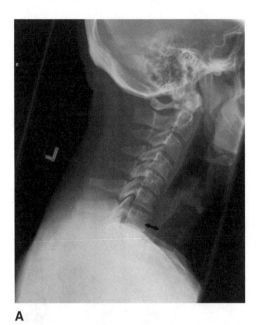

A

Fig 21–5. A. Lateral neck x-ray showing the normal soft tissue width of the retropharyngeal area that abuts C7. *continues*

Epiglottitis

Epiglottitis (also called supraglottitis in adults) is an acute infection involving the region superior to the larynx (supraglottic area) with resultant edema of the epiglottis, arytenoids, and aryepiglottic folds. It is most commonly caused by *Haemophilus influenzae* in children and adults, but in adults can be caused by *Strep spp.* as well.

Symptoms and Signs

The patients generally will have a rapidly progressive course and will present with difficulty breathing, sore

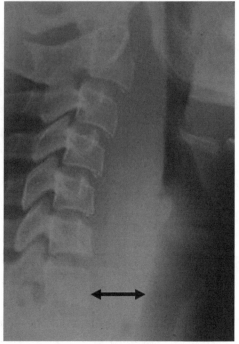

B

Fig 21–5. *continued* **B.** Lateral neck x-ray in a patient with retropharyngeal abscess showing the thickened soft tissue width.

throat, swallowing problems, and at a later stage, drooling. On examination, the patient generally will appear toxic, have a fever, may be sitting with the neck extended (to improve their airway) and drooling, may have stridor (at a later stage), and commonly have a muffled (hot potato) voice.

Diagnosis and What Tests to Order

The diagnosis can be made clinically by the history and flexible laryngoscopy. Given that flexible laryngoscopy generally is not available to the primary care physician, the best method of diagnosis is using a soft tissue lateral neck x-ray. The "thumb sign" seen on the x-ray (Fig 21–6) is a characteristic finding of an edematous epiglottis seen on a lateral film. It is critical that the patient not be rotated as the rotation of a normal patient can cause the appearance of a thumb sign. Therefore, if faced with a lateral neck film that shows a thumb sign in a patient with no signs or symptoms of epiglottitis, emergency intervention is not needed and the x-ray should be repeated.

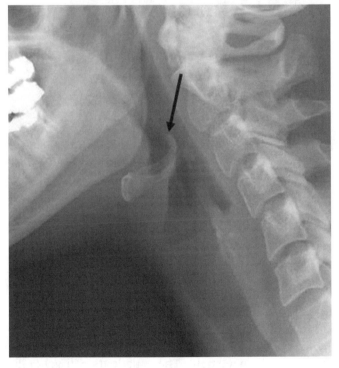

A

Fig 21–6. A. Lateral neck x-ray showing the normal outline of the epiglottis (*arrow*). *continues*

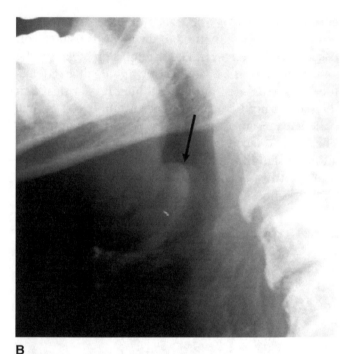

B

Fig 21–6. *continued* **B.** The thumb sign (like a thumbprint on the x-ray) seen in a patient with epiglottitis (*arrow*).

Treatment and When to Refer

A patient suspected of having epiglottitis should be transported via ambulance to the nearest emergency department. The patient should be started on a broad spectrum antibiotic such as ampicillin sublactam 3 g IV q6hrs (children, 300 mg/kg/d IV divided q6hrs). Emergency consultation with an otolaryngologist is needed for airway management. These patients will generally require flexible endoscopic nasotracheal intubation or an emergency tracheostomy.

MECHANICAL OBSTRUCTION

Obstructive Sleep Apnea (OSA)

OSA generally occurs as a result of obstruction of the upper airway during sleep. During sleep, the tongue can fall back and obstruct the pharyngeal airway. This generally will occur most commonly in patients where there is narrowing of the pharyngeal airway due to an enlarged tongue, nasal obstruction, short neck, high body mass index, enlarged tonsils, long soft palate or uvula, or excessive pharyngeal tissue.

Symptoms and Signs

The patients most commonly will present with day-time somnolence and will have experienced a sense of airway obstruction during sleep. The patient (usually the spouse) will complain of loud snoring. The patient generally will need to take naps during the day and involuntarily may fall asleep. On examination, the pharyngeal airway will be small due to an elongated soft palate/uvula, enlarged uvula, tonsils, tongue, or a combination thereof. Patients with a higher body mass index and those with shorter necks are at a higher risk for OSA. Children who snore regularly have a 45% likelihood of having sleep apnea.

Diagnosis and What Tests to Order

The diagnosis is made by performing an overnight polysomnogram (sleep study) in adults. A respiratory distress index (a combination of apneic and hypopneic events per hour) of greater than 15 indicates a diagnosis of OSA. In children, the diagnosis is based on the history of loud snoring, apnea, and enlarged tonsils. A sleep study is necessary in children only if the history of sleep apnea exists in the absence of enlarged tonsils.

Treatment and When to Refer

If nasal obstruction is present, the treatment of nasal obstruction can oftentimes improve the severity of sleep apnea (see Nasal Congestion, Chapter 11 for more details on diagnosis and treatment of nasal obstruction). Having the patient sleep on his or her side will also help reduce the likelihood of the tongue falling back and obstructing the airway. A continuous positive-airway pressure (CPAP) device helps most adult patients with their sleep apnea. Patients who are unable to use a CPAP machine or do not wish to use such a device will sometimes benefit from surgical therapy. An otolaryngologist referral for evaluation for surgical therapy may be appropriate. Children with sleep apnea will have relief of symptoms in 95% of cases after tonsillectomy and adenoidectomy.

NEOPLASTIC OBSTRUCTION

Tumors of the Upper Respiratory Tract

Benign or malignant tumors of the base of the tongue, tonsil, pharynx, hypopharynx, or larynx can all present with acute airway obstruction. These patients generally will have a long smoking or alcohol abuse history.

Symptoms and Signs

The patient generally will have a chronic sore throat, dysphagia, or hoarseness which led to the airway obstruction. The patient commonly will be hoarse or have a hot potato voice because of the mass in the airway. Examination of the oral cavity and pharynx may not reveal the mass, but mirror or flexible fiberoptic laryngoscopy will reveal the mass lesion. Rarely, the mass lesion can be located in the trachea.

Diagnosis and What Tests to Order

The diagnosis is made by examination. In a case of impending airway obstruction, airway management as discussed below under the allergic angioedema section, should be performed. A mass lesion in the pharynx will make intubation greatly difficult as the anatomy will be distorted. Intubation under fiberoptic guidance or an emergency cricothyrotomy or tracheostomy may be necessary in most cases. In the emergency department, a CT of the neck with contrast should be obtained if the patient's airway is stable.

Treatment and When to Refer

A patient with a suspected mass lesion causing airway obstruction should be referred immediately to an emergency department where an otolaryngologist would be available for consultation.

Allergic

Allergic angioedema can occur as a result of response to a variety of sources (Table 21-1) and can be IgE-mediated, histamine-related, mast cell degranulation-related, complement-mediated, or hereditary. Patients on ACE-inhibitors may suddenly develop angioedema even after years of use. ACE-inhibitors can cause isolated edema of the larynx or the supraglottic area (epiglottis, arytenoids, etc).

Table 21–1. The Most Common Causes of Angioedema

Shellfish

Bee sting

Iodine-based radiocontrast agents

Penicillins

Angiotensin-converting enzyme (ACE) inhibitors

Aspirin

Symptoms and Signs

The patients generally will present with an acute onset of edema of the face, tongue, and airway obstruction. The patient may have a hoarse voice, stridor, or have difficulty swallowing secretions. The patient may have cutaneous urticaria, erythema, warmth, or even signs of impending shock.

Diagnosis and What Tests to Order

The diagnosis is made based on the acuity of the symptoms and the exposure to the offending agent preceding the symptoms. In the acute setting with airway obstruction, generally there is no time to obtain tests and securing the airway is of utmost importance. Once the airway is secured in a patient without a clear history of a causative agent, C1 esterase inhibitor level and function should be obtained to evaluate for hereditary angioedema.

Treatment and When to Refer

First, the patient's airway should be assessed. If there is impending airway obstruction, a nasotracheal intubation should be performed. If that is unsuccessful, a cricothyrotomy or an emergency tracheostomy should be performed. For a cricothyrotomy, the patient's neck should be extended and the thyroid cartilage should be palpated (the most prominent cartilaginous structure in the neck). Then by marching inferiorly slowly in the midline with a finger, the first depression that is palpated is the cricothyroid membrane (Fig 21-7). For confirmation, the cricoid cartilage can be palpated immediately below the cricothyroid membrane. The cricoid cartilage is a hard thick ring of cartilage below the membrane. A vertical skin incision is made (to avoid some of the subcutaneous veins that run vertically)

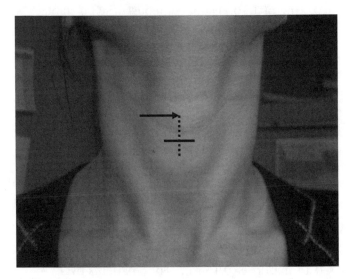

Fig 21-7. Anterior neck in the extended position. The most prominent area of the anterior neck is the thyroid (laryngeal) cartilage (*arrow*). The vertical dashed line indicates the vertical skin incision to be made for a cricothyrotomy. The horizontal solid line indicates the approximate location of the cricothyroid membrane that has to be incised horizontally.

and then a horizontal incision is made in the cricothyroid membrane. An endotracheal tube can be inserted into the opened membrane. In extreme situations, a large bore needle (12, 14, or 16 g) can be used in the midline trachea to allow some movement of air by the patient. It is often difficult to bag the patient through a needle, but it allows for some oxygenation.

If the airway appears secure, then the following medications should be given:

Corticosteroid: dexamethasone 10 mg (children, 0.2 mg/kg) or methylprednisolone 40 mg (children 0.5 mg/kg) IM/IV.

Subcutaneous injection of epinephrine: 0.3 to 0.5 mg of 1:1000 subcutaneously (SC) if stable; 0.3 to 0.5 mg of 1:10,000 IV or via ET if signs of shock: in children, epinephrine is given 0.15 to 0.3 mg (depending on patient weight) of 1:1000 solution SC. If signs of shock are present in a child, 0.01 mg/kg/dose (0.01 mL/kg/dose 1:1000 [1 mg/mL]) IM q5 to 20 min up to 3 doses (dose range, 0.1–0.5 mg/dose). If significant hypoperfusion is present, 0.01 mg/kg/dose IV (0.1 mL/kg/dose 1:10,000 [0.1 mg/mL]) is given. Autoinjectors can be used in the thigh intramuscularly. For a 10 to 20-kg child, EpiPen Jr (1:2000 [0.5 mg/mL]) delivers 0.15 mg/dose (0.3 mL) or Twinject 0.15 mg (1:1000 [1 mg/mL]), which delivers 0.15 mg/dose (0.15 mL). For a patients over 20 kg in weight, EpiPen (1:1000; 1 mg/mL), which delivers 0.3 mg/dose (0.3 mL) or Twinject 0.3 mg (1:1000; 1 mg/mL), which delivers 0.3 mg/dose (0.3 mL).

H1: (eg, diphenhydramine 50 mg IV/IM/PO, children 1 mg/kg IV/IM/PO) and H2 blockers (ranitidine 50 mg IV/IM, children 1 mg/kg IV/IM) can also be given after securing the airway.

The patient with an impending airway obstruction should be transported to the nearest emergency department via ambulance. Treatment with epinephrine and corticosteroids should be started before transportation. Airway management should be performed in the outpatient setting if necessary. A referral to an allergist/immunologist is warranted after an episode of angioedema.

CHAPTER 22

Chronic Cough

ROBERTO L. BARRETTO
HAMID R. DJALILIAN

BACKGROUND

Cough is an explosive force of air through the larynx for the purpose of clearing the airway. Physiologically, cough results in an abrupt, forceful expulsion of air after deep inspiration and closure of the larynx. As a defense mechanism, cough results in the clearance of excess airway secretions as well as particulate foreign material from the airway. The three phases of cough are inspiratory, compressive, and expulsive.

Cough is triggered by chemical and mechanical irritant receptors that are heavily concentrated at the larynx, lower trachea, carina, and larger bronchioles via the vagus nerve as the afferent pathway, to the cough center located in the medulla. The efferent pathway consists of vagal efferents to the larynx and tracheobronchial tree as well as phrenic nerve (diaphragm) and spinal motor nerves (thoracic, abdominal, and pelvic floor muscles) resulting in airflows at the mouth up to 12 L/sec in adults, and up to 2 vital capacities in children.[1] Other important irritant receptors are located in the nose and paranasal sinuses mediated by trigeminal nerve afferents, pharynx mediated by the glossopharyngeal nerve, and external auditory canal and tympanic membrane mediated by the auricular branch of the vagus nerve. Diaphragmatic irritation leading to cough is mediated by afferents of the phrenic nerve.

Although coughing generally is voluntary, chronic cough most commonly occurs from a stimulation of cough receptors in the upper or lower airway. Most acute viral respiratory tract infection lasts less than 2 weeks. Postviral respiratory tract inflammation can last 8 weeks. The guidelines published by the American College of Chest Physicians has defined chronic cough as cough that lasts more than 8 weeks. The most common causes of chronic cough are listed in Table 22–1, the most common of which is smoking. The incidence of chronic cough in smokers increases with increased number of smoked cigarettes per day. This incidence reaches 25% with one pack per day of smoking and close to 50% with two packs per day of smoking. All patients with a chronic cough must undergo chest radiography to rule out the presence of a chest mass, infection, effusions, or other abnormali-

Table 22–1. The Most Common Causes of Chronic Cough with a Normal Chest X-Ray in Adults

Smoking	Postnasal drainage
Postviral reactive airway disease	Pertussis
Laryngopharyngeal reflux	Environmental irritants
Asthma	Eosinophilic bronchitis
Medications (ACE-inhibitors)	Atypical pneumonia

ties (eg, congestive heart failure, etc). The discussion in this section concentrates on chronic cough in the presence of a normal chest radiograph.

CHRONIC COUGH IN ADULTS

See Figure 22–1.

Postinfectious Cough (Postviral Reactive Airway Disease)

Postinfectious cough is defined as a cough lasting more than 3 weeks and less than 8 weeks after an acute

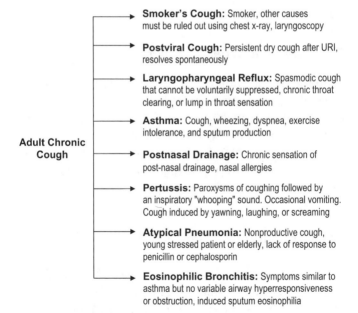

Adult Chronic Cough

Smoker's Cough: Smoker, other causes must be ruled out using chest x-ray, laryngoscopy

Postviral Cough: Persistent dry cough after URI, resolves spontaneously

Laryngopharyngeal Reflux: Spasmodic cough that cannot be voluntarily suppressed, chronic throat clearing, or lump in throat sensation

Asthma: Cough, wheezing, dyspnea, exercise intolerance, and sputum production

Postnasal Drainage: Chronic sensation of post-nasal drainage, nasal allergies

Pertussis: Paroxysms of coughing followed by an inspiratory "whooping" sound. Occasional vomiting. Cough induced by yawning, laughing, or screaming

Atypical Pneumonia: Nonproductive cough, young stressed patient or elderly, lack of response to penicillin or cephalosporin

Eosinophilic Bronchitis: Symptoms similar to asthma but no variable airway hyperresponsiveness or obstruction, induced sputum eosinophilia

Fig 22–1. The most common causes of chronic cough in adults.

respiratory disease. Pathologies suggested for post-infectious cough are inflammation of upper and lower respiratory airways, mucus hypersecretion, and aggravation of pre-existing gastroesophageal reflux disease due to high abdominal pressure during cough.

Symptoms and Signs

The patients generally present with a chronic dry cough that persists after a URI. The examination is generally normal.

Diagnosis and What Tests to Order

Diagnosis is clinical and is based on persistence of cough more than 3 weeks after an acute respiratory disease. Chest x-ray is normal in these patients and the cough resolves spontaneously.

Treatment and When to Refer

Antibiotics are shown not to be effective. Trials of inhaled ipratropium (2 puffs inhaled QID) has shown efficacy in patients with postinfectious cough. Inhaled corticosteroid therapy has not been found to be effective in reducing postinfectious cough. Occasionally, oral corticosteroid therapy starting with 0.5 mg/kg/day of prednisone for 5 days may help.

Laryngopharyngeal Reflux (LPR)

LPR is a common cause of chronic dry cough in adults. The patient may complain of chronic throat clearing or spasmodic cough. Other complaints may include a cough that they cannot stop, which can lead to laryngospasm and temporary airway obstruction.

For diagnosis and treatment of LPR, please see Chapter 18 on sore throat.

Asthma

Asthma is a disease that is characterized by hyper-responsiveness of the airways to various stimuli, which results in reversible airway obstruction. The airway obstruction is from variable components of bronchial smooth muscle spasm and inflammation of the respiratory mucosa and hypersecretion of mucous. Cough variant asthma is defined as a history of cough at night, during or after exercise, in cold air, or precipitated by aerosol sprays.

Symptoms and Signs

The most common presenting symptoms include cough, wheezing, dyspnea, exercise intolerance, and sputum production. Symptoms may be present during the entire year which is called perennial or be seasonal and become aggravated with seasonal allergens. Allergens, exercise, drugs, and occupational exposure may aggravate the symptoms. Patients may have a family history of allergic rhinitis, atopic dermatitis, and asthma. On chest examination end-expiratory wheezing, rales, and prolonged expiratory phase will be found in some lung fields. More severe exacerbation may show decreased respiratory rate and wheezing in all fields. Patients are divided into four groups based on the severity of the disease. Intermittent asthma is when exacerbation occurs less than once a week and nocturnal symptoms are present less than twice a month. In mild persistent asthma symptoms happen more than once a week but less than once a day and nocturnal symptoms occur more than twice a month.

Moderate persistent asthma manifests with daily symptoms and nocturnal symptoms more than once a week. In severe persistent asthma patients have continuous symptoms and frequent nocturnal symptoms.

Diagnosis and What Tests to Order

To confirm diagnosis during acute attacks spirometry before and after administration of β2-agonists is used. Increase in FEV1 more than 15% after inhalation of β2-agonist is diagnostic. Methacholine challenge test is diagnostic for patients without exacerbation. Asthmatic patients show more than 20% decrease in FEV1 after methacholine. CBC may show eosinophilia. Sputum eosinophilia and increased immunoglobulin E are also suggestive. Chest x-ray is usually normal. Arterial blood gas examination in primary stages of acute exacerbation shows increase in pH due to tachypnea that alternates with acidosis and decreased pH later in the course of disease. Allergen skin testing is useful in detecting allergens responsible for exacerbation.

Treatment and When to Refer

The treatment of asthma is beyond the scope of this chapter. If the asthma is previously undiagnosed, then starting appropriate therapy with short acting β2-agonists, ipratropium bromide, inhaled steroids, combination inhalers (eg, fluticasone/salmeterol), leukotriene inhibitors (eg, Montelukast, Zafirlukast), or even oral steroids can be used depending on the severity of the disease.

Adult-onset asthma without a known history of asthma or allergies especially in a smoker needs further workup if initial treatment fails. Smokers (current or previous) are at risk of laryngeal or bronchial carcinoma that can present with shortness of breath. Laryngopharyngeal reflux can also cause a reactive airway by causing spillage of acid into the airway at the level of the larynx. Oftentimes, treatment of the underlying reflux with proton-pump inhibitors (eg, omeprazole 40 mg QAM before breakfast, children 1 mg/kg/d QAM before breakfast or before dinner) will resolve the asthma symptoms.

Postnasal Drainage

See Nasal Discharge, Chapter 13.

Pertussis

Pertussis is a bacterial infection caused by *Bordatella pertussis*. It has been an under-recognized cause of chronic cough. In multiple studies looking at patients with chronic cough, the incidence of pertussis infection diagnosed by culture or PCR studies has been found to be between 7.5% and 17%. Therefore, it is important to consider pertussis as a cause of chronic cough.

Symptoms and Signs

Pertussis has a 2-day incubation period and is followed by mild upper respiratory infection (URI) symptoms of rhinorrhea, cough, and sneezing. Two weeks after the onset of the URI symptoms, the cough changes into paroxysms of coughing followed by an inspiratory "whooping" sound (paroxysmal stage). Coughing fits can cause vomiting when violent. The cough is generally induced by yawning, laughing, or screaming. The cough can decrease over the next 1 to 2 months.

Diagnosis and What Tests to Order

The diagnosis of pertussis is made using a nasopharyngeal culture, polymerase chain reaction (PCR) of the nasopharyngeal swab, immunofluorescence, or serology (anti-pertussis IgG). Serology requires an IgG level in the acute phase (acute serum) followed by testing at 4 weeks (convalescence serum). The convalescence serum generally will be lower than the acute serum. The nasopharyngeal culture or immunofluorescence will only be positive for the first 3 weeks of the infection. The PCR test can be positive for an additional 3 weeks. Serology is the best method of detecting a pertussis infection for most adults and adolescents who present with chronic cough.

Treatment and When to Refer

Erythromycin 40 to 50 mg/kg for 14 days is recommended for children divided into four doses. Adults receive 250 to 500 mg of erythromycin QID for 14 days. Alternatives for patients who can not tolerate erythromycin are trimethoprim sulfamethaxazole (8 mg TMP/ 40 mg SMX BID in children or one tab BID in adults for 14 days) or azithromycin (10–12 mg/kg/day for 5 days in children or 500 mg daily for 5 days in adults).

Atypical Pneumonia

A full discussion of pneumonia is beyond the scope of this book, but atypical pneumonia should be considered in the differential diagnosis of chronic cough.

Eosinophilic Bronchitis

Eosinophilic bronchitis is characterized by an eosinophilic airway inflammation (similar to asthma) in the absence of variable airflow or airway hyperresponsiveness. Although in some patients occupational exposure to allergens can cause this condition, in many, no true etiology is found.

Symptoms and Signs

The patients will present with a chronic dry cough and will have a normal head, neck, and chest examination.

Diagnosis and What Tests to Order

The diagnosis of eosinophilic bronchitis is made in chronic cough patients when induced sputum eosinophilia is found in the presence of a normal chest x-ray (CXR), normal spirometry, and no evidence of variable airflow obstruction or airway hyperresponsiveness.

Treatment and When to Refer

Eosinophilic bronchitis is best treated with inhaled corticosteroids (eg, budenoside 360 μg inhaled BID) for 4 weeks. The patients should be referred to a pulmonologist if there is no response to a 4-week course of inhaled steroids for bronchoscopy and possible oral steroid therapy.

Throat Clearing

Chronic throat clearing most commonly occurs as a result of irritation of the larynx by laryngopharyngeal reflux. When part of the refluxate from the stomach spills onto the vocal cords (folds), the patient will involuntarily clear his or her throat or cough to clear the secretions from the larynx.

Treatment and When to Refer

The patient should be started on a proton-pump inhibitor (eg, omeprazole 40 mg po QD for one month) and make dietary and lifestyle change to reduce reflux. If there is no improvement with the above measures the patient should be referred to an otolaryngologist for evaluation and laryngoscopy.

PEDIATRIC CHRONIC COUGH

Cough is a common symptom of respiratory tract illness in children and is one of the most frequent reasons for ambulatory care visits. Cough, along with the gag reflex, mucociliary clearance, and the immune system, is an important protective mechanism for the respiratory system.

Physiologically, cough results in an abrupt, forceful expulsion of air after deep inspiration and closure of the larynx. As a defense mechanism, cough results in the clearance of excess airway secretions as well as particulate foreign material from the airway. The three phases of cough are inspiratory, compressive and expulsive.

Cough can be a sign of an underlying illness or may be nonspecific but nonetheless be quite distressing to the child and the child's family. Parental worries include fear of the child dying from choking, as well as anxiety about asthma exacerbations, sudden infant death syndrome or permanent chest injury. Children with cough are commonly sent home from school or daycare in fear of a communicable illness. Cough is a leading reason for the use of over-the-counter medications, which have been proven to be ineffective in young children and even dangerous.[2] Parents are often required to take time off from work to care for their child or to bring them for a visit to the doctor. Doctors are pressured to prescribe antibiotics and/or cough suppressants. Continued cough may disrupt sleep for the entire family, contribute to secondary irritation of the laryngotracheobronchial tree or lead to vomiting and failure to thrive. A thoughtful, practical approach to cough can assist the clinician in correctly diagnosing and treating a pediatric patient and ultimately reassuring their families. Figure 22–2 outlines the most common causes of pediatric chronic cough.

The assessment of cough, starting with the age of a child is helpful. For example in the neonatal period, congenital anomalies such as tracheoesophageal fistula are worthwhile considerations on a list of differential diagnoses, but not so for a 10-year-old. Infants and toddlers tend to be more prone to witnessed or unwitnessed aspiration or ingestion of foreign bodies. The duration of a cough is also important in aiding to formulate a diagnosis and treatment plan. Acute cough is classified as <3 week's duration, chronic cough >4 week's duration. A brief discussion on acute cough follows, but the majority of the chapter focuses on the more challenging problem of chronic cough.

ACUTE COUGH: HISTORY AND PHYSICAL EXAMINATION

Acute cough (<3 week's duration) is most often associated with a respiratory viral illness, such as the common cold, but may also be associated with croup, bronchiolitis, bronchitis, pneumonia, or an asthma exacerbation. It may also be associated with laryngitis, pharyngitis, sinusitis, allergic rhinitis or postnasal drip.[3] Especially in young children, cough may also be indicative of an aspirated or ingested foreign body.

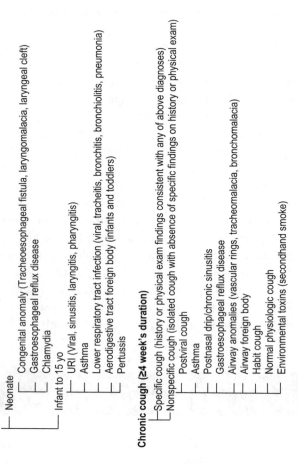

Acute Cough (≤3 week's duration)

Neonate
- Congenital anomaly (Tracheoesophageal fistula, laryngomalacia, laryngeal cleft)
- Gastroesophageal reflux disease
- Chlamydia

Infant to 15 yo
- URI (Viral, sinusitis, laryngitis, pharyngitis)
- Asthma
- Lower respiratory tract infection (viral, tracheitis, bronchitis, bronchiolitis, pneumonia)
- Aerodigestive tract foreign body (infants and toddlers)
- Pertussis

Chronic cough (≥4 week's duration)

- Specific cough (history or physical exam findings consistent with any of above diagnoses)
- Nonspecific cough (isolated cough with absence of specific findings on history or physical exam)
  - Postviral cough
  - Asthma
  - Postnasal drip/chronic sinusitis
  - Gastroesophageal reflux disease
  - Airway anomalies (vascular rings, tracheomalacia, bronchomalacia)
  - Airway foreign body
  - Habit cough
  - Normal physiologic cough
  - Environmental toxins (secondhand smoke)

Fig 22–2. The most common causes of chronic cough in the pediatric patient.

Key points to elicit on history and examination are whether the condition is life-threatening (severe asthma, aspiration, pneumonia, heart failure) or non-life-threatening (viral respiratory illness, asthma exacerbation, or allergic rhinitis). Witnessed choking episodes may indicate an aspirated or ingested foreign body. Fever may indicate an infectious cause.

An ear examination is important to assess for the possibility of an ear canal foreign body or hair that may be stimulating the auricular branch of the vagus nerve. Nasal examination may lead to a suspicion for a viral upper respiratory infection, allergic rhinitis or sinusitis. Acute bacterial sinusitis may be difficult to differentiate from a viral illness, but a useful guide is to consider acute bacterial sinusitis if a cold is worsening or seems to be prolonged beyond 10 days. Sinus x-rays are not useful in differentiating a bacterial sinus infection from the common cold. Examination of the throat may indicate pharyngitis, tonsillitis, adenotonsillar hypertrophy, or postnasal drip.

Auscultation of the upper airway for stridor (a whistling-type noise caused by narrowing at the level of the larynx and/or upper trachea) and listening for a hoarse voice may indicate croup or laryngitis, or even a laryngeal or pharyngeal foreign body. A sudden inability to tolerate oral feeding or sudden loss of voice is very suspicious for an acutely aspirated or ingested foreign body. Auscultation of the lungs is important to assess for wheezing, rales, or rhonchi as well as the presence or absence of breath sounds. Asymmetric findings (especially a unilateral wheeze) may indicate a bronchial foreign body or pneumonia. Diagnostic tests that are useful for these specific findings include spirometry and chest x-ray. Treatment for the above conditions should include appropriate referral to a pulmonologist or otolaryngologist depending on the suspected diagnosis causing the acute cough.

CHRONIC COUGH: HISTORY AND PHYSICAL EXAMINATION

The remainder of the section focuses on chronic cough which is defined as daily cough present for 4 weeks or greater. In children less than 15 years old, chronic cough often has a different etiology and approach to diagnosis and treatment than in adults.

Cough can be associated with specific findings or may be nonspecific. Cough caused by suppurative lung disease may be linked to specific findings such as digital, productive cough, or hemoptysis. Dyspnea or tachypnea can be associated with any parenchymal lung or pulmonary airway disease. Hypoxia or cyanosis may indicate pulmonary, airway, or cardiac disease. Immune deficiency can lead to recurrent pneumonias or atypical lung infections. Recurrent pneumonias, on the other hand, may indicate the presence of a tracheoesophageal fistula or an undiagnosed immune deficiency. Neurologic impairment is a risk factor for aspiration pneumonia. Feeding difficulties may indicate aspiration, anatomic abnormalities of the aerodigestive tract, or foreign body. Failure to thrive may indicate a systemic illness such as cystic fibrosis.

Nonspecific chronic cough is defined as daily cough in the absence of specific signs and symptoms, namely, cough is the only symptom. Etiology of nonspecific cough is more difficult to ascertain, and most cases are thought to be related to postviral cough and/or increased cough receptor sensitivity. Cough may also be a normal physiologic behavior and is termed normal or expected cough. Normal, specific, and nonspecific cough can overlap, and on further investigation a nonspecific cough may prove to have a specific cause, for example, an unsuspected bronchial foreign body. Even though the cause of most nonspecific cough is thought to be benign, a thorough evaluation is necessary to prevent serious sequelae, for example, permanent lung damage from a delay in diagnosing a bronchial foreign body.

DIAGNOSTIC MODALITIES

A chest x-ray and CBC with differential are reasonable tests to obtain in any child with acute or chronic cough, and may point to infectious and/or pulmonary disease. Tuberculosis (TB) testing is warranted if exposure to TB or infection is suspected. Spirometry is advocated in children greater than 3 to 6 years of age. Abnormal spirometry with reversible airway obstruction indicates a diagnosis of asthma. If obstruction is nonreversible, referral to a pediatric otolaryngologist is indicated to assess the need for further workup such as CT scan of the chest and/or diagnostic bronchoscopy. CT scan of the sinuses, and/or referral to a pediatric otolaryngologist should be obtained if there are concerns about the development of chronic sinusitis. CT scans in children should be utilized with caution because of the increased lifetime risk in developing cancer of 1 in 1,000 to 2,500, which is 10 times that of adults.

NONSPECIFIC ETIOLOGIES

Asthma (Cough-Variant Asthma)

Asthma is rarely the cause of isolated cough, and would produce a dry cough in the absence of a coexisting respiratory infection. Complicating the picture is that viral respiratory infections which on their own can cause chronic cough are also the cause of 80% of childhood asthma exacerbations.

Sinusitis/Postnasal Drip

Upper airway cough syndrome (postnasal drip syndrome) is a common cause of cough in adults, but a cause and effect relationship between chronic sinusitis and cough in children has not been definitively established, although cough is a common symptom of children with chronic sinusitis. Cough is not associated with sinusitis once atopy and allergic rhinitis are controlled for.[3] Treating allergic rhinitis in adolescents and adults with mometasone furoate showed a significant improvement in daytime cough versus placebo.[4] There have been no randomized controlled studies on therapies for upper airway disorders in younger children with nonspecific cough.

Gastroesophageal Reflux Disease (GERD)

The relationship between GERD and cough is well established in adults, but not in children. Chronic cough can exacerbate GERD in adults, but it is unclear if respiratory symptoms may exacerbate GERD in children leading to a complex cause and effect relationship that is unclear. A recent study of children with chronic cough showed GERD in 4 of 49 pts.[5]

Airway Abnormalities

Tracheobronchomalacia and congenital vascular anomalies or rings may present with persistent cough. Asthma often is misdiagnosed in children with congenital airway narrowing. Inspissated secretions can build up distal to an airway narrowing and can lead to pneumonia or recurrent infections. Yet, the manner in which congenital airway abnormalities such as tracheobronchomalacia and vascular anomalies such as an aberrant innominate artery cause isolated cough is still not well understood. Airway or vascular anomalies should be suspected when there is no resolution of the cough after conservative management or if there is associated feeding abnormalities.

Environmental Irritants

Increased environmental tobacco smoke increases susceptibility to respiratory infections and increases coughing illnesses. Still, there is some conflicting evidence against the effects of parental smoking and coughing in the first decade of life.[6] Additional studies looking at exposure to other airway pollutants such as general particulate matter, nitrogen dioxide and gas cooking and their association with chronic cough also have mixed findings.

Treatment

In October, 2007 the United States Food and Drug Administration advised against the use of over-the-counter (OTC) cough and cold medicine in children age 2 and younger. The use of these medications in children over 2 is still being debated today, as to their safety and efficacy. The treatment of chronic specific cough should be directed to the underlying etiology and referral to a specialist is warranted for cough that is not improving.

For chronic nonspecific cough, referral to a pediatric pulmonologist or otolaryngologist should be considered early on. A short (2–4 week) empiric treatment for asthma with beclomethasone 400 mcg/d or the equivalent dosage with budesonide may be warranted in children with risk factors for asthma. Treatment should be withdrawn if the cough does not improve.

Treatment can be started empirically for upper airway cough syndrome (postnasal drip, mometasone 1 puff each nostril QD) and even GERD (omeprazole 1 mg/kg/d), but must be monitored closely and the treatments withdrawn or modified if no benefits are noted. One example of a low-risk empiric trial is to start with nasal steroid sprays and GERD preventive measures, adding GERD medication if the index of suspicion for GERD is higher. Extended courses of antibiotics should be reserved for children with a diagnosis of chronic sinusitis. Daily nasal saline irrigations followed by the use of nasal steroid sprays are also important in managing chronic sinusitis.

Bronchoscopy and other tests such as an immunologic workup should be performed on a case-by-case basis. Identification and control of environmental factors such as secondhand smoke exposure should not be forgotten. Recognizing and addressing the concerns and expectations of parents regarding their child's cough also goes a long way in resolving the anxiety surrounding the diagnosis and treatment of this condition. The indications of bronchoscopy and esophagoscopy include unilateral wheezing, witnessed cough with cyanosis (possible foreign body aspiration), feeding abnormalities (eg, recurrent vomiting, failure to thrive), recurrent pneumonias, and chest x-ray findings indicating foreign body aspiration, among others. The patient should be referred to a pediatric otolaryngologist for a full evaluation when conservative therapy fails.

FURTHER READING

Chang AB, Glomb WB. Guidelines for evaluating chronic cough in pediatrics: ACCP evidence-based clinical practice guidelines. *Chest.* 2006;129(1 suppl):260S–283S.

Chang AB, Phelan PD, Sawyer SM, Robertson CF. Airway hyperresponsiveness and cough-receptor sensitivity in children with recurrent cough. *Am J Respir Crit Care Med.* 1997;155(6):1935–1939.

Johnston SL, Pattemore PK, Sanderson G, et al. Community study of role of viral infections in exacerbations of asthma in 9–11 year old children. *Br Med J.* 1995;310(6989):1225–1229.

Munyard P, Bush A. How much coughing is normal? *Arch Dis Child.* 1996;74(6):531–534.

REFERENCES

1. Eigen H. The clinical evaluation of chronic cough. *Pediatr Clin North Am.* 1982;29(1):67–78.

2. Carr BC. Efficacy, abuse, and toxicity of over-the-counter cough and cold medicines in the pediatric population. *Curr Opin Pediatr.* 2006;18(2):184–188.

3. Lombardi E, Stein RT, Wright AL, Morgan WJ, Martinez FD. The relation between physician-diagnosed sinusitis, asthma, and skin test reactivity to allergens in 8-year-old children. *Pediatr Pulmonol.* 1996;22(3):141–146.

4. Gawchik S, Goldstein S, Prenner B, John A. Relief of cough and nasal symptoms associated with allergic rhinitis by mometasone furoate nasal spray. *Ann Allergy Asthma Immunol.* 2003;90(4):416–421.

5. Thomson F, Masters IB, Chang AB. Persistent cough in children and the overuse of medications. *J Paediatr Child Health.* 2002;38(6):578–581.

6. Stein RT, Holberg CJ, Sherrill D, et al. Influence of parental smoking on respiratory symptoms during the first decade of life: the Tucson Children's Respiratory Study. *Am J Epidemiol.* 1999;149(11):1030–1037.

CHAPTER 23

Disorders of the Salivary Glands, Thyroid, and Parathyroid

WILLIAM B. ARMSTRONG

SALIVARY GLAND DISORDERS

Key Points

- Inflammatory lesions of the parotid are more commonly acute in onset, or are recurrently episodic.
- Neoplasms of the salivary glands are generally slow growing and painless.
- Clinical characteristics of the salivary gland mass are unreliable for predicting whether the mass is benign or malignant.
- A mass of the parotid gland is abnormal and evaluation to determine its etiology is required.

Introduction

The salivary glands are divided into the major and minor salivary glands. The minor salivary glands line the mucosal surface of the oral cavity including the lip, buccal mucosa, and the palate. The disorders of minor salivary glands are covered in the chapter on oral lesions (Chapter 17). This chapter discusses major salivary gland disorders (Fig 23–1). The glands produce approximately one liter of saliva per day, which is important for taste, swallowing, digestion, and maintaining mineralization of the teeth and health of the gums and mucosa in the oral cavity. The bulk of saliva is produced by three sets of major salivary glands. The parotid glands and the submandibular glands produce the majority of saliva. The parotid glands are located between the mandible and the ear, partially overlying the masseter muscle. They are divided artificially into superficial and deep lobes by the facial nerve passing through the gland, and drain into the buckle mucosa through the parotid (Stensen's) duct which opens by the second maxillary molars. The submandibular glands lie below the mandible, draining through the paired Wharton's ducts into the anterior floor of the mouth. Also lying in the floor of the mouth are the sublingual glands situated in the submucosal tissues in the lateral floor of the mouth. Finally, a number of minor salivary glands are distributed through the oral cavity.

A variety of acute and chronic pathologic conditions affect the salivary glands, and swelling of the salivary glands has an extensive differential diagnosis. Nevertheless, salivary gland pathology can be classified accurately with a relatively thorough history, physical examination, and focused diagnostic studies. Acute viral infection generally causes bilateral swelling of the parotid glands, and is most commonly caused by

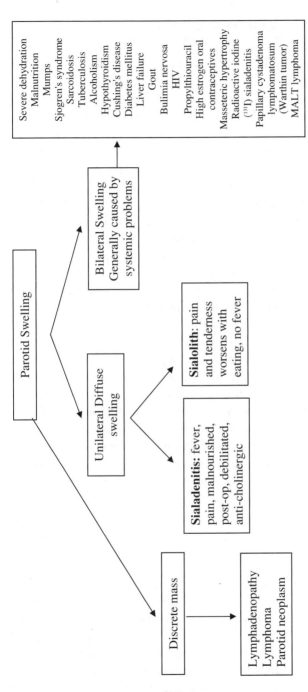

Fig 23–1. The most common pathology of major salivary glands.

mumps infection. In debilitated patients, acute unilateral parotid swelling is often the result of acute suppurative sialadenitis caused by stasis of salivary flow, with bacterial infection and retrograde spread of infection and inflammation to the gland parenchyma. The salivary glands can form stones that block the ductal system resulting in acute and generally recurrent parotid or submandibular pain and swelling. This is often episodic, brought on with eating. The glands can become acutely or chronically infected, leading to permanent gland dysfunction and need for surgical excision. Sjögren's syndrome is a chronic autoimmune disorder that can involve the salivary and lacrimal glands primarily or secondarily in conjunction with systemic rheumatologic disorders.

Masses in the salivary glands are not normal, and warrant further evaluation. A number of benign and malignant tumors affect the salivary glands. In the parotid gland, approximately 80% of parotid tumors are benign. In the submandibular gland about half of the masses are malignant, and in the minor salivary glands the majority will be malignant. It should also be noted that there may be difficulty distinguishing masses in the parotid and submandibular glands from cervical lymphadenopathy. Figure 23–1 shows the most common causes of major salivary gland pathology.

History

The history of the onset and duration of symptoms along with associated symptoms are very helpful in guiding the diagnostic workup of salivary gland disorders. Acute onset, presence of pain or soreness, and development of pain and/or swelling are associated with inflammatory or obstructive disorders. The location of the pain and swelling will distinguish between parotid and submandibular disorders. Recurrent parotid or submandibular swelling point toward chronic inflammatory disease of the gland, and/or presence of salivary stones. Acute bilateral (and occasionally asymmetric or unilateral) swelling with systemic features points toward viral or bacterial sialadenitis. Mumps is decreasing in incidence with vaccination, but remains prominent in the differential diagnosis. Acute swelling of the parotid gland with induration, erythema, and tenderness in the elderly, malnourished, postoperative, debilitated patient, or those on anticholinergic medications points toward suppurative sialadenitis.

Associated symptoms such as dry eyes, rheumatologic disorders, facial nerve paralysis, and pulmonary disorders draw attention to salivary manifestations of sarcoidosis (Heerfordt's syndrome), and Sjögren's syndrome. HIV status should be assessed, as lymphoepithelial cysts are associated with HIV infection. Other diagnoses to be considered include tuberculosis, diabetes, bulimia, and alcoholism, which are associated with parotid swelling. Rarely, medications such as iodine preparations or hypertensive medications can be associated with parotid swelling.

Physical Examination

Careful head and neck examination can be very revealing. The swelling should be accurately classified. Is it unilateral or bilateral? Is it diffuse or discrete? Tenderness should be assessed. The size of discrete mass(es) should be documented. Associated signs of facial asymmetry, eye closure, drooling, and overlying skin changes should be assessed. An attempt to massage the gland and look for purulent discharge from the parotid duct or the submandibular duct is revealing. Presence of cloudy or purulent discharge from the ducts points toward bacterial sialadenitis or chronic obstruction of the glandular ductal system. No salivary flow points to a possible stone in the duct or loss of gland function (eg, Sjögren's syndrome). Facial nerve weakness is an ominous sign associated with parotid gland malignancy, or far advanced parotid infection. The ear should be examined to exclude extension of ear pathology to the salivary glands. If a discrete mass is visible in the floor of the oral cavity, consider transillumination to identify a mucus retention cyst, or a ranula, filled with saliva, which will transilluminate light from an otoscope placed on the surface of the mass.

Additional Diagnostic Studies

History and physical examination findings drive the diagnostic workup. If acute parotid swelling is felt to be of inflammatory or viral origin, complete blood count and mumps titers are obtained. If salivary duct stones are suspected, plain films of the submandibular gland or parotid gland are suspected and, in selected cases, sialography or MRI sialography to characterize the salivary ductal system is indicated. When there are associated dry eyes or xerostomia, or other connective tissue disorders, ANA, rheumatoid factor, ESR, and SS-A and SS-B antibodies should be obtained to evaluate for Sjögren's syndrome. If Sjögren's is highly suspected, referral to otolaryngology for a biopsy of a minor salivary gland from the lower lip is warranted. In a patient with known Sjögren's syndrome, development of new swelling or mass raises the possibility of presence of lymphoma, which is greatly increased in patients with Sjögren's syndrome.

Suspected parotid tumor is generally evaluated by fine needle aspiration of the parotid gland. Incisional biopsy is rarely if ever indicated, and in cases where FNA is nondiagnostic, removal by sub-mandibular gland excision or superficial parotidectomy is indicated.

Indications for Referral

In many cases, history and physical examination will point the practitioner to the correct diagnosis. Disorders like mumps, acute suppurative sialadenitis, or a salivary duct stone often are accurately diagnosed and managed initially by the primary care physician. When the diagnosis is in question, or response to initial treatment is not appropriate, then referral to an otolaryngologist for further evaluation and management is warranted. If a parotid tumor is palpated, referral for diagnostic evaluation and management is necessary. If Sjögren's syndrome is suspected, appropriate referrals include otolaryngology evaluation for minor salivary gland biopsy, rheumatology if associated systemic disorders are present, and possibly ophthalmology if there are significant eye symptoms.

Unilateral Diffuse Swelling of Parotid or Submandibular Gland

Diffuse swelling of a salivary gland most commonly is due to ductal stone or an acute bacterial infection of the gland, termed sialadenitis.

Sialadenitis

Sialadenitis generally occurs in the elderly, malnourished, postoperative, debilitated patient, or those on anticholinergic medications. Its causative organism is most commonly *Staph aureus* or *Streptococcos spp.*

Symptoms and Signs. The patient will complain of pain and tenderness in the parotid area (anterior to the ear or behind the angle of the mandible) or in the submandibular area. A fever may be present. The patient will have increased pain and swelling after eating. These patients have decreased salivary flow which will allow bacteria to travel retrograde through the duct and into the gland causing the infection. There will be tenderness of the gland and there may be erythema of the skin overlying the gland. Visualization of the parotid duct opening (next to the second maxillary molar tooth) or the submandibular duct opening (sublingually, near midline) may show purulent drainage with massaging of the gland.

Diagnosis and What Tests to Order. The diagnosis is based on the history and physical exam. A culture of the purulent drainage is generally not indicated, unless antibiotic therapy has failed. A CT scan of the neck with contrast is indicated if there is evidence of abscess formation (significant edema and erythema overlying the area).

Treatment and When to Refer. The treatment of sialadenitis is with rehydration, massaging the gland, warm compresses on the glands, sialagogues (eg, lemon-flavored candy), and antibiotics. Medications with anticholinergic side effects should be changed if possible. Antibiotic therapy is directed against gram positives with cephalexin 500 mg po TID × 10 days (children, 10 mg/kg TID). For penicillin allergics or suspected methicillin-resistant *S. aureus* (MRSA), order clindamycin 300 mg po QID (children, 20 mg/kg/d divided TID or QID). The patient should be followed up to ensure that the swelling has resolved and that there is no underlying mass that may have created the initial problem. Admission to the hospital with an oto-laryngology consultation is warranted in patients with severe edema and erythema of the gland. Recurrent sialadenitis or a mass in the gland warrants a referral to an otolaryngologist.

Sialolith

Ductal stones are uncommon occurrences, but when they occur, are most common in the sub-mandibular duct(s).

Symptoms and Signs. The patients generally will present with pain and tenderness of the gland that worsens after eating (due to increased salivation). Unlike sialadenitis, there is no evidence of erythema or inflammation on the gland. Palpation of the duct bimanually (one finger on duct and one outside of the mouth, potentially will reveal the ductal stones. Sometimes, milking the duct toward the opening bimanually may express the stone.

Diagnosis and What Tests to Order. Diagnosis is based on the history and examination revealing a stone in the duct.

Treatment and When to Refer. Treatment includes increasing hydration, massaging the gland, warm compresses on the glands, and sialogogues (eg, lemon-flavored candy). Antibiotics should only be given if evidence of an infection is seen (eg, pus from the duct). If the stone is felt to be large or it does not pass through the opening, then a referral to an otolaryngologist is warranted. Recurrent stone formation also warrants a referral to an otolaryngologist.

Bilateral Swelling of the Glands

Bilateral diffuse swelling of the salivary glands has a long differential diagnosis list (Table 23–1). The workup of the patient will generally require evaluating all the diseases on the list in Table 23–1. Routine

Table 23–1. Causes of Bilateral Swelling of the Parotid Glands

Severe dehydration

Malnutrition

Mumps

Sjögren's syndrome

Sarcoidosis

Tuberculosis

Alcoholism

Hypothyroidism

Cushing's disease

Diabetes mellitus

Liver failure

Gout

Bulimia nervosa

HIV

Propylthiouracil

High-estrogen oral contraceptives

Masseteric hypertrophy (especially in the Asian population)

Radioactive iodine (^{131}I) sialadenitis

Papillary cystadenoma lymphomatosum (Warthin tumor)

MALT lymphoma

tests would include a thorough history and start with a blood sugar, ESR, and TSH. If other disorders are suspected, other tests should be obtained to rule out the specific diseases.

Salivary Gland Mass

A noninflammatory unilateral mass in the salivary glands can be benign or malignant neoplasm of the gland or a benign or malignant enlargement of the embedded (parotid) or adjacent (submandibular) lymph nodes. Salivary gland masses in children are more likely to be malignant. Masses in the parotid gland most commonly will occur behind the angle of the mandible. Palpation of the parotid area may only reveal a fullness or asymmetry behind the angle of the mandible. These patients will require a fine needle aspiration as discussed earlier and should be referred to an otolaryngologist for evaluation.

THYROID NODULE

Key Points

- Thyroid nodules are clinically present in approximately 5% of the adult population
- Radiographic and ultrasound prevalence is much higher than clinically palpable nodules
- The majority of thyroid nodules are benign
- TSH and ultrasound are initial diagnostic studies
- Palpable fine-needle aspiration (FNA) or ultrasound-guided FNA are indicated in almost all cases of palpable nodules

- Radioiodine scanning has limited indications in cases of nodules with hyperthyroidism or in indeterminate nodules on FNA with low probability of cancer diagnosis

Background

Thyroid nodules are common, present in approximately 5% of the adult population. The majority are benign, with approximately 10% harboring malignancy. The majority of thyroid nodules are slow growing. The rate of growth does not necessarily predict malignancy, as the majority of thyroid malignancies have a slow-growth pattern. The presence of a palpable thyroid nodule is abnormal, and warrants further investigation. The incidence of thyroid nodules is higher in females, but the incidence of malignancy is higher in males. Papillary carcinoma is the most common type of thyroid cancer, and has the best prognosis overall. Follicular carcinoma is the second most common variant, with a prognosis nearly as good as papillary carcinoma. Medullary thyroid carcinoma forms from the parafollicular C cells. It is not iodine sensitive, has high incidence of nodal metastases, and significantly worse prognosis compared with papillary and follicular carcinoma. Finally, anaplastic carcinoma is an extremely aggressive cancer that is almost uniformly fatal. Figure 24–2 in Chapter 24 shows an algorithm for the workup of a thyroid mass.

Symptoms and Signs

Age and gender are important characteristics to consider. Malignancy is more likely in males. In addition, nodules in childhood and in those over 65 years of age are more likely to be malignant tumors. The duration of the mass should be considered. Although the majority of benign and malignant lesions demonstrate slow growth, rapid growth raises the likelihood of malignancy. Patients should be asked about associated pain, odynophagia, dysphagia, voice changes, and symptoms of hyperthyroidism (tachycardia, sweating, tremor) and hypothyroidism (bradycardia, coarse hair, fatigue, myxedema).

A complete physical examination to identify signs of hyperthyroidism and hypothyroidism must be performed. Additional attention is paid to the head and neck region. Note is made of the vocal quality, and presence or absence of stridor to indicate airway impingement. The neck is carefully palpated to assess for nodal enlargement that could portend lymph node metastases from papillary or medullary thyroid cancer, or lymphoma. Gentle palpation of the thyroid is performed, and patients are asked to sip water to help assess the thyroid gland. If hoarseness is detected, laryngeal examination is indicated to assess for airway compromise, and vocal fold mobility, which can be impaired by thyroid malignancy.

Diagnosis and What Tests to Order

After performing physical examination, thyroid stimulating hormone (TSH) levels are obtained to assess for hyper or hypothyroidism. The majority of thyroid nodules have normal associated thyroid function, but autonomous hyperfunctioning nodules are occasionally seen, and in the face of autoimmune (Hashimoto's) thyroiditis, or multinodular goiter, TSH may be abnormally elevated or depressed.

Thyroid ultrasound is the primary imaging modality to characterize thyroid nodules, and has replaced routine thyroid radionuclide imaging, which is recommended in only select indications. Lesions less than 5 mm are not biopsied. For lesions between 5 mm and 1 cm biopsy is only performed if ultrasound features suspicious for malignancy are identified. Lesions >1 cm are generally sampled cytologically. Ultrasonography can be combined with ultrasound-guided fine needle aspiration (US-FNA) to obtain cytologic diagnosis. Manual FNA without ultrasound guidance can be performed in predominantly solid nodules, larger nodules, and nodules that are not situated posterior within the gland. The diagnostic yield of ultrasound guided FNA is higher than nonguided FNA.

Radionuclide studies are used to evaluate nodules in the face of hyperthyroidism. If there is not an autonomously functioning nodule, then surgery is indicated. Thyroglobulin levels are not routinely measured. Thyroglobulin is elevated in most thyroid disorders, and thus is not sensitive or specific for evaluation. Thyroglobulin levels are useful for monitoring for recurrent cancer after thyroidectomy. Calcitonin levels are not routinely measured unless there is suspicion of medullary thyroid carcinoma.

Treatment and When to Refer

If the thyroid nodule is benign on diagnostic biopsy, the lesion may be followed. Repeat ultrasound in 6 to 12 months is performed. If growth is identified, defined as at least 2 mm increase in size in at least two dimensions, rebiopsy is indicated.

If the cytologic evaluation is indeterminate or suspicious for cancer, at minimum, thyroid lobectomy is performed. If cancer is found, total thyroidectomy is performed in almost all situations. After thyroidectomy, radioiodine ablation of remnant thyroid tissue is performed with scanning for metastatic disease using [131]I.

Evaluation of the thyroid nodule involves separation of malignant lesions and indeterminate lesions that require definitive biopsy from benign lesions that can be observed. Initial workup can be completed by the primary care physician, or endocrinologist. Referral to an otolaryngologist experienced in thyroid surgery is indicated for lesions that require thyroid lobectomy for definitive tissue diagnosis, or total thyroidectomy for malignant disease.

PARATHYROID DISORDERS

Parathyroid disorders seen by the primary care physician are the result of benign tumors of the parathyroid (parathyroid adenoma), hyperplasia of the parathyroid glands, or rarely parathyroid carcinoma.

Symptoms and Signs

Classically, hyperparathyroidism presented with the constellation of symptoms of abdominal pain, renal stones, and bone pain, and in rare cases psychiatric symptoms. With the development of the ability to measure serum calcium, the great majority of cases of hyperparathyroidism are identified by finding elevated calcium on routine serum electrolyte panels.

Diagnosis and What Tests to Order

As the majority of patients presenting with hyperparathyroidism had elevated calcium as the presenting sign, exclusion of the multiple causes of hypercalcemia is necessary. It is useful to remember the "CHIMPANZEES" mnemonic (Table 23–2). It is also important to recognize that parathyroid hyperplasia is associated with multiple endocrine neoplasia (MEN) I and IIa. In addition, hyperparathyroidism is divided into primary hyperparathyroidism from adenomas, hyperplasia, or carcinoma of the parathyroid glands; secondary hyperparathyroidism associated with chronic renal failure; and tertiary hyperparathyroidism resulting from nonresponsive parathyroid tissue secreting excess PTH after correction of secondary hyperparathyroidism. Symptoms such as bone pain, fatigue or malaise, psychiatric conditions, itching, and dyspepsia, are noted. History focuses on excluding nonparathyroid causes of hypercalcemia. Presence or history of cancer is noted, as is history of renal stones, Addison's disease, or sarcoidosis. A complete medication history is elicited. Calcium, vitamin A or D, thiazide diuretics, estrogens, and

Table 23–2. Causes of Hypercalcemia

C	Calcium (exogenous)
H	Hyperparathyroidism
I	Immobility (bone resorption)
M	Metastasis to bone
P	Paget's disease
A	Addison's disease
N	Neoplasms: Solid tumors (lung, colon, breast, prostate)
Z	Zollinger-Ellison syndrome
E	Excess Vitamin A & D, lithium, thiazides, estrogens, antacids
E	Endocrine disorders: Benign familial hypocalciuric hypercalcemia, hyperthyroidism, pheochromocytoma
S	Sarcoidosis and other granulomatous diseases

lithium can all elevate calcium. Family history of hypercalcemia is elicited, which may identify benign familial hypocalciuric hypercalcemia (BFHH).

Physical examination focuses on general examination, with palpation of the neck. The presence of a neck mass raises the possibilities of parathyroid carcinoma, and coexisting thyroid pathology.

If not obtained, a complete metabolic panel including calcium, phosphorus, and magnesium is obtained, as well as urine creatinine and BUN. Intact parathyroid hormone (PTH) and serum alkaline phosphatase are obtained. Twenty-four hour urine for calculation of calcium excretion is obtained. In selected cases, ACE levels (sarcoidosis), prolactin, gastrin, and urine catecholamine levels are obtained.

For asymptomatic patients, DEXA scanning is performed. Hyperparathyroidism selectively results in cortical bone resorption, best measured on DEXA scanning of the radial bone. Cancellous bone is relatively spared in contrast to changes seen with osteoporosis. Asymptomatic patients with significant bone loss are candidates for surgical management.

If primary hyperparathyroidism is documented by the combination of elevated calcium and parathyroid hormone levels, parathyroid localizing studies are performed. High-resolution ultrasound, MRI, and technetium sestamibi scanning are performed. Ultrasound does not localize mediastinal lesions, whereas MRI and radionuclide scanning have increased costs.

Treatment and When to Refer

Hypercalcemia from causes other than hyperparathyroidism is managed based on the underlying cause. For symptomatic hyperparathyroidism, parathyroidectomy is performed. The great majority of tumors will be solitary adenomas, but 10 to 15% may be caused by hyperplasia, and up to 1% parathyroid carcinoma. In recent years, minimally invasive approaches to treat hyperparathyroidism have been developed, limiting surgical incisions, extent of dissection, and relying on use of rapid PTH analysis, or radionuclide guidance to confirm complete excision.

Asymptomatic patients may be observed. Criteria for surgical management of asymptomatic hyperparathyroidism include age under 50 years, calcium elevation over 1 gm/dl above the laboratory maximum normal range, greater than 30% decrease in creatinine clearance from normal, and a DEXA t-score below −2.5 at any site.

If the patient elects to be observed, then serum calcium is checked every 6 months, with annual creatinine levels, and bone density (DEXA) scanning at all three sites (radius, hip, lumbar spine).

There is overlap in training between primary care specialists and endocrinologists, and indications for referral to an endocrinologist will vary depending on the expertise of the primary clinician, and the referral patterns within the community. In difficult cases that are not clear-cut as to the diagnosis, referral to an endocrinologist is prudent. When symptomatic hyperparathyroidism is found, referral either before or after performing localizing studies to an otolaryngologist is warranted. For asymptomatic disease where the patient is unsure whether to observe or proceed with surgery, surgical referral is helpful. It is also helpful to develop a relationship and rapport with the otolaryngologist who performs thyroid/parathyroid surgeries.

CHAPTER 24

Pediatric and Adult Head and Neck Masses

HAU SIN WONG
JASON H. KIM

HAU SIN WONG
JASON H. KIM

BACKGROUND

Head and neck masses are a common occurrence in children and require a thorough evaluation. Frequently, head and neck masses in children can be divided into three main categories: inflammatory, congenital, and neoplastic. Inflammatory and infectious etiology is the most common, followed by congenital causes, and then finally neoplastic. The algorithm for the pediatric head and neck masses provides a general guideline to evaluating a child with a head and neck mass. This section discusses the most common inflammatory, congenital, and neoplastic causes of pediatric head and neck masses, their presentation, evaluation, and treatment. Figures 24-1A and 24-1B show an algorithm in the workup of pediatric neck masses.

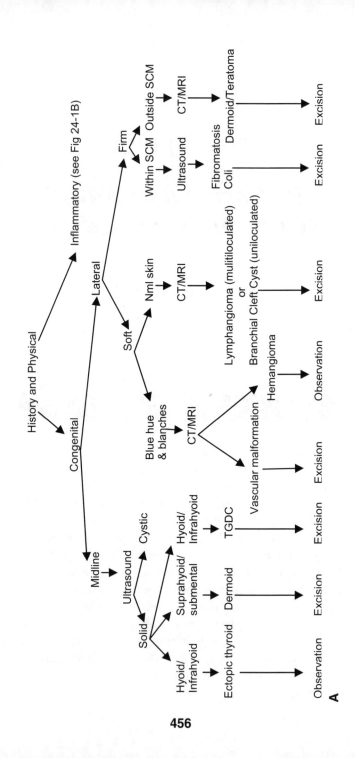

456

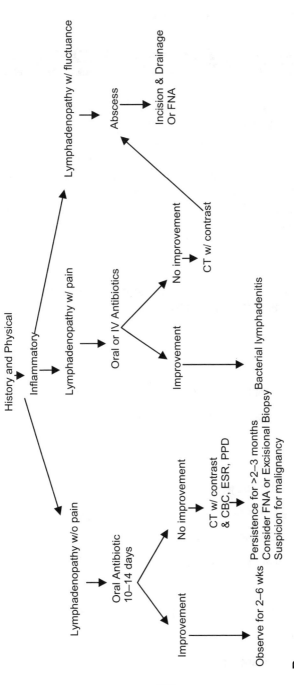

Fig 24–1. Algorithm for the work up of pediatric neck masses (**A**), and, in particular, inflammatory neck masses (**B**).

B

HISTORY

A thorough history is essential in differentiating between various causes of neck masses. The history should elicit the temporal relationship between the mass and upper respiratory infections, trauma, and exposure to animals such as cats, kittens, and farm animals, recent travel, new medications. The rest of the elements of the history and physical examination area outlined in Table 24–1.

Table 24–1. Elements of the History and Physical Examination in Pediatric Neck Masses

History

    Onset, growth of neck mass

    Antecedent trauma or illness

    Tuberculosis contacts

    Fever

    Weight loss

    Productive cough

    Eating problems

    Prior BCG immunization

    Cat exposures/scratches

    Ingestion of unpasteurized dairy products

    Travel history

Physical Examination

    Vital signs and weight

Table 24–1. *continued*

Neck mass

    Location, size, fluctuance, and tenderness

    Overlying skin changes

    Presence of a draining sinus

    Involvement of adjacent salivary glands

Oral cavity

    Teething

    Mucosal breaks

    Parapharyngeal fullness

Chest

    Congestion

Neural examination

    Cranial neuropathies

    Ancillary testing

Radiology

    Chest radiograph

    CT

    MRI

    Ultrasound

Antigen test

    PPD-T

Laboratory

    Complete blood count with differential

    Epstein-Barr virology

    HIV

Microbiology

    Aerobes

    Anaerobes

    AFB

    Fungal stains and culture

PHYSICAL EXAMINATION

A comprehensive head and neck evaluation will provide clues to the pathogenesis. Not only is size important, but also its location (midline, lateral neck, posterior neck), consistency of the mass (soft, firm, fluctuant), association with nearby skin and muscles, namely, fixed to the skin and/or muscles and any associated dimple on the skin suggestive of a sinus tract. The color of the skin overlying the mass can also give a clue to the cause. For instance, a violacious appearance may suggest mycobacterial infection.

DIAGNOSTIC STUDIES

Radiologic studies should be utilized judiciously based on a thorough history and physical exam. They assist in narrowing further the differential diagnosis. Useful imaging studies include: ultrasound, computed tomography (CT) of the neck with contrast, and magnetic resonance imaging (MRI) with contrast. Laboratory studies are also useful in the evaluation of pediatric head and neck masses. A complete blood count with differential is helpful to differentiate between malignancy and a systemic infection. Serologic testing for Esptein-Barr virus (EBV), cytomegalovirus, toxoplasmosis, and *Bartonella henselae* may also be helpful based on the history and physical exam. A purified protein derivative (PPD) may be warranted in a patient suspicious for tuberculosis. A fine needle aspiration (FNA) is warranted in patients where the mass persists beyond 6 weeks. Gram stains and acid-fast bacillus (AFB) stains should be obtained on all FNA specimens. The specimen should also be sent for aerobic, anaerobic, fungal, and mycobacterial culture.

INFLAMMATORY MASSES

Viral Lymphadenopathy

These reactive lymph nodes occur after a viral upper respiratory infection such as adenovirus, rhinovirus, or enterovirus. EBV also causes massive bilateral cervical lymphadenopathy with enlargement of the tonsils and adenoids as well as splenomegaly. A monospot test or EBV serology titer can determine if the child has active disease. Management is mainly observation and supportive care. In the case of mononucleosis, avoidance of contact sports is important to prevent any splenic injury.

Bacterial Lymphadenopathy

Reactive cervical lymphadenopathy usually presents after an upper respiratory infection with associated tonsillitis, pharyngitis, or otitis media. The lymph node is tender to palpation and may have cellulitic changes on the skin. Initial management is with antibiotic therapy. The most common causative pathogens are *Staphylococcus aureus* and group A *β-Streptococcus*. In neonates, *Pseudomonas spp.* and other gram-negative bacteria must also be considered. Additionally, children who have been on recent antibiotic therapy may develop bacterial resistant organisms and thus may require a stronger antibiotic regimen. Most suppurative lymphadenopathy responds to antibiotic therapy within 48 hours (amoxicillin/clavulonate 90 mg/kg/d of amoxicillin with 6.4 mg/kg/d of clavulonate; in penicillin allergics, clindamycin 20 mg/kg/d divided Q 6–8H). Failure with antibiotic therapy and development of an abscess will then warrant a fine needle aspiration or incision and drainage. Referral to an otolaryngologist is warranted in cases of abscess formation or when the mass fails to resolve after 6 weeks.

Mycobacterial Infection

Suspicion for mycobacterial cervical adenitis (scrofula) occurs in patients failing standard antibiotic therapy and an underlying concern for exposure. Most mycobacterial infections are of the nontuberculous type *Mycobacterium avium intracellulare*. Placement of a PPD can help differentiate between tuberculous and nontuberculous type; however, a culture is needed to make the diagnosis. PPDs generally will be positive in only 50% of patients with nontuberculous infections in the neck. Patients usually will present with a painless mass in the upper cervical or submandibular region with overlying violaceous skin changes. Treatment consists of initial medical therapy with azithromycin 10 mg/kg/d given QD for 21 days. If the mass is smaller, the treatment is continued for another 21 days. If there is no improvement after the first 21 days, surgical excision is indicated and a referral should be made to an otolaryngologist. Medical treatment with clarithromycin (20–30 mg/kg/d divided BID) and ethambutol (15 mg/kg/d QD) or clarythromycin (15 mg/kg divided BID) and rifabutin (5 mg/kg/d) for 6 weeks has been shown to be effective in various studies. The otolaryngologist may choose to use serial fine needle aspirations, curettage, or excision, and medical chemotherapy.

Cat Scratch Disease

Cat scratch disease generally presents as a red to brown nontender mass, 3 to 10 days after inoculation by the bacteria. Later, the patient may develop a regional lymphadenopathy which lasts 2 to 3 months. The condition is self-limiting. The inoculation usually occurs from a cat scratch in the head and neck area or contamination of a facial wound with a hand that has been in contact with a cat. It is caused by *Bartonella henselae*. Serology testing (immunofluorescent antibody to *B. henselae* titer of <1/64) can establish the diagnosis. Treatment is mainly supportive but antibiotic treatment with azithromycin (initial single dose of 10 mg/kg on day 1 and 5 mg/kg on days 2 to 5 as single daily doses) can decrease the volume of the lymph node. Surgical treatment may be necessary when the node becomes suppurative.

CONGENITAL MASSES

Midline Congenital Masses

Thyroglossal Duct Cyst (TDC)

TDC is the most common congenital neck mass. It is the result of aberrant embryology of the thyroid gland. The thyroid gland begins as an anlage of tissue located near the base of the tongue and descends anteroinferiorly through the hyoid bone to lie just at or below the cricoid cartilage. By 5 to 8 weeks of gestation, the thyroglossal duct obliterates, leaving the foramen cecum at the base of tongue proximally and the pyramidal lobe of the thyroid gland distally. If the duct fails to obliterate, a cyst persists and is at risk of becoming infected.

The majority of the TDC are detected in the first two decades of life, but can present at any age. TDC usually appear as midline cervical masses. Approximately one-third may present as submental or low cervical masses. They appear as a smooth, round, firm mass that may elevate during swallowing or tongue protrusion as a result of its intimate relationship with the hyoid. There is no sex predilection.

The diagnosis can be achieved with a thorough history and physical complimented by radiologic studies. Ultrasonography can identify the cyst and also to confirm the presence of normal thyroid tissue. In rare instances, the TDC can represent the patient's only thyroid and thus removal would require the patient to be on a lifetime of hormonal supplementation. In these instances, additional evaluation with thyroid function assays and radionucleotide thyroid scan assist in determining the activity of the ectopic thyroid.

Because TDC are prone to infection and ulceration, surgical excision is advised before it becomes infected. Once infected, a large incision and drainage is not recommended and can result in increased risk of recurrence at the time of complete excision of the cyst. Instead, antibiotic therapy with the possibility of needle aspiration to decompress the cyst is advised. In addition, there exists a potential for TDC to undergo malignant degeneration with papillary carcinoma as the associated malignancy. Thus timely surgical excision by an otolaryngologist is the mainstay of treatment for thyroglossal duct cysts.

Teratoma and Dermoid Cysts

Teratomas are a group of various type tumors that contain all three germ layers. They occur in 1:4000 births, with approximately 1 to 3.5% affecting the head and neck. The nasopharynx is the most common site of presentation, but they can also present in the lateral or midline neck. If a teratoma develops in the midline or lateral neck during the second trimester and rapidly expand, it can cause esophageal and/or airway obstruction. If airway obstruction is of concern, a coordinated multispecialty approach for the delivery of the infant is necessary. An EXIT (Ex Utero Intrapartum Treatment) procedure is arranged to allow for the maintenance of uteroplacental circulation while establishing a safe airway. A timely surgical excision is then the mainstay of treatment.

Dermoid cyst is the most common teratoma in the head and neck. Although pathologically related to teratomas, dermoid cysts contain only ectodermal and endodermal tissue. These cysts occur as a result of entrapment of epithelial components along embryonic fusion lines. Cervical dermoids present as painless superficial masses that move with the skin. They will gradually enlarge but rarely become infected. Ultrasonography or CT assists in additional diagnostic evaluation. A complete surgical excision is necessary because incomplete resection or intraoperative rupture is associated with an increased rate of recurrence.

Thymic Anomalies

Thymic tissue is an uncommon source of pediatric neck masses, but it should be considered in the differential. Thymic cysts, ectopic cervical thymus, and cervical thymoma have all been described in the neck, with thymic cysts being most common. During embryologic development the thymus traverses the neck between week 6 to 8 prior to entering the mediastinum, thus thymic rests may be deposited along the path from the angle of mandible to the midline of the neck descending between the common carotid artery and the vagus nerve. Thymic cysts often mimic second branchial cleft cysts or lymphatic malformations. They present as a painless neck swelling and a male predominence has been reported. These cysts are found more frequently in the lower portion of the neck and intraopertatively they are found within the carotid sheath. Preoperative CT or ultrasound may reveal the cystic nature of these lesions, but the only definitive diagnostic test is histopathological examination. Excision is the preferred treatment.

Lateral Congenital Masses

Branchial Cleft Anomalies

Branchial cleft anomalies arise from aberrant development of the branchial apparatus. The branchial apparatus consists of four paired arches, which develop during weeks 3 to 7 of fetal life, and generates important structures of the head and neck. Abnormal development of the branchial apparatus results in branchial cysts, sinuses, and fistulas.

Sinuses are those that connect either to the skin or pharyngeal mucosa. Fistulas connect gut to skin and cysts are entrapped remnants of branchial clefts or pouches and usually present as soft, fluctuant neck masses. On exam, sinuses and fistulas can present with a dimple on the skin and exude mucoid secretions. Often these abnormalities become infected after an upper respiratory infection and need antibiotic therapy. Branchial abnormalities usually present in childhood, but may be seen at any age. Branchial abnormalities are classified by their arch of origin in the branchial apparatus. First branchial anomalies are duplications of the external auditory canal. Second branchial anomalies are the most common branchial anomaly and frequently present as fistula or mass anterior to the sternocleidomastoid. Third and fourth branchial abnormalities are rare.

A CT scan of the neck with contrast can assist in the diagnosis. The treatment for all brachial anomalies is elective surgical excision. Abscess formation should first be treated with fine needle aspiration or an incision and drainage followed by a complete course of antibiotics (amoxicillin/clavulonate 90 mg/kg/d of amoxicillin with 6.4 mg/kg/d of clavulonate; in penicillin allergics, clindamycin 20 mg/kg/d divided Q6–8H) for 10 days before planning for removal (generally 6–8 weeks postinfection). Excision of the entire tract of the anomaly is necessary for successful excision to prevent recurrence.

Lymphatic Malformation

Lymphatic malformations are congenital malformations of lymphatic tissues that fail to connect to the normal lymphatic system or are growth of primordial lymph channels. Several terminologies and classifications have been used to describe these malformations and thus confuse its understanding. Lymphangiomas are classified as macrocystic, microcystic, and mixed. Macrocystic lymphangiomas have large cystic compartments and are responsive to sclerotherapy, whereas microcystic lymphangiomas are more invasive to surrounding tissue with its smaller cystic lesions and are less responsive to sclerotherapy.

Lymphatic malformations can present at birth and the majority are found by age 2. They commonly present as painless soft tissue masses that are slow to grow. On physical examination they are fluctuant and can be transilluminated. They may rapidly enlarge with upper respiratory infections and regress with the resolution of the infection. They involute rarely and eventually recur and enlarge. Due to its large size and/or infiltrative nature, these masses can cause not only cosmetic but also an anatomic dysfunction with associated dysphagia or respiratory compromise. Its involvement with normal anatomic structures is best evaluated with either a CT or MRI of the neck with contrast.

The patients should be referred to a pediatric otolaryngologist for management. Surgical excision is the mainstay of therapy, but it needs to be appropriately timed in young children. Aspiration of the malformation can serve as a temporizing measure while waiting for definitive treatment. More expeditious resection may be necessary when there is recurrent infection, obstruction of the aerodigestive tract, or significant cosmetic deformity. Although surgical excision is the main treatment option, additional medical therapy is emerging. The use of sclerotherapy to create an inflammatory response within the lymphangiomatic cyst and cause and involution of the cyst is currently being investigated.

Hemangiomas

Hemangiomas are true neoplasms of epithelial cells. They will present shortly after birth and tend to rapidly grow in the 1st year of life and will start to involute at 18 to 24 months. By 9 years of age, 90% have involuted. Hemangiomas are red or blue in hue, are compressible, and will blanch with compression. Ten percent of children with cutaneous midline hemangiomas also may present with airway hemangiomas causing stridor. Generally, observation is only needed as most hemangiomas will involute. However, if they are associated with complicated bleeding, thrombocytopenia, cardiac failure, or airway and vision compromise, earlier intervention is necessary. Treatment options range from injection of steroid into the lesion to promote involution, to systemic steroids, to laser removal of airway hemangiomas. If large or complication exists the patient should be referred to a pediatric otolaryngologist for evaluation and treatment.

Fibromatosis Coli

Fibromatosis coli, also known as pseudotumor of infancy or sternocleidomastoid tumor of infancy, results from edema and fibrosis of the sternocleidomastoid with torticolis. This is important in the consideration of congenital neck masses because infants present most commonly between birth to 3 weeks of age with a hard, mobile mass within the sternocleidomastoid. The mass is usually nontender and ultrasound imaging is diagnostic. Treatment is conservative with 50 to 70% resolving spontaneously within the first year of life. If neck rotation is limited, early physical therapy should be initiated to prevent plagiocephaly and craniofacial asymmetries. Surgical lengthening of the muscle is indicated for resistant cases of those diagnosed after the age of one.

NEOPLASTIC MASSES

Lymphomas

Hodgkin's Lymphoma

Hodgkin's lymphoma is a lymphoreticular malignancy with peak incidence at 15 years and 34 years. There is a 2:1 male to female ratio and a 40% association with Epstein-Barr virus. Eighty percent present as asymmetric, firm, rubbery, nontender lymphadenopathy with systemic features like fever, weight loss, and night sweats. Diagnosis is made by excisional biopsy of the lymph node in order to see the architecture of the lymph node and identify the Reed-Sternberg cells within it. Additional workup would include a complete blood count, erythrocyte sedimentation rate, and possible CT scan of the neck with contrast. Staging of the lymphoma will require CT of the neck, abdomen, and pelvis. The patient should be referred to a hematologist-oncologist for management after the mass is excised by an otolaryngologist for tissue diagnosis.

Non-Hodgkin's Lymphoma

Non-Hodgkin's lymphoma is a lymphoreticular malignancy whose incidence increases with increasing age. It is more common in whites and there is a 2:1 to 3:1 male to female ratio. In children, non-Hodgkin's lymphoma presents as rapidly enlarging extranodal disease such as enlarging asymmetric tonsils and adenoids. Dissemination occurs hematogenously and is usually found during late stages. Non-Hodgkin's lymphoma should be especially suspected in a child with a past history of an organ or bone marrow transplantation who presents with enlarging tonsils or adenoids. Definitive diagnosis requires an excisional biopsy, along with blood workup, bone marrow biopsy, and bone scan under the care of a hematologist/oncologist.

Rhabdomyosarcomas

Rhabdomyosarcoma is the most frequent soft tissue malignancy in children and 50% present in children less than 5 years old. Forty percent of the tumors present in the head and neck region in the following descending order: orbit, nasopharynx, middle ear/mastoid, and sinonasal cavity. The presenting symptoms are based on the location of tumor, namely, orbital

rhabdomyosarcomas will present with unilateral proptosis or facial maxilla fullness whereas nasopharyngeal
lesions have nasal obstruction and epistaxis. An incisional biopsy is needed for diagnosis and for typing
via immunohistochemistry and electron microscopy.
Treatment is multimodal requiring a balance of surgery, radiation therapy, and chemotherapy. The patient
should be referred to a pediatric otolaryngologist for
tissue diagnosis and to a hematologist-oncologist for
treatment planning.

NECK MASS IN ADULTS

Introduction

Differential diagnosis of a neck mass in adults is rather
extensive and can be overwhelming (Table 24-2).
They may include infectious, inflammatory, neoplastic, or even congenital etiologies. However, in young
adults over the teenage years, it is most commonly of
inflammatory or congenital process. In adults over the
age of 35 years, any mass that does not disappear
within 3 weeks is considered neoplastic until proven
otherwise. The most common cause of a malignant
neck mass in adults is a metastatic lesion from an
upper aerodigestive tract carcinoma. In addition to the
age of the patient, the location of the mass can further
assist in narrowing the differential diagnosis. Otolaryngologists often work closely with internists, pediatri-
cians, family practioners, oncologists, and infectious
disease specialists in treating patients with neck masses.
Most often, primary care specialists play an important
role in the initial evaluation and timely referral of
patients with neck mass to otolaryngologists.

Table 24–2. Differential Diagnosis of Neck Mass in Adults

Congenital

   Branchial cyst

   Thymic cyst

Inflammatory

   Adenitis—bacterial, viral, granulomatous

   Sialadenitis—parotid, submandibular

Neoplastic

   Primary

      Thyroid

      Lymphoma

      Vascular—carotid body, glomus, hemangioma

      Neurogenic—schwannoma, neuroma

      Salivary—parotid, submandibular

   Metastatic

      Nasopharynx

      Sinonasal cavity

      Oropharynx

      Oral cavity

      Larynx

      Hypopharynx

      Thyroid

      Skin

Age of the patient, location of the mass, and a thorough history and physical examination can usually delineate whether a mass is a primary tumor or a metastatic disease. A primary tumor would be a tumor that arises from the organ itself. For example, a thyroid mass would be considered a primary thyroid pathology. A mass within the parotid gland may be considered a primary tumor of the parotid gland. A mass in the neck that is proven to be carcinoma, most often metastasized from an identifiable primary site in the head and neck region. Commonly, it spreads from the oropharyngeal region. An otolaryngologist or head and neck surgeon would be able to evaluate these specific regions and proceed with appropriate imaging studies and tests.

History

Eliciting a thorough history is extremely important in initiating the evaluation of a patient with a neck mass. Any events that may possibly be related to the emergence of the mass would need to be investigated. These events may include history of trauma, any upper respiratory or upper aerodigestive illness or symptoms, or recent travel. In essence, any symptoms associated with head, eyes, ears, nose, and throat need to be described. For example, any changes in hearing or otalgia can represent nasopharyngeal or oropharyngeal etiology if the neck mass has a high suspicion for metastatic disease. Symptoms of dysphagia and odynophagia along with the neck mass may suggest a primary oropharyngeal etiology. Nasal obstruction or recurrent epistaxis may suggest sinonasal or nasopharyngeal pathology leading to the neck mass. Voice changes, coughing, choking, or breathing difficulties suggest a laryngeal process. Any changes in or associated symptoms of any one of the cranial nerve functions are important part of history taking and may suggest a more ominous sign.

Usually when there is pain associated with a neck mass, it suggests an inflammatory process. But it need not be. The size of the mass and rate of growth can also help to narrow the differential diagnosis. For example, a rapidly growing mass over short time duration may very well suggest lymphoma. A slowly or rapidly enlarging low midline mass usually suggests thyroid pathology.

Careful history can guide one's physical examination and ordering appropriate studies. Again, included in the history would be the associated symptoms, size of the mass, growth of the mass, location of the mass, associated pain or tenderness, referred pain, inciting events, prior treatments, history of skin cancer, unexplained weight loss or gain, drinking and smoking history, and family history of tumors.

Physical Examination

After thoroughly eliciting the patient's history, a complete physical examination is the next step. Although, the history can guide one to concentrate more on certain areas of the head and neck, it should not be used to neglect any other areas. We rely on all of our senses in examining a patient: eyes to inspect the patient, nose to note any odor, ears to note any breathing issues, and tactile sensation to palpate. Most important would be visualization and palpation, however.

It is important to include the patient's vital signs, weight, and general appearance as part of the examination. Cancer patients may appear thin or cachectic. Upper aerodigestive tract carcinomas commonly will have a bad odor similar to halitosis (bad breath) that occurs from the growth of anaerobic bacteria in necrotic tumor. One would also note any unusual breathing noise or pattern as part of the general examination. The head and neck examination then usually continues with overall skin examination, which includes the scalp. Sometimes, there can be lesions in the scalp that can be missed. The eye examination will check the pupils, extraocular movement, and any other findings such as proptosis or enophthalmos. External ear examination inspects the auricle for any lesions. With an otoscope, one looks at the ear canal and the tympanic membrane into the middle ear space if possible for any infection or effusion. The nasal examination is done with a nasal speculum evaluating the nasal cavity, septum, and the turbinates. Oral cavity examination at times can be difficult secondary to the patient's sensitivity but also because there is wide variety of oral pathology. If at all possible, the examination should be done with both hands free with tongue depressors using a headlight or lighted mirror. This allows one to navigate the oral cavity freely in order to examine both sides, especially for symmetry. Two-handed technique also facilitates manipulation of the lips and tongue. In select patients, manual palpation of the gingiva, floor of mouth, tongue, tonsillar areas, and base of tongue is also performed, especially if there is a visible mass or suspected pathology.

The most important part of the examination would be to carefully examine the neck. Again, two-handed technique is used to palpate both sides of the neck simultaneously. This allows one to discern any asymmetry between the two sides. For example, when examining the parotid gland, both glands are palpated at the same time to note for asymmetry. Once the mass or asymmetry is identified or palpated, then a more careful and focused one-handed examination can be performed to better characterize the mass. Firmness, fluctuance, mobility, tenderness, skin status or involvement, and size are noted. If a vascular lesion is suspected, then thrill or bruit is also noted.

For the next part, a trained otolaryngologist would normally perform a laryngoscopy, either indirect or direct. With an indirect (using a mirror) laryngoscopy one can visibly inspect the base of tongue, larynx, and hypopharynx. A direct flexible laryngoscopy would give more details about the nasal cavity, nasopharynx, oropharynx, hypopharynx, and larynx.

Imaging Studies

The most common radiographic study that is ordered to evaluate a neck mass is a CT scan of the neck with contrast. An MRI with gadolinium enhancement is used when giving contrast is not feasible. Any imaging without contrast enhancement has little value in assessing a neck mass and would need to be repeated. Often, an ultrasound is a great option to evaluate the thyroid gland. However, in general, its use is limited to the thyroid gland. Most of the time, for any thyroid process, a CT with iodine-based contrast would not be practical and may potentially jeopardize possible treatment with radioactive iodine. CT scan is perhaps better for evaluating lymph nodes and salivary glands, especially in delineating spatial relationship. CT scan is also superior to MRI for bony pathology. On the other hand, MRI normally provides much better soft tissue details than CT. Most of the time, the initial scan is usually a CT scan as it is easier to obtain and can be performed within just a few minutes.

Regular x-rays are not used much for evaluating neck masses. In specific cases, PET/CT or angiogram may be useful. Angiogram is used in evaluating vascular lesions, usually. PET/CT is normally used in cancer surveillance and evaluating for distant metastasis or primary location of the cancer especially in cervical metastasis with unknown primary site. In general, when in doubt, a trained specialist can order the appropriate studies. This would obviate the unnecessary duplication or repeated imaging studies with more specific instructions or guidelines.

Laboratory Studies

Blood tests are usually targeted to one's suspicion about the neck mass. If an inflammatory of infectious etiology is suspected, then comprehensive metabolic panel, complete blood count, ESR, as well as an infectious panel may be considered. Toxoplasma, coccidiomycosis, *Cryptococcus*, and cat scratch titers may be included. PPD and a chest x-ray can assist in suspected mycobacterial infections. Atypical mycobacterial infections can have normal PPD and chest radiography.

If thyroid malignancy is suspected, then a thyroid function test, thyroglobulin, and antithyroglobulin antibody would be checked. If thyroiditis is suspected, given the history of painful enlargement of the thyroid gland, then aside from the thyroid function test, an anti-TPO assay would be ordered. For suspected malignancy, either primary or metastatic, CBC, comprehensive metabolic panel, and liver function tests are ordered. Further tests can be ordered depending on the biopsy result.

Biopsy

After a thorough history, complete examination, and imaging and laboratory studies, the next step is the evaluation of the mass with a biopsy. In all circumstance, a fine-needle aspiration biopsy should be performed first. This is the standard of care. An open biopsy for metastatic cancer can lead to deleterious consequences. It has been discussed that an open incisional or excisional biopsy of metastatic cancer can lead to increased wound necrosis, regional neck recurrence, and distant metastasis.

Fine-needle aspiration (FNA) biopsy can provide rather quick answers to whether something is cystic or solid, infectious or inflammatory, benign or cancerous. Cultures also can be sent from the aspirated specimen as well. Most of the time, FNA can differentiate between lymphoma, carcinoma, benign tumors, and thyroid pathologies. This differentiation avoids unnecessary formal endoscopy, open biopsy, and guided biopsy under general anesthesia. For lymphoma or suspected lymphoma on FNA, an incisional biopsy can be performed next for further classification. Sometimes, the FNA result is inconclusive or nondiagnostic. In these cases, a repeat FNA should be considered before an open biopsy.

FNA is performed using a 25-g needle and a 10-cc syringe with multiple passes through the mass. This procedure generally is performed by an otolaryngologist or a pathologist. An FNA should not be performed on a mass suspected to be vascular in origin. Most of the time, FNA is considered after the imaging studies. FNA can lead to complete aspiration of a cystic mass, cause hemorrhage into the mass, introduce infection, or even alter the anatomy. In such cases, the imaging studies would not capture the true nature of the neck mass and surrounding anatomical relationship, if performed afterward.

General Approach to Adult Neck Mass

Most of the time, a thorough history and complete physical examination can provide a general sense of the neck mass and raise suspicion (Fig 24–2). If the physical examination fails to show a suspected primary tumor and the mass is thought to be inflammatory, a 2-week course of antibiotics (amoxicillin clavulonate 875 mg po BID, penicillin allergics, clindamycin 300 mg PO QID) should be given. If 3 weeks after initiation of

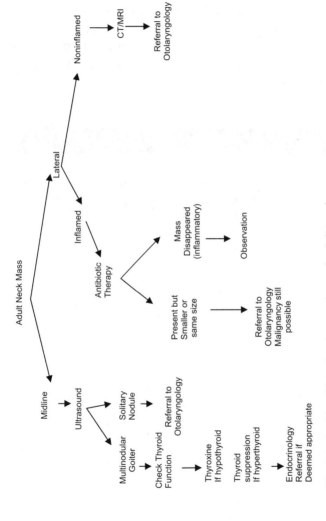

Fig 24–2. Algorithm for the workup of adult neck masses.

antibiotic therapy a mass is still seen, the patient should be referred to an otolaryngologist promptly with a CT scan of the neck with contrast. If the mass is in the midline and in the area of the thyroid, an ultrasound of the thyroid would suffice in place of a CT. A thyroid mass generally will not require antibiotic therapy and should be referred with an ultrasound to an otolaryngologist-head and neck surgeon.

FURTHER READING

Albright JT, Pransky SM. Nontuberculous mycobacterial infections of the head and neck. *Pediatr Clin North Am.* 2003;50:503–514.

CHAPTER 25

Neck Pain

HAMID R. DJALILIAN

Neck pain can be divided into pain in the anterior and posterior aspects of the neck. Figure 25–1 displays the most common causes of neck pain.

Musculoskeletal/Cervical Disk Disease

Symptoms and Signs

Posterior neck pain is most commonly caused by musculoskeletal problems. The most common cause of posterior neck pain is problems with the patient's posture, sleep habits, migraine headaches, or as a sign of psychological stress. Cervical arthritis (degenerative or traumatic) or disk disease can cause posterior cervical pain which occasionally may manifest as radiculopathy or paresthesias in the shoulder, arm, or hand. This can occur as a result of trauma (eg, sports or whiplash injury) or have gradual onset such as degenerative and misuse. Neck stiffness in the presence of a high fever

Posterior Neck Pain
- **Musculoskeletal/Cervical Disk Disease:** spasm of posterior neck muscles
- **Meningitis:** fever, nuchal rigidity, positive Kernig sign

Anterior Neck Pain
- **Neck Mass:** mass palpable in neck
- **Sternocleidomastoid (SCM) Fasciitis:** radiation into postauricular area, SCM tenderness, tenderness on mastoid attachment of SCM
- **Carotidynia:** h/o migraines, tenderness on carotid bulb
- **Thyroiditis:** severe pain and tenderness in thyroid region
- **Laryngopharyngeal Reflux:** lump in throat sensation, chronic cough or throat clearing, chronic sore throat
- **Neck Trauma:** recent trauma history

Neck Stiffness
- **Musculoskeletal:** spasm of neck muscles
- **Meningitis:** fever, nuchal rigidity, positive Kernig sign
- **Deep Neck Space Infections:** fever, toxic, oropharyngeal infection
- **Atlantoaxial Instability:** recent trauma or surgery, especially in Down syndrome patients
- **Dystonia:** phenothiazines, haloperidol, carbamazepine, metoclopramide, phenytoin, reflux in neonate
- **Congenital Torticollis:** shortening of sternocleidomastoid muscle

Fig 25–1. The most common causes of neck pain.

482

(>102°F) may be an early sign of meningitis. A history of migraine headaches (classical or nonclassical) should be solicited. Other signs pointing to migraine include light or sound sensitivity, unilateral headaches, auras, or retro-orbital headaches.

On examination the patient with musculoskeletal pain will have stiffness and tenderness on the posterior cervical musculature and point tenderness on the insertion of the muscles in the occipital area. Fibromyalgia can also cause similar symptoms.

Diagnosis and What Tests to Order

Diagnosis is by history and examination. Cervical spine MRI is indicated in the presence of radiculopathy or paresthesia.

Treatment and When to Refer

Patients with posterior cervical musculoskeletal pain will respond well to a combination of NSAIDs (eg, ibuprofen 600 mg po TID for 2 weeks) and muscle relaxants (eg, cyclobenzaprine 10 mg po TID for 2 weeks; in elderly start at 5 mg po QD). Patients with radiculopathy or paresthesia of the upper extremities should be referred to a spine surgeon. A short course of corticosteroids (prednisone 0.5 mg/kg/d po for 7 days) may reduce the symptoms in patients with radiculopathy or paresthesia.

ANTERIOR NECK PAIN

Neck Mass

Anterior neck pain can be a manifestation of an underlying neck mass. Painful neck masses are generally inflammatory or infectious in nature. These masses are most commonly in the lateral aspect of the neck and can be deep to the sternocleidomastoid muscle. The patient will present with pain and tenderness in the neck. The pain may radiate to the ear or the pharynx. The onset of the pain is generally less than 2 weeks in duration. An earlier history of a sore throat or dental work may be present.

On examination, the patient will have tenderness and a mass deep or anterior to the sternocleidomastoid muscle. Viral lymphadenitis will have a short duration of pain with acute onset of the neck mass development. A bacterial lymphadenitis generally will have evidence of inflammation (warmth and erythema) on the skin overlying the enlarged lymph node. The oral cavity, pharynx, hypopharynx, and larynx should be examined to rule out a primary carcinoma of the upper aerodigestive tract that may have metastasized to the neck. Nasopharyngeal carcinoma should be suspected especially in patients of East/Southeast Asian descent.

Diagnosis and What Tests to Order

A recent history of dental work may indicate a gram-positive or anaerobic infection. Recent pharyngitis may indicate a gram-positive infection (most commonly, Group A Strep). A nonhealing mucosal ulcer or mass in the upper aerodigestive tract may indicate a metastatic mass in the neck. If the mass is present for more than 3 weeks in an adult, a CT scan of the neck with contrast must be obtained to evaluate the mass and the patient should be referred to an otolaryngologist.

Treatment and When to Refer

Viral lymphadenitis can be treated expectantly or with a short course of prednisone (0.5 mg/kg/day for 4–5 days). Bacterial lymphadenitis is best treated with clindamycin 300 mg (in children, 20 mg/kg/day divided TID) po TID for 7 to 10 days. If a neck mass is greater than 1 cm in its width and is present for more than 3 weeks in an adult or for more than 6 weeks in a child, the patient should be referred to an otolaryngologist.

Sternocleidomastoid Fasciitis

The patient with sternocleidomastoid (SCM) fasciitis will present with nonspecific unilateral neck pain with radiation into the postauricular area. On examination, tenderness of the SCM is found in the absence of a mass. The patient will also have point tenderness at the mastoid attachment of the SCM muscle.

Diagnosis and What Tests to Order

The diagnosis is made by history and examination. Tenderness limited to the SCM muscle belly and insertion on the mastoid is diagnostic.

Treatment and When to Refer

The treatment is with nonsteroidal anti-inflammatories (NSAIDs) (eg, ibuprofen 600 mg po tid for 14 days). The patient should be referred to an otolaryngologist if persistent pain is present despite NSAID therapy.

Carotidynia

Carotidyna is a migraine-related condition which generally presents as unilateral neck pain that radiates to the face and ear on the same side. The pain is characterized by its continuous, dull, and throbbing nature.

The patients may feel the pain in all the areas supplied by the external carotid artery, for example, the ipsilateral mandible, face, eye, and ear. On examination, the patient will have exquisite tenderness over the carotid bulb. The carotid bulb is distinguished by its pulsatile nature and its location anterior to the SCM at the level of the angle of mandible.

The diagnosis is made by history and examination. Point tenderness on the carotid bulb is diagnostic. Patients over the age of 60 who present with carotidynia and have a carotid bruit present on examination may have a variant of carotidynia called atherosclerotic carotidynia. Patients suspected of having atherosclerotic carotidynia should undergo an ultrasound of the carotid to evaluate for stenosis.

Treatment and When to Refer

The treatment is with nonsteroidal anti-inflammatories (NSAIDs) (eg, ibuprofen 600 mg po TID for 14 days). Prophylactic migraine treatment (propranolol 20–40 mg po bid) for a 14-day period also can be of benefit in the patients with migrainous carotidynia. The patient should be referred to a neurologist if persistent pain is present despite NSAID and migraine prophylaxis therapy. Patients with atherosclerotic carotidynia with carotid stenosis may need neurosurgical or vascular surgery consultation.

Thyroiditis

Pain in the region of the thyroid can be secondary to subacute thyroiditis or infectious thyroiditis. Subacute thyroiditis will present with severe pain in the thyroid region. There generally is an antecedent history of upper respiratory infection. The patient may have associated dysphagia or odynophagia with radiation of pain into the ear. The patient with infectious thyroiditis will present with similar symptoms with the exception of a concomitant or recent bacterial pharyngitis in the previous week—this condition is less common than subacute thyroiditis. On examination, the painful thyroiditis patient will have exquisite tenderness in the region of the thyroid gland. Bacterial thyroiditis can rarely develop into an abscess. This condition generally will manifest as continued pain despite antibiotic therapy. Bacterial thyroiditis or abscess generally will occur in the presence of underlying thyroid cysts or a branchial cleft anomaly.

Diagnosis and What Tests to Order

A check of thyroid hormone levels at diagnosis of subacute thyroiditis will show a thyrotoxic state due to the release of the stored thyroid hormone. After 1 to 3 months from the acute painful stage, the patient will be in a hypothyroid state. The diagnosis is by history and the examination. Laboratory studies (thyroid hormone levels) and an erythrocyte sedimentation rate (ESR) will help to confirm the diagnosis. T4 concentration is generally more elevated relative to the T3 level and TSH level is low. Thyroglobulin is elevated. A normal ESR and thyroglobulin level essentially rules out the diagnosis of subacute thyroiditis. Subacute thyroiditis generally has four phases. In the acute phase, thyroid pain is present and the patient will commonly be hyperthyroid or thyrotoxic for 3 to 6 weeks. This stage may last longer, but generally is followed by a transient euthyroid state. Hypothyroidism generally will follow that and may last weeks to months. In a small group of patients (~5%) the hypothyroidism may be permanent. After the hypothyroid stage, most patients will revert back to a euthyroid stage.

Patients with bacterial thyroiditis generally will have normal thyroid function tests in the acute setting. They will, however, have an elevated ESR level. Thyroid auto-antibodies will be absent in bacterial thyroiditis.

Treatment and When to Refer

During the acute stage, 50% of patients with subacute thyroiditis will be hyperthyroid. Antithyroidal treatment is not indicated in the acute stage, but beta-blockers can be used in thyrotoxic patients. NSAIDs (indomethacin 50 mg po TID) will provide relief. In severe thyroid pain, prednisone 20 to 40 mg po QD for a 2-week period with taper will help in symptomatic relief. Some patients (~20%) may have recurrence of thyroid pain after stopping the prednisone. Endocrinology consultation will be beneficial in patients with prolonged hyper- or hypothyroidism.

Patients with bacterial thyroiditis should be treated with antibiotics against *Staph* and *Strep spp.* (eg, clindamycin 300 mg po TID × 10 days) and suspected thyroid abscess should be referred to an otolaryngologist for drainage.

Laryngopharyngeal Reflux (LPR)

LPR may present with symptoms of chronic pain in the region of the larynx. The patient will have discomfort in the neck which is worse upon swallowing. The etiology is the inflammation caused by the stomach refluxate onto the larynx and pharynx. Please see the chapter on Sore Throat (Chapter 18) for more detail on the diagnosis and treatment of LPR.

Trauma to the Neck

Occasionally, a patient with trauma to the neck may present to a primary care physician. Patients with penetrating trauma should all be referred to an emergency department. The management of penetrating trauma to the neck is beyond the scope of this book. The patient generally will complain of pain in the anterior neck and over the thyroid cartilage area. Dysphagia, dysphonia, hemoptysis, and/or difficulty breathing may be present. A history of domestic abuse should be sought. The patients generally will have some ecchymosis in the anterior neck skin. Examination of the cervical spine is essential as neck trauma can lead to cervical spine injury. A complete cranial nerve and neurologic examination will rule out significant injuries.

Diagnosis and What Tests to Order

The diagnosis is by history. Cervical radiographs (AP and lateral) and soft tissue x-ray of the neck will assist in examination of the cervical spine and check for subcutaneous air, tracheal deviation, or hyoid fracture.

Treatment and When to Refer

Minor blunt trauma without a carotid bruit, subcutaneous air, dysphagia, dysphonia, hemoptysis, and/or difficulty breathing can be treated symptomatically with acetaminophen with or without codeine.

Crepitus or subcutaneous air in the neck is an ominous sign indicating violation of the upper aerodigestive tract and requires immediate referral to an emergency department via ambulance. A carotid bruit or Horner syndrome (ipsilateral eyelid ptosis, ipsilateral myosis, and anhydrosis of ipsilateral facial skin)

may indicate an intimal tear of the carotid with resultant dissection and injury to the sympathetic nerves
traveling with the carotid artery. A patient with a
carotid bruit or Horner syndrome after trauma to the
neck should be referred to an emergency department
via ambulance.

NECK STIFFNESS

Neck stiffness can occur from a variety of factors that
cause neck pain. The patient will hesitate in moving
the neck to reduce pain. Aside from neck stiffness in
meningitis, other conditions that can cause inflammation in the deep neck spaces can also cause stiffness.
For example, a deep neck space abscess or cellulitis,
namely, parapharyngeal or retropharyngeal space infections, can cause stiffness of the neck. See Chapter 18
on sore throat and Chapter 21 on airway obstruction
for those disorders, respectively. In addition, neck stiffness after an adenoidectomy procedure can be caused
by inflammation of the anterior transverse ligament
that can cause atlantoaxial instability or subluxation
(Grisel syndrome). This will occur about 7 days postoperatively and is most common in children with
Down syndrome. Down syndrome patients generally
have laxity of the atlantoaxial joint and are at a higher
risk of C1-C2 subluxation. Cervical spine x-rays will
help in the diagnosis of C1-C2 subluxation.

Congenital (due to a shortened sternocleidomastoid muscle) or aquired torticollis can cause neck stiffness. The treatment of congenital torticollis is physical
therapy and rarely surgical. Congenital torticollis
patients who are untreated at birth will have asymmetric facial features due to their chronic head tilt. Aquired
torticollis can be caused by a variety of factors includ-

ing muscle spasm after poor sleep position (treated with stretching, massage, warm packs, and ibuprofen 600 tid, and cyclobenzaprine 10 tid for 5–7 days); post-traumatic, or as a side effect of medications (eg, phenothiazines, haloperidol, carbamazepine, metoclopramide, and phenytoin). Medication-induced dystonias are treated with diphenhydramine (25–50 mg po/IV) or benzodiazepines (eg, diazepam 2–10 mg po/IV). Rarely, patients with a cranial nerve IV or VI palsy may present with a neck tilt to compensate for their diplopia that may be misinterpreted as torticollis. Finally, Sandifer syndrome is a disorder characterized by gastroesophageal reflux with torticollis as part of a posturing and can occur in infants.

FURTHER READING

Farwell AP, Braverman LE. Inflammatory thyroid disorders. *Otolaryngol Clin North Am.* 1996;29:541–556.

CHAPTER 26

Trauma to the Neck

JOHN F. MCGUIRE
HAMID R. DJALILIAN

Injury to the neck is always dangerous and most frequently will present to trauma centers with full ancillary support. This chapter outlines basic considerations when evaluating a patient with neck trauma, with the understanding that the majority of neck trauma patients should be treated by an experienced trauma team.

MECHANISMS OF INJURY

With penetrating trauma to the neck, the most common injuries will be secondary to gunshot or knife wounds. There is a proclivity for direct injury to the great vessels and other structures in the neck with penetrating injuries. Importantly, signs and symptoms of vessel injury may not become apparent until an hour after the traumatic event. Laryngeal or esophageal injuries are also possible with penetrating trauma. The potential for injury to these vital structures necessitates close monitoring in a trauma setting.

Blunt trauma to the neck most often occurs with assault, sports injuries, motor vehicle accidents, strangling, or attempted suicide by hanging. Patients with isolated blunt neck trauma frequently present to ambulatory care centers, but a high degree of caution must be observed nevertheless. In these cases, vessel injury is also possible, but the mechanism is usually from stretch or shear forces. The potential for laryngeal framework injury with blunt trauma to the neck must always be kept in mind.

ZONES OF INJURY

Anatomic zones of injury have been used to help classify types of neck trauma.

Zone I is the lowest zone, spanning from the thoracic inlet inferiorly to the cricoid cartilage. Structures at risk include the great vessels, the trachea, the esophagus, the cervical spine, and the brachial plexus. Zone I wounds are often associated with thoracic injury causing a pneumothorax, hemothorax, or tension pneumothorax.

Zone II spans the midportion of the neck, and spans from the cricoid cartilage to the angle of the mandible. Structures at risk include the great vessels, the laryngeal framework, and the cervical spine. Most carotid injuries occur in Zone II. Zone II injuries carry the best prognosis because the anatomy is surgically accessible.

Zone III is the most superior zone, and encompasses all structures from the angle of the mandible to the skull base. The deep lobe of the parotid, the great vessels, cranial nerves IX to XII, the sympathetic ganglia, and other vital structures traverse this zone. Zone III injuries are the most difficult to access surgically.

TREATMENT IN THE TRAUMA BAY

In the trauma setting, the patient history usually is relayed simultaneously during the transfer from the ambulance gurney to the trauma bay. Key history items that are relayed by the prehospital personnel include:

- Time that the injury occurred, estimate blood loss, level (or loss) of consciousness, evidence of intoxication.
- If a motor vehicle accident, determine if there was seat belt use, airbag deployment, the magnitude of car damage, and if there were any fatalities at the scene.
- If this was assault, get details on the type of weapon used (if a knife, how big; if a gun, the range and caliber).

Primary Survey

While this transfer is being performed, the "primary survey" is started. The "primary survey" refers to the most essential elements of the patients status; airway, breathing, and circulation (the "ABCs"). The following outlines special considerations in the ABCs when evaluating a patient with neck injury

Airway

Evaluation of the airway in a patient with neck injury always presents a problem. Airway instability usually is addressed by intubation. However, in the context of neck injury, attempting intubation may cause further compromise. Gagging or coughing may dislodge a clot and cause severe hemorrhage. Direct laryngeal or pharyngeal injury can be made worse through attempted intubation. If there is cervical spine damage, standard neck maneuvers to access the airway may cause further damage. In cases of laryngotracheal separation, attempted intubation can be fatal. Therefore, only in cases of total airway compromise should intubation be attempted. Here are some considerations when establishing an airway in the patient with neck injury:

- Use all other possible means of securing an airway before intubation. This includes first the use of supplemental oxygen. First, clear the airway of any debris, dentures, foreign bodies, and blood, and reassess ventilatory status. Bag mask ventilation can be used, but it can also exacerbate subcutaneous emphysema in cases of airway injury (suspected in cases of subcutaneous emphysema or bloody sputum in the absence of nasal or oral cavity bleeding).
- If attempting intubation, always use the modified jaw thrust technique, never the head-tilt chin-lift maneuver, because of the possible instability in the spine after neck trauma.
- Other strategies to establish the airway include the use of fiberoptic intubation, gum elastic bougies, and percutaneous jet ventilation, and emergency tracheotomy.
- Emergency surgical airway (ie, tracheotomy) is also a possibility and is preferred in cases of suspected laryngotracheal separation or significant laryngeal framework trauma.
- See Chapter 21 Airway Obstruction, for the technique of cricothyrotomy.

Breathing

Respiratory difficulties with an adequate airway should raise suspicion for a hemothorax or a pneumothorax. This is more likely with Zone I injuries. Emergency placement of a chest tube may be necessary. For tension pneumothorax, needle decompression may be attempted at the second intercostal space at the midclavicular line.

Circulation

Most bleeding from neck injuries can be slowed via direct pressure. However, massive bleeding can lead to hypovolemic shock. Fluid resuscitation and adequate venous access are essential and should be addressed before any further workup is attempted.

Secondary Survey

The "secondary survey" in the trauma setting is a more detailed examination of each organ system. Focused evaluation of the neck should now be performed. Examination requires head stabilization and removal of the cervical stabilization collar. If there is penetrating injury, characterize the point of entry and the direction of the wound. If possible, determine if the playtysmal layer has been violated. Platysmal violation generally will require a surgical exploration of the neck to rule out great vessel or neural injury. However, never explore or probe a neck wound in the trauma bay as this may dislodge a clot that is stabilizing an injured vessel. Palpate the laryngeal architecture. Feel for crepitus, which would indicate laryngeal or pharyngo/esophageal injury. Auscultate for bruits near the great vessels.

The mechanism of injury should further inform you as to what to pay attention to on examination.

The following are signs and symptoms that should raise suspicion for corresponding injuries:

- Larynx/Trachea: voice alteration, hemoptysis, stridor, drooling, bubbling through the neck wound, subcutaneous emphysema and/or crepitus, dyspnea, distortion of anatomic landmarks, odynophagia.
- Vessels: hemorrhage, hemothorax, hypotension, hypovolemic shock, cardiac tamponade, weak carotid pulse, bruit, hematoma, upper extremity ischemia, neurologic deficits (contralateral hemiparesis, decreased level of consciousness).
- Aerodigestive: hematemesis, odynophagia, crepitus (subcutaneous emphysema), blood in the saliva.
- Nerves: paresthesias, weakness, hoarseness, plegia, and paresis

Imaging Studies

All imaging studies should be ordered in the context of patient stability. Often, severe injury to the neck will require emergent exploration before any imaging is ordered. Indeed, to send an unstable patient to the CT suite can end in disastrous results, and only patients who are deemed to be stable should get ancillary studies.

- Neck x-ray: Standard x-ray films to evaluate for cervical spine injury are routine (AP, lateral, and odontoid views).

- Chest x-ray: Helps with the evaluation of for occult subcutaneous emphysema, widened mediastinum and pneumothroax.
- CT scan: CT angiography (CTA) is a common standard study for stable patients.
- Standard angiography: Has an advantage over CTA in that it can be both diagnostic and therapeutic. Embolization of injured vessels in Zone III is often necessary.
- Gastrograffin study: Useful in the evaluation of potential esophageal injuries, but sensitivity is much higher when combined with endoscopy.

OUTSIDE THE TRAUMA SETTING

Occasionally, patients will present with neck injuries to ambulatory care settings. This happens, for instance, when a family member drives someone to the nearest urgent care center. The following is a list of points and principles to remember when placed in a position of being a first responder to a neck injury outside the trauma setting.

1. Airway first: Always keep the airway in mind in the context of neck trauma. Even if the airway seems stable at first, delayed bleeding can lead to airway compromise. Indeed, even the irritation caused by blood around laryngeal tissues has been known to lead to respiratory compromise.
2. Avoid intubation: Try to avoid intubation, if possible. Providing supplemental oxygen and clearing the airway will often prove to be sufficient until the patient can be transported to a trauma center.

If intubation is necessary, use the chin-lift maneuver and do not tilt the head back to avoid exacerbating a potential cervical spine injury.

3. Impaled foreign bodies: Any foreign body in the neck should be left in place until a patient reaches a trauma center. To take it out before then may disrupt a clot and cause massive hemorrhage.

4. Cervical spine stabilization: Always assume the potential for cervical spine damage or instability. Institute cervical spine immobilization as soon as possible.

5. Active bleeding: It is always best to use direct pressure with gauze in the case of active bleeding. Never blindly clamp into the neck, as vital structures are everywhere and injuries can be massively compounded.

CHAPTER 27

Common Otolaryngology Procedures

HAMID R. DJALILIAN
GURPREET S. AHUJA
ROBERTO L. BARRETTO
HAU SIN WONG
DAVID M. STONE

Otolaryngology procedures are among the most common procedures performed in the United States. It is important for the primary care physician to understand the relative and absolute indications of these procedures, a bit about the procedure, and the expected postoperative course.

TONSILLECTOMY

Tonsillectomy is an operation in which both tonsils are removed. The indications for tonsillectomy have been defined by the American Academy of Otolaryngology-Head and Neck Surgery (AAO-HNS):

- Enlarged tonsils that cause upper airway obstruction, severe dysphagia, sleep disorders

(eg, obstructive sleep apnea), or cardiopulmonary complications
- Peritonsillar abscess that is unresponsive to medical management and drainage
- Tonsillitis resulting in febrile convulsions
- Tonsils requiring biopsy to define tissue pathology
- Three or more tonsil infections per year despite adequate medical therapy
- Persistent foul taste or breath due to chronic tonsillitis that is not responsive to medical therapy
- Chronic or recurrent tonsillitis or pharyngitis in a streptococcal carrier not responding to beta-lactamase-resistant antibiotics
- Unilateral tonsil hypertrophy that is presumed to be neoplastic.

The patient generally will have pain in the pharynx for 1 to 2 weeks postoperatively, which is treated using acetaminophen or acetaminophen with codeine. Amoxicillin (clindamycin in penicillin-allergic patients) is given also postoperatively, as it has been found to reduce postoperative pain. There is a 2 to 4% chance of bleeding postoperatively which can occur up to 14 days post-op. The patients are asked to eat soft foods, refrain from strenuous physical activity, and to not travel for 14 days postoperatively. The patient should immediately report to their primary surgeon if bleeding occurs.

ADENOIDECTOMY

In the adenoidectomy operation, the adenoid pad located in the nasopharynx is removed through the oral cavity. It is most commonly performed in children and is only performed in adults in cases of obstructive sleep apnea, recurrent adenoiditis, HIV, or lymphoma for diagnostic or therapeutic purposes. Indications for adenoidectomy include:

- Recurrent or persistent middle ear effusion (usually performed with the second set of myringotomy and tubes)
- Chronic sinusitis in a child
- Nasal obstruction due to enlarged adenoids
- Obstructive sleep apnea symptoms, and chronic mouth breathing.

The procedure is commonly performed either in conjunction with a tonsillectomy for obstructive sleep apnea or a myringotomy and tube placement for chronic otitis media. Adenoidectomy alone is performed for nasal obstruction or chronic sinusitis in a child. The postoperative course is similar to tonsillitis with shorter duration of pain and no dietary restrictions. The likelihood of bleeding is less than 1%.

MYRINGOTOMY AND TUBE PLACEMENT (PRESSURE EQUALIZATION [PE] TUBE PLACEMENT)

Myringotomy and tube placement is a procedure in which a small opening is made in the tympanic membrane (TM) and a small tube is placed into the TM which allows continued communication between the outside and the middle ear. In adults, the procedure is performed in the clinic with topical anesthesia, but children require general anesthesia due to their inability to tolerate discomfort. The function of the tube is to allow air to enter the middle ear space and for middle ear fluid to drain. The tubes generally stay in the TM for 6 to 12 months and come out on their own. After extruding from the TM, 1% of the time there will be a small perforation that remains in the TM which may require patching. Should the perforation persist, there is a risk of acquiring cholesteatoma. Absolute indications for PE tube placement are acute otitis media in the presence facial nerve paralysis, meningitis, or labyrinthitis (hearing loss and vertigo).

Relative indications for PE tube placement include:

- Otitis media with effusion that is present for 3 months that is associated with a hearing loss, earlier if speech or language delay exists
- Severe retraction of the TM that lasts more than 3 months and does not reverse
- No response to 3 courses of antibiotics for acute otitis media
- Mastoiditis not responding to antibiotics
- Recurrent episodes of acute otitis media (more than 3 episodes in 6 months or more than 4 episodes in 12 months)
- Persistent middle ear effusion for 6 months in one ear
- Autophony (hear body sounds such as breathing) due to patulous (abnormally open) eustachian tube
- Craniofacial anomalies (eg, cleft palate) that predispose to middle ear dysfunction
- Middle ear dysfunction due to head and neck radiation and skull base surgery.

The patient may have drainage from the ear for the first few days which can be treated with topical drops (eg, ofloxacin or ciprofloxacin/dexamethasone 3 gtt

TID for 5 days). There is generally minimal discomfort with the procedure and acetaminophen suffices for pain. The patients are seen in 4 to 6-month intervals until the tube extrudes.

TYMPANOPLASTY

Tympanoplasty is an operation where the surgeon uses some fascia (commonly from the temporalis muscle) to patch a tympanic membrane perforation. The procedure which takes 1 to 2 hours usually is done on an outpatient basis. It is performed when there is a persistent tympanic membrane perforation with no recurrent drainage from the ear. The ear canal is generally packed for a few weeks after the surgery. The hearing result will be known after 8 to 12 weeks, when the middle ear packing has resorbed. The patient is asked to not blow his or her nose and to not perform heavy activities for 2 weeks postoperatively. The patient should not allow water to enter the ear until the ear canal has healed entirely (usually 4 weeks). The patients generally will require narcotic pain medicines for the first 3 to 7 days postoperatively.

MASTOIDECTOMY

A mastoidectomy is an operation in which the surgeon removes the mastoid air cells to remove infection in the air cells or to remove cholesteatoma. Surgeries for cholesteatomas sometimes have to be done in 2 stages to remove the cholesteatoma in the first operation and to recheck for recurrence and to reconstruct the hearing (ossicular chain) in the second operation. This outpatient procedure is generally performed in conjunction with a tympanoplasty and takes 2 to 3 hours to complete. The postoperative course is similar to a tympanoplasty.

STAPEDECTOMY

A stapedectomy operation is an outpatient procedure performed for reconstruction of hearing in otosclerosis. In this condition, the stapes bone becomes fixed and has to be replaced with a mobile prosthesis. The procedure is performed through the ear canal and is outpatient. The patient will generally experience some dizziness postoperatively which improves after 1 to 2 weeks. The patient is asked to not blow his or her nose or perform heavy activities for 2 weeks postoperatively. Hearing results are known soon after the surgery.

COCHLEAR IMPLANTATION

A cochlear implant is a device that restores hearing to the deaf. It is most commonly indicated in children who are born deaf or those who lose hearing at a later point in life in whom hearing aids are no longer of benefit. The procedure is performed using an incision behind the ear. The device is placed and the stimulation is first performed typically 3 weeks after surgery. The patient generally takes a few months to completely learn how to understand speech with the device. The procedure can be performed on an outpatient or inpatient basis. In children who are born deaf the implant generally is performed at the age of 1 year. It is performed at a younger age if the hearing loss is due to meningitis. The postoperative care is similar to the tympanoplasty operation. Cochlear implant recipients must be vaccinated for *Streptococcus pneumoniae* (Prevnar for children younger than 2 years; Prevnar and Pneumovax in children between 2 and 5 years; and Pneumovax for patients over the age of 5) to reduce the chance of meningitis from acute otitis media. The implant provides a conduit for middle ear infections to enter the inner ear and from there to the subarachnoid space. Patients under the age of 5 years should be vaccinated for *Haemophilus influenzae b* (Hib vaccine) if not already vaccinated.

SEPTOPLASTY

Septoplasty is a surgery to correct the deviation of the nasal septum to improve nasal breathing. This outpatient procedure generally is performed along with a turbinate reduction (fracture, partial removal, and/or cauterization). The procedure takes 30 min to 2 hours depending on the complexity and anatomy. The patient may have packing or silicone splints placed in the nose postoperatively for the first few days (depending on surgeon preference) and will need to be treated with anti-*S. aureus* antibiotics postoperatively until the packing/splints are removed. The patient should not perform any heavy activities for the first 2 weeks postoperatively. The patient generally will require narcotic pain medications for the first 5 to 10 days postoperatively. The patient is treated with saline spray or irrigation of the nose for the first 6 weeks after the surgery.

RHINOPLASTY

A rhinoplasty is an outpatient cosmetic procedure performed to improve the appearance of the nose. The surgery can be done by making an incision inside the nose or with a small incision outside the nose on the nasal columella. The procedure may be performed in conjunction with a septoplasty. The surgery is outpatient and depending on complexity can take from 1 to 5 hours. Occasionally, cartilage from the ear or the rib must be obtained to reconstruct the nose. Tape and casting material is placed on the nasal dorsum (bridge) for immobilization and to keep the edema down, which is removed about 1 week postoperatively. The postoperative course is similar to a septoplasty.

FACELIFT

A facelift or rhytidectomy is an operation designed to reduce signs of aging in the face and neck area. With the aging process, there is increased laxity and redundancy of skin and tissues in these areas. The facelift operation involves incisions placed in front and behind the ears and in the hairline. An incision is often used under the chin (the submental region). Via these well-camouflaged incisions, the temple, cheek, jowls, and neckline can be lifted, tightened, and rejuvenated. The procedure takes 2 to 5 hours and can be done under local or general anesthesia on an outpatient basis. The results are usually quite favorable with relatively low risk by experienced surgeons. Most patients are between 40 to 75 years old. Prospective patients should not be taking blood thinners or aspirin products, as postoperative bleeding and/or hematoma formation is possible. Most patients can be back in social function within 2 weeks.

BLEPHAROPLASTY

Blepharoplasty is the aesthetic surgical rejuvenation of the upper and lower eyelids. This outpatient procedure usually involves removal of excess and redundant skin, tissue, and even fat from the eyelids, with the attempt to restore these structures to a more youthful form. There are multiple modifications of blepharoplasty, which is designed to improve the appearance of "saggy-baggy" eyelids. Incisions can be placed on the eyelids themselves and also on the lower eyelid mucous membrane (transconjunctival approach). Preoperative assessment of vision, tear function, and extraocular movement are required. There is usually very little discomfort postoperatively and patients can return to work and social function within 7 to 10 days. Patients are usually 30 to 80 years of age.

SINUS SURGERY

A functional endoscopic sinus surgery (FESS) is generally performed when sinus disease (eg, recurrent sinusitis, chronic sinusitis, or nasal polyposis) has become refractory to medical therapy. The procedure is performed with endoscopes through the nostrils to remove disease and to open drainage ports of the sinuses. The procedure generally takes 1 to 4 hours depending on complexity and disease extent. The postoperative course is similar to a septoplasty.

NECK DISSECTION

A neck dissection generally is performed to remove cancerous lymph nodes from the neck. The surgeon makes an incision in the neck and removes the lymph node groups in the neck. It is most commonly performed in conjunction with removal of cancer from the upper aerodigestive tract. The procedure commonly has to be performed bilaterally. The procedure is labeled as "radical" if the cancerous lymph nodes are adherent to the jugular vein, sternocleidomastoid, and the spinal accessory nerve (cranial nerve XI) and these structures are removed. The term modified radical dissection is used when one or more of these structures are saved. The procedure is performed on an inpatient basis and requires drains in the neck for the postoperative period to prevent a hematoma. The patient who has had other cancers removed from the upper aerodigestive tract may need a tracheostomy. The patient will generally be admitted to the hospital for 1 to 14 days postoperatively depending on the extent of the other cancer resection. Antibiotic therapy (anti-*Staph aureus*) is continued until the drains are removed.

THYROIDECTOMY

A thyroidectomy is most commonly performed using an incision in the lower neck to remove half or the entire thyroid gland. More recently at some academic medical centers, endoscopic thyroidectomy is performed using small incisions. It is most commonly performed for a neoplasm of the gland. If a fine needle aspiration of a mass shows a follicular lesion, the lobe of the gland with the mass should be removed. If there is evidence of carcinoma on pathology (which generally takes a few days), a completion thyroidectomy operation is performed a few days after the first operation. A papillary thyroid carcinoma or a goiter with compressive symptoms that does not respond to medications is another common indication. The patients are generally admitted for 1 to 3 days for observation and to check for serum calcium levels, which may drop from inadvertent parathyroidectomy. Drains are generally placed and anti-*Staph aureus* antibiotic is continued until the drains are removed. A total thyroidectomy patient will require thyroid replacement therapy.

PAROTIDECTOMY

A parotidectomy generally is performed for an enlarging parotid mass or one that is found to be malignant on fine needle aspiration. The procedure is performed using an incision in front of the ear in the crease and extends to the neck. The surgeon has to define the facial nerve as it travels through the parotid gland to ensure its safety and integrity. The patient is admitted postoperatively with a drain and is kept in the hospital for 1 to 3 days. Antibiotic therapy (anti-*Staph aureus*) is continued until the drains are removed.

PEDIATRIC BRONCHOSCOPY

Pediatric bronchoscopy is generally performed in patients with a suspicion of an airway abnormality or a foreign body. It is also performed in patients who fail extubation or those who have feeding problems. The procedure is generally performed in conjunction with a direct laryngoscopy for evaluation of the larynx and an esophagoscopy for evaluation of the esophagus. The patient may have to be admitted to the hospital for observation postoperatively.

MICROSCOPIC-ASSISTED DIRECT LARYNGOSCOPY (MDL)

The MDL operation generally is performed when an abnormality of the larynx is seen on flexible laryngoscopy in the clinic. The surgeon visualizes the larynx with a microscope and biopsy, resection of mass, or injection of the vocal fold (cord) is performed depending on the pre-existing pathology. The procedure generally is outpatient and the patient is treated with antireflux medications and a short course of corticosteroids postoperatively.

UVULOPALATOPHARYNGOPLASTY (UPPP)

A UPPP operation is performed for patients with sleep apnea or those with severe snoring. The surgery is performed by removing redundant tissue that obstructs the pharyngeal airway in the patient. If tonsils are present, they are removed as well. Occasionally, a septoplasty, tongue base reduction, or other adjunctive procedures (eg, geniohyoid advancement) have to be performed for improvement of the upper airway. The procedure requires a 1 to 4 day hospitalization (may require intensive care observation if severe sleep apnea exists). The procedure is only curative in mild sleep apnea patients. The moderate or severe sleep apnea patients generally will require continuous positive airway pressure (CPAP) therapy postoperatively. The procedure is performed to reduce the pressure needed on the CPAP and allow the patients to tolerate the CPAP mask better. The patient will need narcotic pain medications for 1 to 2 weeks postoperatively.

FACIAL FRACTURE REPAIR

Facial fracture repair generally is performed using incisions hidden in the lower eyelid, hairline, or intraorally to repair midface or mandible fractures. A fracture repair is warranted for the mandible if the fracture is deemed to cause long-term dental occlusion abnormalities. Midface fractures are repaired if they are thought to destabilize the face and cause facial deformity. The procedure generally requires a 1- to 3-day hospitalization. The patients are treated with antibiotics postoperatively (gram-positive and anaerobe coverage, eg, clindamycin). Narcotic pain medications and mouth washes are used for the first week after surgery. Mandibular fracture repair must be performed within the first 3 days after injury and other facial fractures must be performed within 14 days of trauma.

TRACHEOSTOMY

The tracheostomy operation is performed to obtain an alternative airway. Its indications are different in a child versus an adult. In a child, the indications are as follows:

1. Upper Airway Obstruction

   Craniofacial anomalies or other structural abnormalities of the upper airway

Laryngotracheal stenosis (congenital vs acquired)

Choanal atresia

Pierre Robin sequence

Congenital high airway obstruction syndrome (various causes)

Macroglossia

Neoplastic (eg, hemangioma)

Traumatic: Laryngeal trauma/fracture; burns with inhalation injury;

Bilateral vocal fold paralysis

Tracheomalacia

Neuromuscular disorders with hypotonia

Infectious (eg, acute epiglottitis, diphtheria, Ludwig's angina)

Inflammatory (acute angioedema, Wegener's granulomatosis with laryngotacheal cicatrization)

2. Chronic Ventilatory Failure (usually considered after 6 weeks of intubation)

Bronchopulmonary dysplasia

Myopathies/muscular dystrophy

Head trauma

Cervical spine injuries

3. Chronic Aspiration

Primary

Secondary

Posterior laryngeal cleft

Tracheoesophageal fistula

In adults, tracheostomy is most commonly performed for chronic ventilatory failure (usually considered after 7 days of intubation if it is anticipated that the patient will be intubated for more than 10 days). If a patient is intubated for longer than 10 to 14 days, she or he is at risk of developing a stenosis of the trachea below the level of the larynx, termed subglottic stenosis. This problem is very difficult to treat and sometimes will require lifelong tracheostomy dependence. Therefore, a temporary tracheostomy is performed and the patient is decanulated after ventilatory support is no longer needed. If surgeries in any part of the body are planned in the near future, the tracheostomy is kept in place and removed after all surgeries have been completed. Tracheostomy also allows the patient to wean off the ventilator faster given that the patient does not have to overcome the resistance of the long endotracheal tube when breathing. Other reasons are all similar to the indications in the pediatric age group, with the exception of Pierre Robin sequence, craniofacial anomalies, and macroglossia which generally are not problematic in adults. The tracheostomy tube should remain in place for the first 3 days postoperatively until a tract develops between the skin and the trachea. After that point, the tube can be changed. The inner cannula of the tracheostomy tube (in adults) should be changed intermittently and washed. Suctioning is necessary to keep the tube open.

In a trach-dependent patient who has a cardiac arrest, it is common to assume that the patient has an adequate airway through the trach tube. However, most commonly, the trach tube may have been slightly dislodged and be sitting under the skin in a false tract and cause respiratory arrest, and secondarily cardiac arrest. Therefore, it is critical to first assess the trach tube in these situations by passing a suction catheter down the trach tube to check if it is located in the trachea. In adults, the suction catheter must pass easily at least 15 cm (10 cm in children) into the tube to indicate that the tube is in the airway. If the tube is not in the airway, it must be removed and replaced. The tube is replaced by holding the curvature perpendicular to the way it would normally sit in the airway and placing it into the tracheostoma. After the tube is halfway in, it is turned to go down into the airway. Alternatively, Seldinger technique can be used by inserting a suction catheter into the stoma and into the trachea and sliding the trach tube over the suction into the airway. If all these efforts fail, the patient can be intubated from above (unless the patient has a history of a laryngectomy, in which case there is no communication between the oral cavity and the trachea).

CHAPTER 28

Danger Signs in Otolaryngology

HAMID R. DJALILIAN

DANGER SIGNS IN OTOLARYNGOLOGY AND DISORDERS NOT TO BE MISSED BY THE PRIMARY CARE PHYSICIAN

- Tonsillar hypertrophy in a patient after solid organ or bone marrow transplantation can be the first manifestation of lymphoma. An otolaryngology referral is warranted for tonsillectomy.
- Unilateral tonsillar enlargement can be a sign of lymphoma or a squamous cell carcinoma. The patient should be referred for a tonsillectomy to an otolaryngologist.
- A neck mass in an adult over the age of 35 is cancer until proven otherwise. An inflammatory mass rarely will last more than 3 weeks in an adult (or more than 6 weeks in a child). The patient should be referred to an otolaryngologist for a full head and neck examination and fine

needle aspiration. An excisional biopsy of a neck mass in adults should never be performed as it is likely to spread the carcinoma if the mass is carcinomatous.

- A salivary gland mass (eg, parotid or submandibular glands) in children is more likely to be cancerous than benign. If resolution does not occur within 6 weeks, an otolaryngology consultation is warranted.
- Hoarseness that lasts more than 3 weeks in an adult should be evaluated by an otolaryngologist for laryngoscopy to rule out a carcinoma. This is especially true if the patient has a smoking or drinking history.
- An oral cavity mass or ulcer that does not resolve in 3 weeks in an adult should be evaluated for biopsy by an otolaryngologist to rule out a carcinoma.
- A neck mass in a child that lasts more than 6 weeks should be evaluated by an otolaryngologist for carcinoma.
- Unilateral wheezing in a child can be a sign of a bronchial foreign body. An evaluation by a pediatric otolaryngologist is warranted especially in toddlers where the foreign body aspiration may have been unwitnessed.

EAR

- Tympanic membrane redness that does not improve with antibiotics in an adult should be evaluated by an otolaryngologist to rule out a glomus tumor of the middle ear.
- Unilateral otitis media or unilateral middle ear effusion in an adult needs an evaluation by an

otolaryngologist with nasopharyngoscopy to rule out a nasopharyngeal mass that could be obstructing the eustachian tube opening. This is especially important in a patient who is of Asian descent. These patients have a much higher likelihood of nasopharyngeal carcinoma.

- Sudden hearing loss a patient with a normal tympanic membrane is a medical emergency which should be evaluated using tuning fork examination. The patients most commonly will present with plugging of the ear, tinnitus, or state that they have hearing loss. Not all patients will notice the hearing loss initially and it may be attributed to a plugged ear. If the Weber examination (tuning fork on the forehead) is heard in the opposite ear, the patient needs to be started on prednisone and sent for an audiogram and an otolaryngology visit the same day or the next day. If the tuning fork is heard in the ear with hearing loss, the likely cause is conductive hearing loss, which is not an emergency. Sometimes, the hearing loss may be high frequency only and may manifest as plugging or high-pitched tinnitus. In this case, the tuning fork test (256 or 512 Hz) will be normal as it only tests low-frequency hearing. Suspicion should be high and the patient should be referred for an audiogram the same day. All patients with a sudden hearing loss need to obtain an MRI of the internal auditory canals to rule out an acoustic neuroma.

- Asymmetric sensorineural hearing loss or unilateral tinnitus can be an early sign of an acoustic neuroma. An audiogram with follow-up with an otolaryngologist is warranted.

- Pulsatile tinnitus can be an early sign of a glomus tumor, arteriovenous malformation, or other vascular abnormalities. An otolaryngologist referral is warranted.
- A white mass behind the tympanic membrane in a child can be a congenital cholesteatoma and needs to be evaluated by an otologist/neuro-otologist.
- Yellow or brown-appearing crusting that appears like cerumen (earwax) that is on a very retracted tympanic membrane (negative pressure on tympanometry) can be a cholesteatoma. An otologist/neuro-otologist referral is warranted.
- Slow onset facial paralysis that occurs over more than a week is a possible sign of a tumor involving the facial nerve. An MRI of the temporal bone and parotid gland with gadolinium should be obtained.
- If there is a sudden partial weakness of the facial nerve (part of the facial nerve is paralyzed), a tumor of the facial nerve should be suspected. An MRI of the temporal bone (internal auditory canal sequence) and parotid gland with gadolinium should be obtained.
- If facial paralysis does not involve the forehead but all other branches are paralyzed, then a cerebrovascular accident should be suspected.

NOSE

- Unilateral nasal mass most commonly is a malignancy. If a unilateral nasal mass is seen, the patient should be referred to an otolaryngologist for nasal endoscopy.

- Nasal polyps (gray glistening smooth masses) in a child under 18 years of age are commonly associated with cystic fibrosis. A sweat chloride test is warranted.
- Unilateral watery nasal drainage that worsens when the patient bends forward can be caused by a CSF leakage. The patient should be referred to an otolaryngologist for evaluation urgently.
- Recurrent epistaxis (nasal bleeding) in a peripubertal male should be evaluated by an otolaryngologist with nasal endoscopy to rule out a juvenile nasopharyngeal angiofibroma.
- Recurrent epistaxis or new onset nasal obstruction in an adult with a history of smoking or woodworking or an adult of an Asian descent should be evaluated further by nasal endoscopy. These patients have a higher risk of sinonasal or nasopharyngeal carcinoma.
- Fever and hypotension in a patient with a nasal packing in place must be treated by removal of nasal packing and intravenous antibiotics against *Staphylococcus aureus*. This may represent toxic shock syndrome induced by *S. aureus*. All patients with nasal packing should be treated with an anti-*S. aureus* antibiotic (eg, cephalexin or clindamycin).

Index

A

Acetaminophen, 330, 335, 344
Acetaminophen with/without
  codeine, 489, 502
Achalasia, 359, 375–376
  cricopharyngeal, 359,
    375–376
  esophageal, 381
ACHOO syndrome (autosomal
    dominant compelling
    helio-ophthalmic
    outburst syndrome),
    254
Acoustic immittance overview,
    14–17
Acoustic neuroma
  versus benign positional
    vertigo (BPV), 166
  cerebellar pontine angle
    (CPA) tumor, 86–87
  hearing loss, 80, 82
  imbalance, 174
  versus labyrinthitis, 170
  versus Ménière's disease,
    169
  sudden hearing loss, 83
  and tinnitus, 154
  versus tinnitus, 99
  vertigo, 165–166
Acrania, 78

Acute myelogenous leukemia
    (AML), 350
Acyclovir, 44, 303
Addison's disease, 452
Adenoidectomy, 110, 382, 490,
    502–503
Adenoiditis, 503
Adenoids
  enlarged, 503
  facies, 209, 210, 237
  hypertrophy, 108, 190, 192,
    209–211, 226, 236, 237,
    386
  pediatric, 209–211, 236,
    237, 386
Adenopathy, bilateral hilar, 146
Adenotonsillectomy, 382–383
Adenovirus, 326, 327, 343, 344
Adentitis, mycobacterial
    cervical, 462
Afrin, 180
Airway obstruction, 338, 449,
    501–502, 513–514
  allergic angioedema,
    411–415
  causes, 401
  chronic, 340
  infectious, 402–408
  intermittent, 350
  mechanical obstruction,
    409–410